Pelvic Rehabilitation

of related interest

Functional Exercise Prescription
Supporting rehabilitation in movement and sport
Eyal Lederman
Foreword by Robert Schleip and Wilbour E. Kelsick
ISBN 978 1 91208 548 4
eISBN 978 1 91208 549 1

Palpation and Assessment in Manual Therapy—Fourth edition
Learning the art and refining your skills
Leon Chaitow
Foreword by Jerrilyn Cambron
ISBN 978 1 90914 134 6
eISBN 978 1 91208 515 6

Managing the Spino-Pelvic-Hip Complex
An integrated approach
Carl Todd
ISBN 978 1 91342 629 3
eISBN 978 1 91342 630 9

Pelvic Yoga Therapy for the Whole Woman
A Professional Guide
Cheri Dostal Ryba
Foreword by Shelly Prosko and Eve Andry
ISBN 978 1 78775 664 9
eISBN 978 1 78775 665 6

PELVIC REHABILITATION

The manual therapy and exercise guide across the lifespan

Maureen M. Mason DPT, MS, WCS, PYT

Illustrated by Bruce Hogarth
Foreword by Ginger Garner

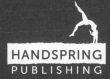

HANDSPRING
PUBLISHING

First published in Great Britain in 2023 by Handspring Publishing, an imprint of Jessica Kingsley Publishers
An imprint of Hodder & Stoughton Ltd
An Hachette UK Company

1

Foreword copyright © Ginger Garner 2023
Illustrated by Bruce Hogarth

Disclaimer: The information contained in this book is not intended to replace the services of
trained medical professionals or to be a substitute for medical advice. The complementary therapy
described in this book may not be suitable for everyone to follow. You are advised to consult a
doctor before embarking on any complementary therapy programme and on any matters relating to
your health, and in particular on any matters that may require diagnosis or medical attention.

A CIP catalogue record for this title is available from the British Library and the Library of Congress

ISBN 978 1 91342 609 5
eISBN 978 1 91342 610 1

Printed and bound in China by Leo Paper Products Ltd

Handspring Publishing
Carmelite House
50 Victoria Embankment
London EC4Y 0DZ

www.handspringpublishing.com

Contents

Foreword

The book is a treasure for anyone who has struggled personally, or who has a loved one, with pelvic health issues. It is also a foundational book for those interested in learning about pelvic health, for students studying anatomy, physiology, and pathology, for parents, teachers, fitness instructors, movement therapists, and working health care providers who want a big picture on pelvic health across the lifespan. Dr. Mason logically introduces the level of information presented, starting with introductory concepts and moving through to advanced paradigms. The progressive knowledge base advances through the chapters, which spikes curiosity and interest as the topics are developed in the book.

The adept presentation at tackling pelvic health issues across the lifespan is apparent throughout the book, and reflected in Dr. Mason and colleagues' extensive clinical experience in pelvic health. This book does a wonderful job of elucidating the team approach, as there are so many medical specialties that may be called upon to treat pelvic health challenges, and there are many interrelationships in teasing out best care practices for pelvic floor dysfunction. From self-care to health care strategies, the reader can glean preventative as well as wellness care knowledge in managing their individual health across the lifespan.

Chapter 1 encourages empowerment toward educating people about how their bodies work, something many feel is missing in our education system today. Chapters 2, 3, 5, and 11 provide a chronological journey across the lifespan of pelvic health, and explore the challenges, from infancy and early childhood through to adolescence, and from pregnancy, birth and midlife through to elder years. Pelvic expert Dr. J. Michelle Martin provides insight as a mother of three, doula, and sexual health educator in her contributions to the pregnancy, birth, and early postpartum chapter. She addresses disparities in maternal care and pelvic health in regard to minority and lower socioeconomic group status, with facts addressing increased maternal morbidity and mortality due to inadequate care, and a call to action to improve skilled care for all. She also includes perinatal fitness programs and safety profiles. These specific chapters are foundational in understanding specific health challenges and solutions in relation to the seasons of life, as well as providing wellness pearls for each life phase. Additionally, pelvic problems may be considered as "part of aging" and must be accepted, which is simply not true.

Chapters 4, 6, 7, and 8 tackle the difficult topics of pelvic pain, postpartum abdominal, pelvic joint, and organ support system challenges. Chapter 13 covers sexual health concerns, well-being, and healing. Pelvic health topics are often regarded as taboo, and overlooked, shamed, ridiculed, or marginalized, especially in the lesbian, gay, bisexual, transgender, and queer (LGBTQ+) communities. Safety, comfort, and pleasure with sexual function can be improved with strategies portrayed in this book, as well as continuing education with the reference list which is provided.

Chapters 9 and 10 address bladder and bowel health and dysfunction, including gastrointestinal (GI) function and the gut microbiome influence on overall health. Providers may take a course on one of these topics, or specialize in one field (urology, gastroenterology), however these two functions are anatomically, structurally, and physiologically interconnected, and the interplay of the two is clarified in this book, including topics such as pressure systems and inflammation.

Chapters 12 and 14 cover meditation, mindfulness, and complementary and integrative approaches to health care. Expert insight on self-care is provided from Dr. Pauline Lucas, pelvic health therapist, yoga, and meditation instructor (Chapter 12) and editing from Dr. Jessica Drummond, founder of The Women's Integrative Health institute (Chapter 14).

An example of the integrative approaches covered in this text is the concept of the "three diaphragms," with sample exercises to sense those connections. I originally presented this concept in my *Medical Therapeutic Yoga* text (Garner 2016). I used the term "thoracic diaphragm" in reference to the laryngeal area (see Figure 1.1); however, the reader may see many other names for the uppermost of the three diaphragms, including cervical, laryngeal, vocal, and cervico-thoracic.

After working in pelvic health and orthopedics for nearly three decades, I have found that one cannot treat pelvic health conditions without using both a biomedical and integrative, biopsychosocial approach. Put quite simply, using mind-body interventions such as yoga, Pilates, and mindfulness make pelvic health physical therapy intervention far more effective, with clients learning insight, self-care, and sustainable nutrition, stress management, and fitness routines. This book does a wonderful job of addressing these topics.

Another important tenet is the treatment of men, women, and non-binary individuals with regard to pelvic health. This population is well recognized as underserved, under researched, and under attended to today. People with pain or other pelvic health challenges are too often disregarded or shuffled through the health care system without being truly listened to. Listening is a hallmark of connection. And because many pelvic health disorders begin with trauma or microtrauma, listening, connection, and compassion is requisite for healing.

This book will take down barriers to receiving pelvic care and help the reader understand that critical topics like environmental contributors to health, including but not limited to clean air, water, soil, food, beauty products, and household cleaners, matter in pelvic health. Additionally, other exciting areas of development addressed are the influence of the gut microbiome, epigenetics, the gut-brain axis, and functional endocrinology. Together, these variables are part of what is evolving pelvic health.

We should all be passionate about pelvic health, and after having served in multiple capacities over the years in policy and academics in pelvic health at state, federal, and global levels, it is deeply satisfying to see this textbook arrive, one that is finally dedicated to empowerment of the individual and the health care system itself through pelvic health education. I expect the reader will delight, as I did, in reading it, in the journey toward their best self, whether for their own self-care, or in providing mind-body client or patient care. This book is a welcome addition for embracing person-led, compassionate pelvic health care.

Dr. Ginger Garner PT, DPT, ATC/L
Living Well Institute & Garner Pelvic Health
Greensboro, NC

Preface

You may wonder why you need this book. Who is the intended audience? What is pelvic health? The information follows, as well as my story in the evolution of my physical therapy profession into a specialty certification, and my mission for pelvic health and healing worldwide.

Here is the scoop.

As a health and wellness enthusiast I'm aware medical facts are severely lacking in health care literacy worldwide. As a physical therapist and medical yoga instructor, I know the lifestyle factors that can create health and, if absent, which can cause distress, suffering, illness, and even disease. This book will promote lifestyle factors that are associated with good health!

Pelvic health is determined by many factors including genetic and environmental influences, personal health history, nutrition, gut microbiome diversity, fitness level, core body strength, flexibility, self-care habits, mindset, and mind–body spirit integration. Pelvic functions ideally are automatic and symptom free. Or pelvic health challenges may occur with a significant impact on health.

This book is for a wide range of readers:

- the general public seeking pelvic health care education across the lifespan
- massage therapists, structural integration practitioners, somatic therapists
- yoga, Pilates, dance, and other fitness instructors
- medical professionals from occupational and physical therapies, psychologists, nurses, MDs in general or specialty practice
- chiropractors, acupuncturists, nutritionists, and health coaches.

WHAT IS PELVIC HEALTH?

Pelvic health is pain-free pelvic joint mobility and stability, ease of bladder and bowel control, and sexual function. Your pelvic functions, from the ability to move from sit to stand, to balance on one leg, to your digestive fire, to absorb nutrients, assimilate, and produce optimum urine and stool output, are all components of pelvic health. From the information in this book, ideally your health will improve, as well as your health care literacy in understanding risk factors and treatment plans for pelvic challenges. And if you, the reader, are a movement therapist, bodyworker, or medical professional, your ability to recognize and provide care or a referral to a pelvic health specialist will be enhanced by this book.

My story is as follows.

I started off my career as a physical therapist (PT) with a master's degree, and I relentlessly attended three or more specialty training seminars per year in neurological, orthopedic, and pain rehabilitation, and attempted to "fix" everyone with my packet of skills. While I loved my treatment successes with improved patient function, I was frustrated and saddened by the lack of improvement by certain patients. With more experience I began to understand the psychology of change behavior and improve my ability for patient interviewing and education.

As I strived to be the best PT I could be for patient health and healing, I encountered my own personal health problems. I was injured from lifting a heavy patient, and began to experience sciatica, with radiating back and leg pain and sleep disruption. At this time, I also journeyed through pregnancy and the postpartum hurdles of urinary incontinence, diastasis rectus abdominis, and pelvic girdle pain (Lee *et al.* 2008). These health challenges were totally unexpected and shocking. Postpartum, I felt embarrassed and thought nobody else had these problems. I felt like an outlier and I suffered in silence.

Through these experiences I developed a sensitivity towards the myriad of pelvic health challenges faced by women and men. Through suffering, I developed compassion and patience. At the time of my own pelvic troubles, I received a request by a hospital manager for the development of a urinary incontinence program. This led me into introductory courses and pelvic program development, and then advanced study in pelvic health with a specialty board certification: women's clinical specialist (WCS), a medical yoga certification (PYT), and my doctorate (DPT).

WHAT I TREAT

I treat pelvic health challenges with individualized programs including lifestyle habits, therapeutic exercise, and manual therapy. Biofeedback and pain relief modalities such as electrical stimulation and meditation/mind–body approaches are also used. These treatment paradigms are the basis of this book on conservative care. Beyond conservative care, pelvic health challenges may require medical specialists for screening and treatment, as discussed in "red flags" in this text.

PELVIC FLOOR DYSFUNCTION

Pelvic floor dysfunction (PFD) is a medical term that encompasses conditions and symptoms that may occur related to the pelvic region, including pelvic pain, bladder and bowel problems, pelvic organ prolapse, and sexual health concerns. This book introduces the profound interrelationships of pelvic anatomy, function, and PFD across the lifespan. It will illuminate paradigms for care providers and ideally improve the integration of conservative care into first line treatments where appropriate.

Concepts that will be introduced and expanded upon include the following:

- pelvic floor muscle and architecture within the bony pelvic bowl
- anatomic principles that illustrate interconnected pelvic functions and physiology
- PFD that occurs at varied points across the lifespan, from birth to senior years
- exercise samples for PFD and general health and wellness

- movement and athletic screening of the lower extremity to the pelvis, spine, trunk, and upper extremity, in the arthro-kinematic "chain"
- yoga and Pilates programs for safe, sustainable fitness and mind–body care
- the biopsychosocial model, with consideration of individual health dynamics, the assets or barriers towards overall health, and pelvic health
- pelvic pain and considerations in screening, and holistic treatment paradigms
- recognition of the role of trauma and supporting recovery and resiliency with multiple methods
- pelvic health and wellness in pregnancy and postpartum
- diastasis rectus abdominis, pelvic girdle pain, and pelvic organ prolapse conditions and sample treatment outlines
- continence mechanisms: how bladder and bowel control occur, and dynamics for elimination
- urinary and gastrointestinal disorders, and the options for lifestyle training and holistic care in improving function
- midlife to senior life phases health and wellness and optimizing pelvic health and vitality
- meditation and the role of mindfulness and mental health in self-care
- sexual medicine principles to optimize comfort and pleasure, and co-morbidities that impact pelvic health
- integrative health and pelvic health care concepts and resources, from socioeconomic, nutrition, gut microbiome, and consideration of the biopsychosocial model.

DEPTH OF MATERIAL FOR GLOBAL HEALTH LITERACY

I have chosen to create a book that reaches the middle ground to speak across disciplines to inspire common sense self-care, client care, and to help identify barriers to care, such as racial, socioeconomic, and environmental factors. Some readers may find the depth of material overwhelming, and need to refer to other textbooks, internet resources, and workshops for clarity, with a journey of both interest and discovery. Movement therapists, bodyworkers, and others wanting to improve pelvic care options can glean vital therapeutic principles and help clients with programs to optimize pelvic health and healing, as illuminated in this text.

Readers who are medical professionals and researchers may want more facts and, where possible, I have presented evidence-based research. Each pelvic condition described in this text is the focus of medical specialty care and

ongoing research and medical education. All the terms and medical conditions that are listed in the book are not completely defined, in order to present general paradigms and program options rather than a massive boring medical dictionary. I am sharing professional knowledge based on published medical research, as well as my expert opinion and insights versus a list of isolated facts. An exact "how to treat" is not possible in this book, as cookbook approaches do not fit unique human beings in all their presentations for care.

My mission is to open the door into the secret world of pelvic health and rehabilitation, as well as to encourage readers to further study via textbooks, internet, and specialty seminars that match their interest. It is my hope for readers that this book will have a positive impact on global health literacy in the varied forms of

PFD, and options for self-care as well as provider intervention to reduce or relieve symptoms, and to promote wellness and healing where possible. Reducing suffering and promoting compassion-based care are global goals. Perhaps this book will inspire careers and research as well. And finally, readers may discover a need for in-person care, telehealth, or the use of resources as listed to further improve their own pelvic health across the lifespan.

Maureen Mason

REFERENCES

Lee, D., Lee, L., and McLaughlin, L. (2008) "Stability, continence and breathing, the role of fascia following labor and delivery." *Journal of Bodywork and Movement Therapies 12*, 4, 333–338.

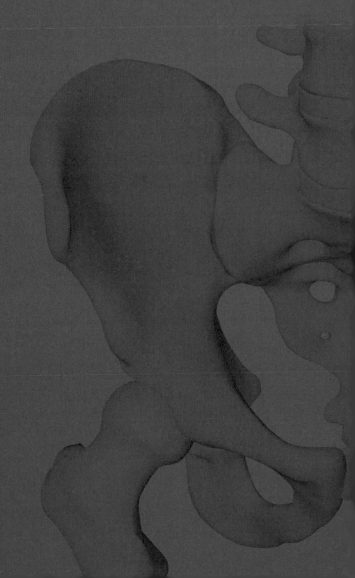

PELVIC ANATOMY, FUNCTION, MOVEMENT FOUNDATIONS, AND PAIN

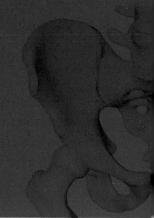

CHAPTER 1

Pelvic Anatomy and Function

INTRODUCTION

Welcome to *Pelvic Rehabilitation: The manual therapy and exercise guide across the lifespan*. This book will guide you through the intersection of primal pelvic body functions, holistic pelvic health care, and portray joys and sorrows that may occur in relation to pelvic functioning.

The purpose of this chapter is to introduce pelvic anatomy and function, and to illustrate the profound interrelationships between structures. Further chapters will define and illustrate more detailed concepts in pelvic anatomy, function and dysfunction, and somato-emotional aspects, across the lifespan.

> For ease of reading, content that is more technical/scientific in detail will be identified in boxes with the eyeglasses symbol ∞. The butterfly symbol will identify therapeutic pearls, insights, and expert, experiential tips 🦋. Client stories with a heart symbol will bring the information to life ♥. The viewpoint in this book will use the term "clients" versus patients to promote a collaborative viewpoint between those seeking care and care providers.

PERSPECTIVES: HOW WE MAY VIEW THE PELVIS AND ITS COMPONENTS

The mystery of pelvic anatomy

Pelvic anatomy can be puzzling to comprehend, as there are multiple terms and nomenclature, and sparse information in most textbooks. Pelvic anatomy terminology is based on illustrations from bodies (cadaver studies) where structures appear as isolated units. Current pelvic anatomy pictures that depict isolated structures help us to understand a mechanistic view, versus living adaptable humans in all their complexity, with linked, contiguous connective tissue, the fascia (Box 1.1). The pelvic structures, from bones to ligaments, nerves, muscles, viscera, and lymphatics, are mysterious to many movement therapists, bodyworkers, and health care practitioners, as well as the general public. Little is mentioned in medical education and rehabilitation unless it is specialty care, and these structures are housed in the most "private" area of the body.

> Box 1.1 We are one fascial body 🦋
> One may consider how our static anatomy pictures that we learn from cause us to isolate areas, rather than to see potential vast interconnections.

We have in the pelvis, a set of structures where everything is connected to every other thing.

(Niall Galloway 2021)

Fluidity of motion

Fluidity of motion may occur through the pelvis and its connections. The pelvic osseous structures may be viewed symbolically as a butterfly, with the sacrum and the lower spine as the body of the butterfly, and the wings, the ilium, ischium, and pubic bones. As the butterfly can move in any direction, so too can human bodies, with the pelvis at the mid-center. The spectrum of pelvic function from movement and flight, leaping into landing, and holding still, are functions that dancers, gymnasts, and anyone that is free to move fully can perform, generally more so in youth to midlife. Pelvic stability and mobility is ideally synchronized with the trunk, spine, hips, and lower extremities. The hips may be viewed as extended wings that bring leg motion into or out of the pelvic center, and the spine as a flowing connected sail that may initiate movement before the pelvis moves.

A biomechanical view

A biomechanical view of the bones of the pelvic region can consider the pelvic bones as an axle that serves as a strut for the wheels, the hips. As the hips and the pelvis turn, our direction changes. This axle has a front center (the pubic bones) and a back center (sacrum and coccyx). When we bend, arch, or rotate the spine and hips we transmit varied loads into the pelvis, from the exterior to all the interior structures. Adding exertion with increased biomechanical loads with work or play, the sacrum, coccyx, and other joints as well as myofascial structures move in ranges for shock absorption and stability, which includes some independent left- and right-sided motions of the pelvic structures.

Housing the organs

This bony pelvis houses and protects the vital organs or viscera: the bladder, bowel, and the organs of reproduction. The organs are anchored into place, yet also have mobility to move and glide upon each other. Loss of pelvic visceral mobility may create symptoms locally, as well as referred out to other regions in the pelvis, abdomen, spine, and legs. Pelvic viscera mobility and stability will be elaborated in manual therapy/visceral mobilization concepts in the following chapters.

More than one diaphragm

The "pelvic diaphragm" is a general term for the pelvic muscles and fascia that course from side to side, and front to back, and support the pelvic organs (Figure 1.1). Readers may have heard of the Kegel muscles; the muscles are housed in the "pelvic diaphragm" region, along with supportive connective tissue (Donmez and Kavlak 2015). The function of this pelvic diaphragm is dependent on local as well as distant myofascial, nerve, vascular, and lymphatic function, including ideally a piston or pump type pressure system. The pelvic diaphragm works in coordination with two regions above, the respiratory diaphragm and the lesser-known vocal or thoracic diaphragm (Box 1.2).

An example of coordination among the diaphragms is singing: as an inhalation brings air into the lungs, the respiratory diaphragm and rib cage expand to increase lung capacity. There is a descent of the respiratory diaphragm during inhalation. Next, during exhalation, the pelvic and respiratory diaphragms contract and rise. The respiratory diaphragm rises to provide air flow into the vocal cords, and the pelvic diaphragm rises to support bladder and bowel continence as well as providing stability to the trunk (via connections from the spinal multifidus and transverse abdominis). During exhalation for singing, the vocal cords in the upper thoracic region contract via motor control into the throat, with a steady release of pressure for the desired quality of the sound (Box 1.3).

An opposite portrayal of the three diaphragms is the optimal synchrony that occurs during relaxed belly diaphragm breathing. The throat is relaxed to allow easy inhalation via the trachea, and the abdomen and trunk muscles relax as an inhale is performed, and the pelvic diaphragm descends slightly to allow a downward, or inferior, movement of the abdominal and pelvic organs.

Box 1.2 The three diaphragms

Remarkably, the interrelationships of the "diaphragms" are not yet mainstream thinking in the medical field. However, movement therapists and bodyworkers may help alleviate chronic conditions with integrative treatment to these regions. All three of these diaphragms influence each other for stability and mobility.

Box 1.3 Three diaphragms: humming

Notice the sensations in your body as you make sounds, as this involves all three "diaphragms" of the body. Inhale, and then close your lips and hum to yourself; any note is fine. When humming, your pelvic diaphragm (including pelvic floor muscles) contracts, and your respiratory diaphragm contracts to assist exhalation and sound production. The exhale (during the respiratory diaphragm contraction) generates a pressure into the thoracic diaphragm and vocal cords, which the vocal cords "play with" to generate varied pitches. The length of the exhale and quality of the sound reflect the ability for the diaphragms to work together. Try varied pitches from low to high, and you may note sensations in varied body areas.

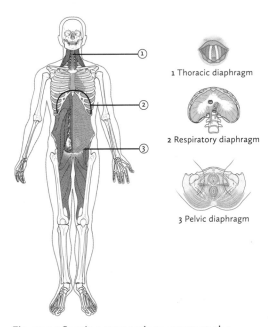

1 Thoracic diaphragm

2 Respiratory diaphragm

3 Pelvic diaphragm

Figure 1.1 Sensing connections amongst the diaphragms, with humming (see Box 1.3).

Courtesy of Garner, G. (2016) Medical Therapeutic Yoga. Three diaphragms and fascial interrelationships, Figure 3.16. London: Handspring Publishing.

Pelvic myofascial functions

Pelvic floor muscles and fascia have multiple functions, which can be viewed as sphincteric, supportive, sexual, piston/pump, and stabilization. These muscle functions occur with little need for our attention, along with automatic postural control, and habits. Pelvic muscle function is sphincteric for bladder and bowel continence and pregnancy, supportive for organs, sexual for orgasm, sump-pump for arterio-vascular and lymphatic flow, and stabilization for all pelvic joints including the spine and hips, and load transfers (Ashton-Miller and DeLancey 2007; Gabelsberg and Tanner 2014; Raizada and Mittal 2008).

Fascia

All the pelvic structures are supported and anchored by fascia, which surrounds, supports, and flows from skin and subcutaneous fat (adipose) into superficial and deep layers around organs, muscles, ligaments, tendons, and bone surfaces (Box 1.4). Large sheets of fascia that support and may exert pressure on surrounding and adjacent structures are termed retinaculum. Nerve, vascular, and lymphatic systems are supported and embedded in fascia (Bordoni and Zanier 2014; Netter 2011).

Box 1.4 Fascia

Fascia, the substance of our connective tissue, can be considered a "soup" of components that provides elasticity and form. It is what we can see with the naked eye. It is produced from specialized fibroblast cells from the embryological mesenchyme and is composed of a ground substance or matrix with collagen, mucopolysaccharides, and varied types of cells in relation to location and function, with varied densities. Fascia has historically been viewed as a structural component that is not influenced by the nervous system, yet newer research has identified myofibroblasts in fascia, as well as contractile properties that may alter stiffness and assist in the stability of body regions (Schleip *et al.* 2019). A body-wide view of fascia can consider that in "a healthy body which expresses a high degree of elastic mobility and tensegrity-like biomechanics, the load bearing elements will tend to become isolated spacers (rather than brick-like building blocks) while the tensional members will tend to interconnect with each other in order to better transmit their loading demands" (Schleip *et al.* 2019).

The layers of fascia

Superficial fascia under the skin that is mobile, and is an adipose layer, is termed Camper's fascia, and a denser, stronger component of the superficial fascia is Scarpa's fascia. Research identifies a continuity from the superficial to deep layers among the abdominal, pelvic, and lumbar fascia (Ramin *et al.* 2015).

Scarpa's fascia in the abdomen is superficial to the external oblique abdominal muscle, and it blends into the midline linea alba, pubic symphysis, the spermatic cord, and scrotum, as dartos fascia. From the scrotal area it is traced into the perineum from superficial to deep. In females this fascia is also traceable from the abdominal region into the perineum at the labia majora (Joshi and Duong 2020).

In men, Scarpa's fascia and Camper's fascia wrap from the lower abdomen into the scrotum and testes, and the superior sites are embryological zones where the testes formed in development and then invaginated and descended from the abdominal wall. In women, the round ligament reaches out from the uterus and descends like octopus arms into the suprapubic region, then the mons, and some anatomists describe it as wrapping around bulbospongiosus, the central vaginal ring muscle. Knowing these profound fascial connections can help readers understand how compression, shortening, spasm, or scar tissue in one region can create far-reaching symptoms!

Manual therapists and movement educators ideally work with local and distal reaching fascial networks in assessment and treatment of dysfunction. Recognizing the fascial structures in their inter-related links is critical for understanding optimum organ alignment, sphincteric and support systems, pressure systems, stability, mobility, dysfunction, and pain (Chaitow and Lovegrove Jones 2012; Joshi and Duong 2020; Killens 2018; Myers 2011). The far-reaching extent of myofascial connections is the basis for pain and dysfunction occurring across broad expanses in the body. Bodyworkers may assess myofascial function with a vast tool kit of skills, and consider the broad, layered myofascial networks such as depicted in Tom Myers' *Anatomy Trains* (Myers 2011).

FOUNDATIONS: PELVIC STRUCTURES

Bones

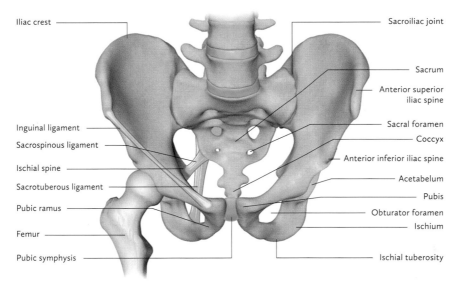

Figure 1.2 Anterior view of pelvic bones.

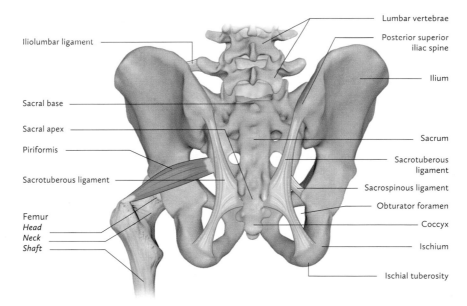

Figure 1.3 Posterior view of pelvic bones.

The bony structure of the pelvis includes the paired innominate bones and the sacrum (Figures 1.2 and 1.3). The innominate bones are formed from three bones embryologically, which become fused in infancy into the ilium, ischium, and pubis. The triangular-shaped sacrum and its tip, the coccyx, are wedged into place at the ilium with irregular interlocking articulations, the sacroiliac joints. Bony anatomy as well as ligaments, tendons, and myofascial structures that weave throughout the pelvis and into the trunk and lower extremities provide structural support to the pelvis. The bones of the pelvis surround the organs of the urinary and digestive systems, and the reproductive organs.

Bony landmarks include: the iliac shelf, crest, the anterior superior and anterior inferior iliac spine, the pubic bone, pubic symphysis, pubic tubercle and pubic ramus, acetabulum, the ischium, ischial spine, ischial tuberosities, the lumbosacral junction, transverse and spinous processes of lumbar vertebra 5, sacral base, sacroiliac joints, posterior superior iliac spines, sacrococcygeal joint, and the coccyx (Box 1.5).

> **Box 1.5 Freeing up the pelvic area: the pelvic clock**
>
> Sit tall in a chair; imagine you are sitting on a clock, with 12:00 towards the pubic bone, the front, and 6:00 towards the tailbone, the back. (See Figures 2.3–2.7 and Box 2.6.) Consider 3:00 your right sitting bone, or right ischial tuberosity, and 9:00 your left sitting bone, your left ischial tuberosity. Sit comfortably upright and imagine you are centered on the clock with equal pressure throughout. Notice gravity, the sense of skin, and deeper, to the muscle layer, and then a sense of the bones of the pelvis, and your "sit bones" that help support your weight. Take a breath and adjust if needed, to center. Then sit tall like a king or queen about to look out proudly towards a happy crowd outside a window, and lightly try lifting your breast bone (sternum) high and arching your back, rocking the pelvic area towards 12:00, as a bowl tipping out forward; notice how this feels, then slowly move back to the center, stacking the spine comfortably upright. Next, allow a spinal bend or slump as if tired, tucking the tailbone under towards pressure at 6:00. Notice how this feels, to tuck under and round the back. Slowly come back to center. Next, explore a motion towards the left or right sitting bone, moving to the side and keeping the ribs lifted up over the pelvis, as if going around a traffic circle in a car ... how does the ease feel, or any restriction, going to each side? Finally, explore small circular motions around the clock, clockwise or counterclockwise, and larger circles as desired, and then come back to the center. Finish with a few breaths in the center, and perhaps thank your pelvis for helping you get around in the world. (This pelvic clock exercise can be explored sitting on large bolsters that are like a saddle, or on a rolled towel or other item from front to back ... in order to sense the bones of the pelvic area, and a sense of pressure, stretch, or other sensation in the surface muscles of the pelvic area.)

ORGANS: PELVIC VISCERA

Pelvic viscera include the bladder, bowel, and reproductive organs. The bladder is a reservoir for urine storage, as well as a muscular system for emptying urine. The bladder is situated behind the pubic bone, yet it rises up towards the abdominal cavity with filling. It receives urine via the ureters at the ureterovesical junction and, with appropriate filling, the detrusor muscle of the bladder, a smooth muscle, is stimulated to contract and empty while the pelvic muscles relax (Shemadou, Rahman, and Leslie 2020).

The urethra allows passage of urine from the bladder to the urethral meatus or outlet in the external pelvic floor muscles. The urethra is anatomically divided in relation to four distinct regions: 1) the proximal origin in the bladder wall, or intramural, 2) the mid urethra, 3) the urethra in the deep part of the anterior pelvic muscles (urogenital diaphragm), and 4) the most distal section at the superficial urogenital diaphragm (DeLancey 1986). Each region provides support for urinary continence, and laxity or deficiency at one area may challenge other areas to provide more support.

The colon is considered part of the abdominal, gastrointestinal system, and the colon is the final system involved in digestion and elimination, where it terminates in the distal pelvis as the bowel, rectum, and anus. The colon originates at the right lower quadrant, at the ileocecal valve, and becomes the ascending, transverse, and then descending colon in the left lower quadrant,

which turns posterior and inferior as the sigmoid colon, rectum, anal canal, and the internal and external anal sphincters. The distal colon, rectum, and anal canal are the final structures of the digestive system for solid waste. The rectum is directly posterior to the vaginal canal in women, and the lower bladder in males.

The reproductive organ system includes the vagina, fallopian tubes, uterus, and ovaries in the female (Figure 1.4), and the penis, testes, epididymis, vas deferens, spermatic cord, seminal vesicles, and prostate in the male (Figure 1.5). These organs are regulated by the endocrine, cardiovascular, neurological, and lymphatic systems (O'Rahilly and Muller 2008; Shermadou *et al.* 2020).

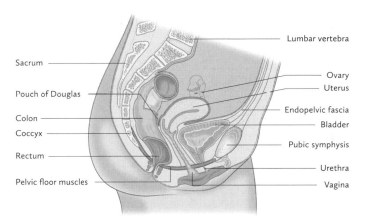

Figure 1.4 Lateral view of female pelvis and organs.

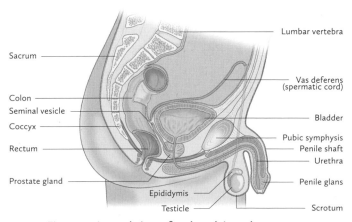

Figure 1.5 Lateral view of male pelvis and organs.

The pelvic organs are nestled against each other and have muscular as well as fascial attachments between organs and into the bony skeletal frame (Petros 2011). Pelvic viscera and the associated outlets of the rectum to the anal sphincter, bladder to urethra, and reproductive structures to the external genitals contain an array of smooth and striated muscle fibers. Smooth muscle fibers are part of autonomic function, and they are automatic controllers for cardiovascular and organ functions. Striated fibers are under our conscious control such as "winking" an eye, or "winking" the circular anus muscle. (Humor helps pelvic education!) Pelvic organs and smooth and striated muscles ideally work in synchrony, at rest, and in movement (Box 1.6).

functions, and pelvic muscles and ligaments ideally maintain closure and integrity during all body maneuvers, yet those that have lost the support may suffer discomfort, strain, pain, pressure, or even bladder, gas, or bowel leaks with bending or other motions. Consider standing up from sitting; perform this now if possible, and if it is effortless, you may not bend forward very much as you move to erect standing. But if one bends over forward before getting up, and needs arms to push up, and there is perhaps a breath hold or even bearing down (Valsalva), consider what is happening at the hips, spine, and all the diaphragms. How are the pelvic organs impacted by a weakened sit to stand maneuver, and maximum downward pressure? If the bladder is full, is there still an automatic maintenance of continence? General body strength, organ mobility, and pelvic floor myofascial support are all components of pelvic health, of symptom-free life.

> **Box 1.6 Sit to stand function**
>
> When viewing sit to stand function, the pelvic viscera require support, as well as mobility. The viscera have to glide upon and around each other for their physiologic

LIGAMENTS

Posterior ligamentous sites in the pelvic region that may be palpated externally include the iliolumbar ligament, the long dorsal ligament, the sacrotuberous ligament, the sacral coccygeal ligament, and the anococcygeal ligament (see Figures 1.2 and 1.3). Anteriorly, palpable structures include the inguinal ligament, and the pubic symphysis ligaments which are defined by their superior, anterior, and inferior locations.

The sacrotuberous ligament starts at the posterior sacroiliac joint, lateral to the long dorsal sacroiliac ligament. The sacrotuberous ligament inserts into the ischial tuberosity and has distal fibers blending with the insertion of the biceps femoris and semitendinosus hamstring muscles (Bierry *et al.* 2013). Anterior to the sacrotuberous

ligament, at the sacral-coccygeal region, is the sacrospinous ligament. A few millimeters of space exists between these two ligaments, of importance to the pudendal nerve that passes between these two structures. The sacrospinous ligament extends from the lateral distal edge of the sacrum, and it runs laterally to the ischial spine. This ligament is the anchor point for fixation in many urogynecologic surgeries. It is in line with the coccygeus muscle.

Anteriorly, the inguinal ligament spans the anterior iliac spine superiorly, into the pubic ramus and tubercle, and it is formed by the aponeurosis of the external oblique muscle. The femoral nerve, artery, and vein pass under the inguinal ligament, and also the psoas minor, iliacus, and pectineus muscles (Netter 2011).

Organ support structures

Internal ligaments of the pelvis are thin web-like fascial structures that reach from organ to organ and into the skeletal framework and/or the abdominal, lateral, and posterior walls. These ligaments may contain elastin and smooth muscle fibers. Surprisingly, anatomists may disagree as to exact origins, insertions, and morphology of some ligamentous structures, and in fact connective tissues vary in individuals in surgical anatomy, radiologic imaging, and cadaveric studies (Box 1.7).

Key ligaments involved in support of the uterus include the round and broad ligaments, the laterally branching transverse cervical (cardinal) ligaments, and anterior to posterior branching pubovesical and uterosacral ligaments.

ROUND LIGAMENT

The round ligament is a rope-like band of tissue that begins at the superior lateral uterus or cornea, and branches to the ventral inguinal ring and pubis at the mons. Anatomists Gorniak and Conrad (2015) describe the round ligament as spanning from the body of the uterus and coursing through the inguinal canal, terminating in the labia majora. Muscle fibers as well as collagen fibers are present in histology of the round ligament. (These findings explain pain and cramping with menses, endometriosis, and pregnancy.)

BROAD LIGAMENT

The round ligament is attached to the more inferior broad ligament, spanning the side walls of the uterus. In its most inferior and lateral reaches the broad ligament becomes the transverse cervical or "cardinal" ligament. The broad ligament is a wide structure like a bird with open wings, and it is a fold of peritoneum that envelops the uterus and bladder, fallopian tubes, ovaries, ovarian and uterine arteries, and round and ovarian ligaments. The broad ligament serves as mesentery with nerves, blood vessels, and lymphatic structures (Chaudhry and Chaudhry 2020; Craig and Billow 2018).

UTEROSACRAL LIGAMENT

The uterosacral ligament (USL) originates in its anterior margins from the upper third of the anterior wall of the vagina to the dorsal cervix. Posteriorly the USL connects to multiple sites, including the sacrospinous ligament, the sciatic foramen and ischial spine, anterior sacral fascia primarily from S2 through S4, and the piriformis muscle. The USL is a mesentery-like structure which contains smooth muscle fibers, blood vessels, and nerve bundles. The cardinal ligament originates at the internal iliac artery which inserts into the cervix and vagina, and it is described as a sheath that is more vascular than a connective tissue structure (Pitt *et al.* 2003; Ramanah *et al.* 2012).

A deep internal fascial site of clinical importance is the arcus tendinous fascia lata (ATFA), identified anatomically as a white line. In its anterior section, ATFA is attached to the pubic bone, traced to the obturator foramen and its membrane, with the medial connection to the levator ani, and laterally the membrane over obturator internus. ATFA in its more superior aspect blends into the levator ani muscles as arcus tendinous fascia pelvis (ATFP) (Pitt *et al.* 2003).

The internal ligaments blend into pelvic fascia, also termed the endopelvic fascia, which surrounds organs and blends into the body walls and skeletal framework. Pouches exist in the endopelvic fascia in folding or junction points between organs, and these are landmarks to note organ positioning in relation to pelvic descent, surgical anatomy, and scar tissue restrictions. Fascia supporting the urethra and the vagina is termed paraurethral and paravaginal fascia (Yavagal *et al.* 2011).

Box 1.7 Ligamentous mobility for fluid motions

Ligaments may be sites of pain, with touch, pressure, or stretch, and this pain may also be traced into myofascial and/or visceral/internal structures as well. Sometimes ligaments that are stiff, or associated with an adjoining muscle spasm, or even instability or hypermobility, will not tolerate stretch. Pain may occur from excess laxity or stiffness and loss of mobility. An example of the need for pain-free myofascial stability and mobility is the "boat pose" that is performed in Pilates and yoga routines (Figure 1.6), as well as the "roll back" maneuver (Figure 1.7). In moving from boat to a roll back, one must tuck the sacrococcygeal joints under, there must be abdominal and trunk control for the spine and pelvic area, and flexibility in the sacrococcygeal joints, the anococcygeal ligament, and the sacrospinous, long dorsal, and sacrotuberous ligaments (Kiapour *et al.* 2020). Difficulties with this exercise sequence may indicate a need to break down the components and screen for where and why the performance is limited.

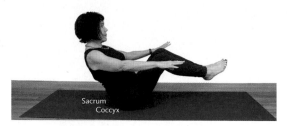

Figure 1.6 Boat pose.

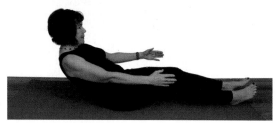

Figure 1.7 Roll back.

MUSCLES

The pelvic floor muscles (PFM) and ligaments have been described as a hammock, and as a boat in suspension (DeLancey 1994; Lee and Meurette 2011). PFM are relatively thin in comparison to larger muscles such as the gluteals, hip adductors, and hip flexors. The muscles are positioned in the region slung between the ischial tuberosities, the pubic bone, ischial spine and ramus, and the sacral-coccygeal area. The PFM intimately weave into myofascial slings and ligaments that support the pelvic viscera, the bladder, bowel, uterus and ovaries, prostate, and testes (Barber 2005). Beyond a simplistic view of the PFM as a hammock, clinically we recognize three levels or layers of the muscles. These levels may be described from superficial to deep as levels I, II, and III for clinical medical evaluation (Gabelsberg and Tanner 2014), or from a surgical perspective level I is the deepest, then level II, and level III is the most superficial (DeLancey 2016) (Box 1.8). (This text will defer to a clinical terminology for rehabilitation care rather than surgical terminology.)

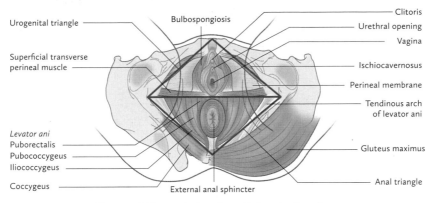

Figure 1.8 Urogenital and anal triangle, female.

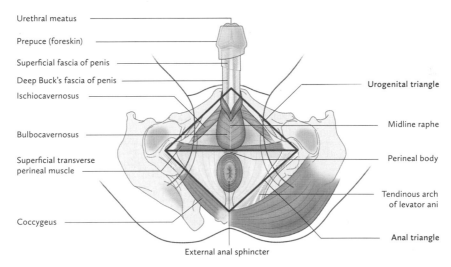

Figure 1.9 Urogenital and anal triangle, male.

Level I

The most superficial muscle layer, level I, is palpable externally, and schematically represented as the urogenital triangle and anal triangle. The urogenital triangle (UGT) includes three muscles, the ischiocavernosus muscle, superficial transverse perineal muscle, and the bulbospongiosus muscle (female) (Figure 1.8) or the bulbocavernosus muscle (male) (Figure 1.9). The perineal body, transverse perineal muscle, and ischial tuberosities are landmarks that divide the anterior triangle from the posterior, the anal triangle. The anal triangle includes the external anal sphincter muscle, and the ischial rectal fascia containing the levator ani muscles. The perineal body is a central anchor point between the urogenital triangle and the anal triangle.

Level II

Level II, the urogenital diaphragm, consists of a sheet of dense fascia, the perineal membrane, and muscles. Level II in the female includes the external urethral sphincter, sphincter urethra-vaginalis, sphincter compressor urethrae, the deep transverse perineal muscle, the perineal body, and the perineal membrane (Figure 1.10). Level II is a site of critical muscle and fascial support for the pelvic organs. Males also have a sheet of dense fascia at the urogenital diaphragm.

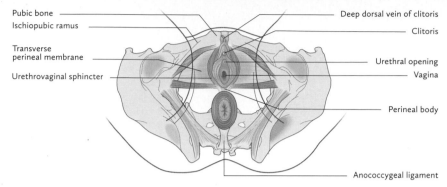

Figure 1.10 Urogenital diaphragm, female.

Level III

Level III, the deepest section of the PFM, is the levator ani muscle group, including the more central puborectalis muscle, the pubococcygeus muscle, as well as the more lateral iliococcygeus muscle (Figures 1.11 and 1.12). The levator ani muscle group is the deepest muscle and fascia support system for the pelvic organs (DeLancey 1994; Gorniak and Conrad 2015; Ramanah *et al.* 2012).

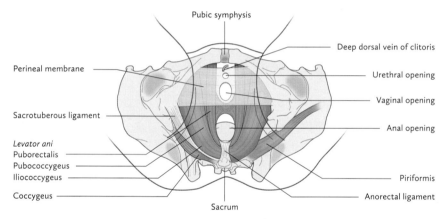

Figure 1.11 Levator ani, female.

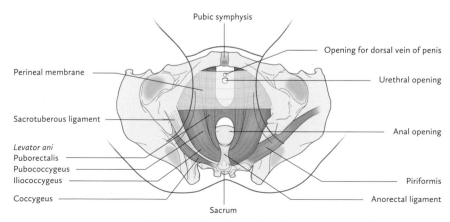

Figure 1.12 Levator ani, male.

Box 1.8 Mobility of pelvic floor muscles

Body check: Do you have a "mobile" pelvic floor muscle (PFM) group? The PFM are a blend between the autonomic/automatic system and the volitional system; they are always holding some tension yet should move up and down a little as well. Consider exploring mobility with external self-palpation over the clothes or on bare skin if desired (Figures 1.13 and 1.14). In sitting, drape your fingers under your pelvic area so that the fingertips move into the inside edge of the ischial tuberosities. (The PFM are medial, towards the midline, compared to the gluteals.) Breathe in; do you feel any motion in the pelvic muscles? (See Figure 1.13.) Next, in side lying, drape your hand over your ischial tuberosity, and softly place your fingertips at the inner edge of the tuberosity, and take a relaxed belly breath, and notice if your fingertips feel any movement during the inhale (Figure 1.14). Ideally, the PFM group relaxes upon a gentle inhale, or "belly breath," yet many individuals "pull up and in" with the PFM group during inhalation. With breathing, you may imagine the PFM as flower petals that drop down and open upon inhalation. Perhaps the reader may sense a lengthening, an opening and letting go in this area as you inhale. PFM relaxation is a key concept that will be explored more in the following chapters.

the piriformis muscle, obturator internus and externus muscles, and superior and inferior gemelli muscles. The gluteals, hamstrings, hip adductors, hip flexors iliacus and psoas, and quadratus lumborum muscles all attach to the pelvis, as well as the abdominal and spinal muscles.

The PFM, transverse abdominis, and spinal multifidus are considered the inner core of the unit for support and function. The PFM, transverse abdominis, and multifidus work with outer muscle groups of the pelvis, trunk, and limbs for function, as elucidated in future chapters. (See Figure 2.12.)

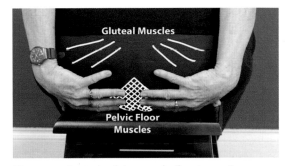

Figure 1.13 Seated pelvic muscle (levator ani) palpation.

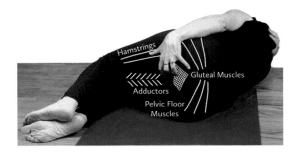

Figure 1.14 Side lying pelvic muscle (levator ani) palpation.

Muscles situated deep in the pelvis (but not included in the pelvic floor muscle group) include

EXTERNAL PELVIC ANATOMY: GENITALS AND PERINEUM

The perineum is the outlet region of the pelvis, with passages for the urinary, gastrointestinal, and reproductive systems. External structures include the vulva to the anus in the females, and the penis, scrotum, and anus in males, with the perineal body in the center. The perineal body is a muscular and fascial landmark between the urogenital and anal triangles (Boxes 1.9–1.10).

The clitoris has one purpose: sexual pleasure. It is the only structure in the human body solely designed for pleasure.

(Jen Gunter 2019)

> **Box 1.9 Gynecologic anatomy**
> External structures observed in an examination with the feet in stirrups (lithotomy) position include the mons pubis, the labia majora and minora, the mons, clitoris, prepuce or hood, the clitoral bulb, the vestibule and glands, the urethral meatus, the perineal body, the skin of the vulva, and the external anal sphincter. Deeper structures in the perineum include the clitoral bulb, Bartholin's glands at right and left lower vaginal outlet, and the lesser Skene's or paraurethral glands, at the urethral outlet. The internal female genitalia that are viewed with a speculum and/or palpated by an examiner include the vagina, the uterus and cervix, and the fallopian tubes and ovaries, and the myofascial support structures (Yavagal *et al.* 2011).

> **Box 1.10 Male genitalia and reproductive system**
> In the male, the external genitals include the penis, from the base of the shaft (bulb) to the tip or glans, and the scrotum. The penile tissue is composed of corpus callosum, and corpus spongiosum, both of which are covered by a firmer tissue, the tunica albuginea, and anchored at the base by Buck's fascia and penile suspensory ligaments. The internal structures include the testes, epididymis, ductus deferens, seminal vesicles, ejaculatory duct, and the prostate (O'Rahilly and Muller 2008).

BLOOD SUPPLY: ARTERIES AND VEINS

The oxygenated blood supply to the pelvis stems from the aorta, then the internal iliac artery and its branches, the anterior and posterior trunk. Anterior bifurcations off the internal iliac artery include the inferior gluteal, internal pudendal, vaginal, rectal, obturator, umbilical, superior and inferior vesical, and uterine arteries. The posterior branches off the internal iliac include the iliolumbar, superior and inferior lateral sacral, and the superior gluteal arteries (O'Rahilly and Muller 2008).

Venous structures follow a path adjacent to the arteries in most cases, with the veins routing deoxygenated blood from organs back to the central vena cava. Major pelvic veins include the external, internal, and common iliac veins. The internal iliac vein is key to most of the venous drainage from pelvic organs. The vein from the internal iliac to the ovary (ovarian vein) may become blocked and create swelling, pain, and pelvic congestion, requiring surgical attention (Rastogi, Kabutey, and Kim 2012).

LYMPHATIC SUPPLY

The lymphatic system is a circulatory and immune system body-wide matrix, consisting of small vessels that are often parallel to arteriovenous structures. The lymphatic system in the pelvis is embedded in the dense fascial network, with small plexus sites termed nodes.

The lymphatic system is the transport sites for lymphatic fluid, which ultimatcly drains into the chest in the thoracic duct, and then the subclavian and the internal jugular veins. Major lymph nodes are identified as the inguinal, sacral, internal, and external and the common iliac lymph nodes (O'Rahilly and Muller 2008).

The nodes in the pelvis may be partially or totally removed in surgeries, or these nodes may be injured from trauma or oncologic processes, with potential sequelae of lymphocele or lymphedema (Dunberger *et al.* 2013; Mikhael and Kahn 2020; Naselli *et al.* 2010).

CENTRAL AND REGIONAL NERVE SUPPLY

Nerve supply to the pelvic area includes local innervations at the level of the pelvis, to structures in the central (brain and spinal cord) and peripheral nervous system (Box 1.11). Two types of nerve innervation exist, the autonomic, and the voluntary or somatic system. The autonomic, or "automatic," nervous system is the regulator for organ function and muscle tone, with reflex regulation of bladder and bowel storage, filling, and emptying, and digestive peristalsis. The autonomic system is not directly under volitional control, and it regulates pelvic viscera homeostasis (Browning and Travagli 2014; Thor and de Groat 2010).

> ### Box 1.11 Nervous system controls of pelvic functioning
>
> The volitional somatic or "voluntary" nervous system is able to control muscle function that can override certain aspects of the autonomic system, such as decision making to delay bladder emptying despite strong sensations of bladder fullness. As an individual reaches full bladder capacity, they may begin to have spontaneous bladder contractions to initiate emptying, via the autonomic system, as the bladder reaches its full capacity. These are termed "bladder urge contractions." The somatic, voluntary system can delay bladder emptying via conscious motor impulses that contract the urethral sphincters to stop urine

loss. Upon reaching maximum storage, leakage may occur as the bladder performs its reflexive emptying function. This illustrates the interplay of pelvic autonomic functioning and human willpower, attention, and decision making.

Two types of nerves are involved in relaying information into and out from the nervous system. The afferent system consists of nerves that convey sensory input such as touch, pressure, stretch, temperature, and pain signals, and therefore relays sensations such as bladder fullness, bowel filling, and sexual appreciation for touch, or pain from a hemorrhoid. The incoming sensory afferent nerves synapse with multiple reflex connections near the spinal cord as well as in the spinal cord and then to higher brain centers.

Junction points for control from the incoming, sensory, afferent input nerves synapse with the outgoing efferent nerves that send signals out from the spinal cord. The efferent nerve system controls muscle contraction, such as signaling sphincters to tighten to stop urine or bowel emptying. The central and peripheral nervous systems have multiple relays for afferent or sensory signal input, and efferent or motor signaling for homeostasis. In optimum health, pelvic functions occur with ease, such as bladder and bowel storage and emptying (Furness 2012; Raizada and Mittal 2008).

INNERVATION

The nerves innervating the pelvic organs, muscles, genitals, and overlying skin zones are from branches from the sympathetic and parasympathetic autonomic system, the central nervous system, and the thoracic (T), lumbar (L), sacral (S), and coccygeal regions. Individual nerve roots supply zones in their dermatome, and autonomic nerves as well as peripheral nerves supply areas in an overlapping distribution (Box 1.12).

> **Box 1.12 Multiple drivers for symptoms**
> Nerves originating several vertebral levels away may create distal systems that require medical examiners to screen multiple

pathways in looking for the "drivers" for symptoms. Organs and myofascial systems can cause symptoms locally as well as distally. For example, anterior upper thigh pain may occur from the hip joint, referred from an ovary or other organ, or from compression of the femoral, or iliohypogastric, nerve or the L2 or L3 nerve root, or simply spasm of the hip flexor or rectus femoris. Irritation of the pudendal nerve in the posterior medial buttock under the sacrotuberous ligament or other sites may produce pain, numbness, tingling, or other sensations in the front body, such as persistent genital arousal with clitoral and vulvar pain, or penile tip, shaft, and testicular pain, anteriorly.

PUDENDAL NERVE

> **Box 1.13 The shame-laden pudendal region**
> Shame! The pudendum is the saddle area that houses the male and female genitals. In ancient Latin, pudenda means "to be ashamed of." Shame is a complex emotion,

associated with a sense of immorality, impropriety, embarrassment, or humiliation, being a dishonor, and often accompanies anxiety and/or depression. The pudendal nerve and the regions it supplies has had a bad rap for hundreds of years.

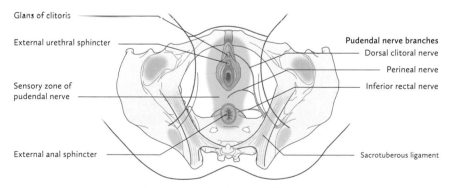

Figure 1.15 Pudendal nerve, female.

The pudendal nerve is formed from the sacral roots 2, 3, and 4, and it is sensory to skin around the anus and genitals, and motor to the external anal sphincter, urogenital triangle, and urethral sphincter (Box 1.13 and Figure 1.15). The pudendal nerve also has autonomic fibers which regulate blood flow and sexual function. The pudendal nerve originates in the sacral plexus and wraps in front of the sacrotuberous ligament and behind the sacrospinous ligament, making it vulnerable to compression and sensitization. It then courses inferiorly and anteriorly into Alcock's canal into three branches, rectal, perineal, and dorsal. The rectal branch supplies the skin and muscle of the external anal sphincter, the perineal branch supplies the skin and muscles of the urogenital triangle and urethral sphincter, and the final dorsal branch supplies the skin and erectile tissue of the clitoris or penis. The pudendal nerve may be irritated with pregnancy and childbirth, prolonged bicycle riding, overstretch or strain from certain sexual practices, and other factors (Apte *et al.* 2011; Hollis, Lemay, and DeBeradino 2019).

NERVES TO THE LEVATOR

A separate innervation exists to the deepest pelvic muscle group, the levator ani. Anatomists find variations in spinal levels, with some contributions from the pudendal nerve, yet also contributions from sacral roots 4 and 5, and sometimes sacral root 3, and possible nerves from the coccygeal plexus (Barber *et al.* 2002). These nerve roots course through or exit anterior to the coccygeus muscle to supply the iliococcygeus muscle, and the pubococcygeal and puborectalis muscle. Intact nerve innervation to the levator is critical for the sphincteric and supportive functions of the PFM, including "the distribution of loads during walking and the movements of the trunk and limbs" (Gowda and Bordoni 2020) (Box 1.14).

Several other nerves innervate areas around the pelvis, hips, and thighs, and these are discussed in Chapter 4 on pelvic pain.

> **Box 1.14 Nerves to pelvic viscera, autonomic controllers**
> Autonomic nerve fibers that supply viscera are termed "splanchnic" nerves, and in the pelvis, these arise from central nervous system sympathetic and parasympathetic fibers, that then synapse with fibers in lumbar as well as sacral and coccygeal regions. A cluster of nerves are termed a "plexus." Sympathetic and parasympathetic splanchnic nerves provide autonomic control of the pelvic organs.

FUNCTION

Functionally, when we view the body as a whole, it appears obvious to note the connections amongst the "three diaphragms" as in the humming exercise in this chapter (Box 1.3). In fact, we can consider a symphony of functions that typically occur with ease, with the pelvis at the base. We can identify connective tissue links traced throughout the pelvic and abdominal areas into the entire body, as considered in structural integration, bodywork, visceral mobilization, and movement therapy.

The pelvic myofascial structures can have a resilience and adaptability for support and stretch for demanding functions such as pregnancy and childbirth, jumping hurdles, dancing, and helping lift, push, pull, and carry heavy loads, as in construction work or cross fit training. In everyday life, ideally the PFM and related systems work in synergy and harmony. The pelvis is the base from which, ideally, we can move in all directions with ease, stability, mobility, power, speed, agility, and flow.

An understanding of myofascial, visceral, arterio-vascular, neurologic, and lymphatic anatomy and function is vital for providing care in pelvic health conditions. Movement therapists and bodyworkers, as well as health care professionals, can help individuals towards improved pelvic health with a vast number of therapeutic interventions as will be covered in further chapters.

Congratulations on the completion of this elaborate material in this chapter. The healing arts are a calling. Detailed anatomy/physiology studies can be intense, demanding, and yet help you to discover new areas for care, including the depths of injury and dysfunction into the deepest parts of a human being.

REFERENCES

Apte, G., Nelson, P., Brismee, J. M., Dedrick, G., Justiz, R., and Sizer, P. (2011) "Tutorial, Chronic female pelvic pain—Part 1: Clinical pathoanatomy and examination of the pelvic region." *Pain Practice 12*, 2, 88–110.

Ashton-Miller, J. and DeLancey, J. (2007) "Functional anatomy of the female pelvic floor." *Annals of the New York Academy of Sciences 1101*, 266–296.

Barber, M. (2005) "Contemporary views on female pelvic anatomy." *Cleveland Clinic Journal of Medicine 72*, 4, S3–11.

Barber, M. D., Bremer, R. E., Thor, K. B., Dolber, P. C., Kuehl, T. J., and Coates, K. W. (2002) "Innervation of the female levator ani muscle." *American Journal of Obstetrics and Gynecology 187*, 1, 64–71.

Bierry, G., Simenoe, F. J., Borg-Stein, J. P., Clavert, P., and Palmer, W. E. (2013) "Sacrotuberous ligament; relationship to normal, torn, and retracted hamstring tendons on MR images." *Radiology 271*, 1.

Bordoni, B. and Zanier, E. (2014) "Clinical and symptomological reflections; the fascial system." *Journal of Multidisciplinary Healthcare 7*, 401–411.

Browning, K. N. and Travagli, R. A. (2014) "Central nervous system control of gastrointestinal motility and secretion and modulation of gastrointestinal functions." *Comprehensive Physiology 4*, 1339–1368.

Chaitow, L. and Lovegrove Jones, R. (2012) *Chronic Pelvic Pain and Dysfunction.* London: Elsevier.

Chaudhry, S. and Chaudhry, K. (2020) *Anatomy, Abdomen and Pelvis, Uterus Round Ligament.* Treasure Island, FL: StatPearls.

Craig, M. E. and Billow, M. (2018) *Anatomy, Abdomen and Pelvis, Broad Ligaments.* Treasure Island, FL: StatPearls.

DeLancey, J. (1986) "Correlative study of paraurethral anatomy." *Obstetrics and Gynecology 68*, 1, 91–97.

DeLancey, J. (1994) "Structural support of the urethra as it relates to stress urinary incontinence: The hammock hypothesis." *American Journal of Obstetrics and Gynecology 170*, 6, 1713–1720.

DeLancey, J. (2016) *Biomechanics of the Female Pelvic Floor.* London: Elsevier.

Donmez, S. and Kavlak, O. (2015) "Effects of prenatal perineal massage and kegel exercise on the integrity of postnatal perine." *Health 7*, 4.

Dunberger, G., Lindquist, H., Waldenstrom, A. C., Nyberg, T., Steineck, G., and Lundqvist, E. A. (2013) "Lower limb lymphedema in gynecologic cancer survivors—effect on daily functioning." *Support Care Cancer 21*, 3063–3070.

Furness, J. (2012) "The enteric nervous system and neurogastroenterology." *Nature Reviews Gastroenterology and Hepatology 9*, 286–294.

Gabelsberg, J. and Tanner, H. (2014) "Pelvic floor function, dysfunction, and treatment level I." Herman & Wallace Pelvic Rehabilitation Institute.

Garner, G. (2016) *Medical Therapeutic Yoga.* Three diaphragms and fascial interrelationships, Figure 3.16. Edinburgh: Handspring Publishing.

Gorniak, G. and Conrad, W. (2015) "An anatomical and functional perspective of the pelvic floor and urogenital support system." *Journal of Women's Health Physical Therapy 39*, 2, 65–82.

Gowda, S. N. and Bordoni, B. (2021) *Anatomy, Abdomen and Pelvis, Levato Ani Muscle.* Treasure Island, FL: StatPearls.

Hollis, M. H., Lemay, D. E., and DeBeradino, T. M. (2019) "Nerve entrapment syndromes of the lower extremity clinical presentation." *Orthopedic Surgery.* Medscape.com.

Joshi, R. and Duong, H. (2020) *Anatomy, Abdomen and Pelvis, Scarpa Fascia.* Treasure Island, FL: StatPearls.

Kiapour, A., Joukar, A., Elgafy, H., Erbulut, D. U., Agarwal, A. K., and Goel, V. (2020) "Biomechanics of the sacroiliac joint: Anatomy, function, biomechanics, sexual dimorphism, and causes of pain." *International Journal of Spine Surgery 14*, 1, 3–13.

Killens, D. (2018) *Mobilizing the Myofascial System.* Edinburgh: Handspring Publishing.

Lee, P. Y. H. and Meurette, G. (2011) *The ASCRS Textbook of Colon and Rectal Surgery.* Berlin/Heidelberg: Springer Science.

Mikhael, M. and Khan, Y. S. (2020) *Anatomy, Abdomen and Pelvic Lymphatic Drainage*. Treasure Island, FL: StatPearls.

Myers, T. W. (2011) *Anatomy Trains, Myofascial Meridians for Manual and Movement Therapists*. London: Elsevier.

Naselli, A., Andreatta, R., Introini, C., *et al.* (2010) "Predictors of symptomatic lymphocele after lymph node excision and radical prostatectomy." *Urology 75*, 3.

Netter, F. H. (2011) *Atlas of Human Anatomy*. London: Elsevier.

O'Rahilly, R. and Muller, F. (2008) "Blood Vessels, Nerves and Lymphatics of the Pelvis." *Carpenter and Swenson Basic Human Anatomy*. London: W. B. Saunders.

Petros, P. (2011) "The Integral System." *Central European Journal of Urology 64*, 3, 119.

Pitt, M. J., De Ruiter, M. C., Lycklama, A., Nijeholt, A. A., Marani, E. and Zwartendijk, J. (2003) "Anatomy of the arcus tendinous fasciae pelvis in females." *Clinical Anatomy 16*, 2, 131–137.

Raizada, V. and Mittal, R. (2008) "Pelvic floor anatomy and applied physiology." *Gastroenterology Clinics North America 37*, 3, 493–762.

Ramanah, R., Berger, M. B., Parratte, B. M., and DeLancey, J. O. L. (2012) "Anatomy and histology of apical support; a literature review concerning cardinal and uterosacral ligaments." *International Urogynecology Journal 23*, 11.

Ramin, A., Macchi, V., Porzionato, A., Caro, R. D. and Stecco, C. (2015) "Fascial continuity of the pelvic floor with the abdominal and lumbar region, review." *Pelviperineology 35*, 3–6.

Rastogi, N., Kabutey, N. K., and Kim, D. (2012) "Incapacitating pelvic congestion syndrome in a patient with a history of May-Thurner syndrome and left ovarian vein embolization." *Annals of Vascular Surgery 26*, 5, 732. e7–732.e11.

Schleip, R., Gabbiani, G., Wilke, J., Naylor, I., *et al.* (2019) "Fascia is able to actively contract and may thereby influence musculoskeletal dynamics: A histochemical and mechanographic investigation." *Frontiers in Physiology 2*, 10, 336.

Shemadou, E. S., Rahman, S., and Leslie, S. W. (2020) *Anatomy, Abdomen and Pelvis, Bladder*. Treasure Island, FL: StatPearls.

Thor, K. B. and de Groat, W. C. (2010) "Neural control of the female urethral and anal rhabadosphincters and pelvic floor muscles, review." *American Journal of Physiology 299*, 2, R416–R438.

Yavagal, S., de Farias, T. F., Medina, C. A., and Takas, P. (2011) "Normal vulvovaginal, perineal, and pelvic anatomy with reconstructive considerations." *Seminars in Plastic Surgery 25*, 2, 121–129.

CHAPTER 2

Pediatric Pelvic Health

Challenges and Optimizing Function

INTEGRATIVE CARE IN PEDIATRICS FROM MANY VIEWPOINTS

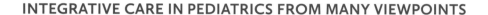

This chapter introduces pelvic health in pediatrics, with examples of genetic and environmental influences, and the whole person view provided by the biopsychosocial model. Pelvic, bladder, digestive, and bowel problems are defined and described, and therapeutic conservative care with movement strategies and somatic/bodywork therapies are presented. Paradigms for medical care in the pelvic region are profiled so all therapists working with these conditions can offer help. Ideally, bridgebuilding in health care can occur where both the "alternative–holistic" practitioners and medical-based therapists can recognize needs and cross refer for teamwork and optimizing client care.

Individuals working in pelvic health must honor their practice standards, guidelines, and laws. Movement therapists and bodyworkers use adaptable programs and formats to help with fitness, wellness, and healing. Medical providers screen, diagnose, and treat specific conditions and often hold a narrow lens in treating disorders and diseases, in part due to medical specialization. Optimum care for individuals ideally includes adequate, pertinent medical screening and testing, as well as the integration of holistic wellness care.

Movement therapy may be achieved with multiple methods from therapeutic exercise, developmental sequencing skill building, yoga and Pilates therapy, and bodywork practices. Bodywork is a broad term that encompasses many types of treatment. "In alternative medicine, bodywork is any therapeutic or personal development technique that involves working with the human body in a form involving manipulative therapy, breath work, or energy medicine" (Thackery and Harris 2003). Chiropractic and massage therapy, somatic experiencing, qigong, tai chi, Feldenkrais method, and craniosacral therapy are also types of bodywork.

In order to not place any therapist or provider reading this material in a box as to individual training and skill set, the terms "movement therapy" and "bodywork" can be recognized as terms that represent a broad spectrum of therapeutic methods and practices, which may or may not include medical certifications as well.

Movement therapy and bodywork can offer clients an overall sense of self, of body awareness and control, and ease of functioning. It can also address trauma and behavioral aspects that may accompany pelvic health conditions. And movement therapy and bodywork can also identify areas of tension or laxity in the myofascial body; here is where an integrative system views the entire body, mind, and spirit as interconnected.

Foundations for pelvic rehabilitation that address the "myofascial body" are profiled in this chapter. Readers need to view the book chapters in sequence to attain a progressive knowledge base of pelvic health anatomy, conditions, and terminology, as they may present at different ages from infancy to senior life.

WHAT PELVIC HEALTH CONCERNS AND PROBLEMS ARE ENCOUNTERED IN BABIES, TODDLERS, AND YOUNG CHILDREN THAT CAN BE HELPED BY THERAPIES?

- Sensory processing disorders, including a lack of sensing bladder or bowel fullness
- A lack of bladder and bowel control along standard timelines
- A lack of nutritional education and poor dietary habits, including insufficient fluid and fiber management
- A lack of physical fitness, overall low mobility
- A body in fight, flight, freeze, flop, or friend; trauma care, from neglect, verbal, physical, or sexual abuse (TRAILS 2022)
- Neurological dysfunction: low tone of the myofascial system, with poor motor control, or high tone, as in spasticity or rigidity
- Respiratory disorders that affect pelvic functioning, shallow respiration, lack of diaphragm and rib mobility, and breath holding
- Trunk and pelvic muscle weakness, and inability of the trunk and lumbopelvic core to be able to stand, or sit, and control mechanics for urination or defecation
- Fascial imbalances, post injury or postoperative scar tissue layers in the endopelvic fascia and visceral-organ systems
- Pelvic pain from myofascial or neurological sources
- Individual and family distress, a need for support and insight for an individual on a spectrum of psychological and/or behavioral disorders, and their care providers
- Pelvic muscle "dyssynergia," with potential pelvic muscle tightening versus relaxation, and the tightening may cause difficulties with bladder/bowel control

This above list is a sample of pelvic health problems and concerns and related factors. The reader will see these topics repeat in varied form throughout this text, with initial presentation here and examples of movement therapies, bodywork, and topics that explain and link to aspects of medical care throughout the lifespan.

NORMAL TIMELINES FOR PELVIC HEALTH

In development from birth into childhood, bladder and bowel control develop along standard timelines, with continence (control of bladder and bowel) most likely achieved between ages 3 and 5 years. Pelvic health conditions may be present at birth, or manifest early in childhood, or later in the lifespan. Some conditions may require surgery. At birth, optimally babies present with normative genitalia and rectal and urethral orifices, and begin passing urine and stool in the first 24 hours (Box 2.1).

PELVIC ANOMALIES AT BIRTH

Box 2.1 Unexpected challenges: pediatric pelvic anomalies

Parents and birth attendants breathe a sigh of relief when everything appears normal in the structure of infant female and male genitalia. Yet genital, urethral, and rectal anomalies may be present, along with other conditions such as hernias and even multisystem organ abnormalities. In the most extreme cases, hospital support and multiple surgeries may be needed.

Potential pelvic health conditions include the following conditions that may need surgery. Males: hydrocele, undescended testes, hypospadias (Springer, van den Heijkant, and Baumann 2016). Females: vestibular and perineal fistulas (Wood and Levitt 2018). Males and females: anorectal malformations such as imperforate anus (Brantberg *et al.* 2006), Hirschsprung's disease (Pini-Prato *et al.* 2010; Solomon 2011; Tjaden Butler and Trainor 2013), and VACTERL/VATER Association (Solomon 2011). Surgeries may be needed over the lifespan in some cases (Schultz-Lampel *et al.* 2011). Additionally, children with medical conditions such as spina bifida, trisomy 21 (Down syndrome), and cerebral palsy (CP) commonly have pelvic health challenges. All the above listed conditions may benefit from movement therapies for motor control improvement and the development of sensory awareness of the "need to go" to transport to the toilet.

Risk factors for pediatric pelvic health conditions that require surgery are genetic, as well as environmental exposure in utero, yet all causative factors are unknown and population studies are ongoing to elucidate the reasons mutations occur (Boxes 2.2–2.3).

Box 2.2 Phthalates and health risks

Phthalates are common chemicals in modern environments that are recognized as endocrine disruptors, with potential alterations in DNA structure and biological processes. Phthalates are used as plasticizers in products such as hair spray, lipstick, mascara, skin care, sunscreen, perfumes, candles, clothing, and packaging materials for many foods. Their chemical constituents are also found in air and water (Wang and Qian 2021).

Altered anatomical development, metabolic pathway signaling, behavioral conditions such as attention deficit disorder (ADD) and autism, changes in puberty timelines, thyroid function, fertility, and other health parameters are associated with the quantity of exposure. Exposure in utero can affect male genital development with risk for hydrocele, undescended testicles, and hypospadias increasing in relation to exposure (Sathyanarayana *et al.* 2016). First trimester diethylhexel phthalate (DEHP) was tested in urinary screening and levels were associated with increased odds of fetal genital anomalies. The most common presentation in research of 371 infants with known exposure to phthalates was 30 with hydrocele, undescended testes in five infants, and hypospadias in three infants.

Box 2.3 Health risks, and healthier options

Ideally, when funds are sufficient, people can wean off the products that are recognized as health adverse. With worry regarding pregnancy, family planning, personal health, and overall exposure to chemicals such as phthalates, education is critical. A shift can be made to use healthier beauty products, food and beverage items, and packaging products with the consumer education guidelines from sites such as the environmental working group (EWG.org).

AUTISM AND PELVIC HEALTH

Autism is a neurodevelopmental brain disorder with impairments in sensory processing, affecting socialization and communication. Repetitive behavior, impaired immune functioning, and gastrointestinal issues can often occur. Children with autism spectrum disorder (ASD) have higher rates of urinary and fecal incontinence compared to typically developing children. Atypical children (those with ASD) are often challenged with pelvic health conditions (Box 2.4).

years compared to age matched controls (0), and daytime urinary incontinence (DUI) of 20.5% versus controls of 4.7% (von Gontard *et al.* 2015). Gastrointestinal (GI) symptoms are more common with individuals with ASD, and may include abdominal pain, gastric reflux, and constipation or diarrhea. Characteristics unique to ASD and the gut microbiome, and dysbiosis (dysfunction), are being studied for their role in pelvic health, behavior, and immune system functioning (Vuong and Hsiao 2017).

> **Box 2.4 Autism and pelvic health**
> Bedwetting (nocturnal enuresis) was found in 30% of ASD children over the age of 5

SOMATO-EMOTIONAL/BEHAVIORAL

Behavioral disorders are found in up to 40 percent of children with urinary incontinence (Zink, Freitag, and von Gontard 2018). Attention deficit disorder, anxiety, depression, sleep disorders, and delays in speech and motor performance are common co-morbidities in association with urinary incontinence. Pediatric pelvic bladder and bowel problems often have a multifactorial etiology which may include genetic or congenital factors, health history, and learned behavior patterns, and possibly delayed emotional, physical, and cognitive development (Chase *et al.* 2010; Franco 2011). Childhood stressors such as a new baby in the household, a change of school or home, and parental divorce are all associated with urinary and fecal incontinence. Medical attention in the form of therapy for delays

(speech, occupational, and physical therapy) may be provided, and bodywork and movement therapies may provide holistic care that addresses myofascial and somato-emotional factors as well (Box 2.5).

> **Box 2.5 A pediatric patient case: Aaron**
> Aaron, age 4 years, had difficulties at preschool per his inability to rest or nap, thereby disrupting the class schedule, and exhibiting hyperactive and inattentive behavior. His parents were concerned regarding his emotional state and restlessness. (He was later diagnosed with attention deficit disorder.) He also had a need to use the restroom for

urination 4–6 times during the day, as well as having monthly bladder accidents requiring clothing changes. He was screened by a cranial-sacral focused pediatric osteopath, and found to have restrictions in the cranium, including the sub-occipital area, likely from enduring a long labor and birth with forceps assistance. Also, he had experienced falls and bumping into furniture with his head during toddler play and appeared to be clumsy. The osteopath provided therapy to myofascial, cranial, and spinal areas over the course of four treatment sessions. She advised the parents in home general relaxation massage therapy, and play activities including crawling, rolling, and relaxed belly breathing, which the parents instituted a few times per week as "family play time." Following four osteopathic sessions and a few months of home family play time, Aaron was calmer, participated better in napping, and reduced his bladder urgency, frequency, and leaks. He was breathing with his diaphragm versus an upper chest pattern. A pre-school teacher asked the parents, "He seems much calmer lately, and is napping now and not having accidents; are you doing anything different at home?"

Aaron's story illustrates expertise in osteopathic pediatric care, how the general status of the nervous system in a case of wound up, sympathetic over-activity can be affected by bodywork, and how calming the system towards balance can help rest, sleep, and bladder habits. Osteopathy uses multiple methods to screen and decipher areas of myofascial dysfunction, with a look towards a primary lesion or imbalance, a place of tension or pull, a restriction in the motion of tissues from superficial into visceral and skeletal structures. Pediatric osteopathy may involve manual care directed at the cranium and the outlet at the cranial base, which in this case above resulted in generalized relaxation (Figure 2.1). (Frontal,

temporal, sphenoid, parietal, and occipital bones ideally have mobility, as well as the sub-occipital area. These regions usually in the healthy individual are not tender to palpation or associated with pain such as headaches.) The holistic care is carried over to improved rest and napping for the child, improved diaphragm mobility, as well as reduced urinary urgency, frequency, and continence control.

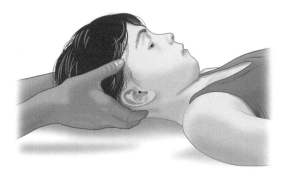

Figure 2.1 Cranial base release in pediatrics.

What is happening in the body that allows bladder or bowel leaks/constipation to occur? And why is it happening?

Why do children have delays in their ability to control bladder and bowel? In the case of sensory processing disorders and developmental delay, they may be unable to sense, process, and respond to bladder and bowel filling. The central and peripheral nervous systems and organ systems may not "communicate" with the mind to prompt a response, and spontaneous emptying may occur as in infancy. Additionally, retention of urine or stool may occur, with insufficient/ inadequate emptying.

Aside from congenital disorders or anomalies, children may simply not pay attention to their signaling from pelvic organs, such as bladder or bowel filling. At the simplest level, they may be solely focused on a task such as a video game, reading, or playing (Figure 2.2). And yet, with either congenital problems or habit-based concerns, therapy may help a child to tune into a sense of bladder or bowel pressure or fullness and to self-prompt to toilet. Therapies addressing the somatic system and cuing into body signals and sensations is required (Boxes 2.6–2.7).

a star." The pelvic clock exercise was useful in the pediatric case of Jaquelyn below, in her introduction to pelvic therapy.

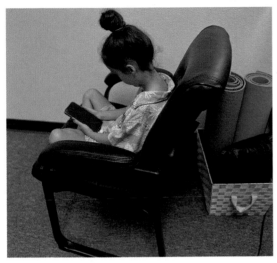

Figure 2.2 Child on computer with legs crossed and the body flexed.

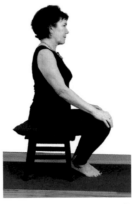

Figure 2.3 Seated neutral spine on bolster.

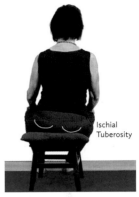

Figure 2.4 Rocking right.

Ischial Tuberosity

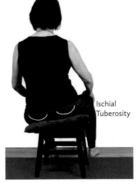

Ischial Tuberosity

Figure 2.5 Rocking left.

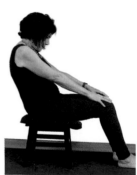

Figure 2.6 Slump.

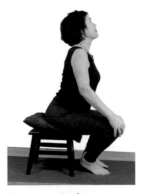

Figure 2.7 Arch.

Box 2.6 Bodily signs of stress, and pelvic centering

There are so many interconnections in pelvic health in the myofascial body, and most medical training focuses on isolated evaluation of "problem areas." Yet observing posture, respiration, and movement can offer clues for therapy. General stress and anxiety may be considered with crossed arms and legs in sitting, and shallow respiration. The seated experience of the "pelvic clock" and "pelvic rocking" can begin to help children tune into their pelvic area and promote a natural body scanning (see Figures 2.3–2.7). Cues may be provided as to "notice where you are making pressure" or "notice the bones you sit on, the sit bones" while holding up a pelvic model, or "make circular motions like the hands on a clock, or to the points on

Box 2.7 A pediatric patient case: Jaquelyn

Jaquelyn, age 10, was referred to physical therapy (PT) for constipation that was resistant to laxatives. She had stopped her dance classes due to her problems, which included abdominal pain, bloating, and random bowel and bladder leaks requiring pads and clothing changes at school and home. Her mom reported that she had occasionally needed suppositories as an infant and even a few enemas, and in middle school she started having stomach pains. Her parents did not know that she was avoiding toilet use due to painful defecation, and only passing one or two stools per week. A visit to the emergency room three months prior had involved an X-ray showing she was "very backed up" and an enema was performed, which was painful for her, yet it resulted in a large amount of stool elimination. Jaquelyn's physician recommended twice daily laxative use (polyethylene glycol) and sitting on the toilet for 15 minutes after each meal. After starting laxative use, she had almost daily episodes of loose stool, including the need for pad use and occasional clothing changes. Jaquelyn sat with her arms crossed at her waist and her head down in the waiting room. She turned away from the PT and said, "I do not want to be here." On her intake paperwork, her mom had written in "autism, picky eater," and checked "urinary incontinence, fecal incontinence, and constipation." Her first session introduced her to the "pelvic clock" exercise. (Jaquelyn's pelvic program outline is listed in more detail in the therapy section in this chapter.)

PARENT/CAREGIVER STRESS

Parents may be overjoyed with an infant who quickly learns "potty training" and develops autonomy with bathroom use. Yet parents can experience a phenomenal amount of stress and need for expert intervention, including social/emotional support, in the case of a child's failure to meet continence goals. Prolonged dependency on diapers, clothing changes, and hygiene assistance may occur. Other household members, from siblings to other relatives, need to help with continence training. From occasional bedwetting to the more serious condition of daily urinary or fecal incontinence, parents may consult multiple providers for assistance. Disruptions in work attendance, school, and playtime occur with pediatric continence issues, and/or pelvic pain.

LEARNED WITHHOLDING BEHAVIOR

The experience of straining and pain with passing large stools may lead children to withhold stool, and to avoid toilet use, and even reduce food and water intake to limit the need for bathroom use. Constipation creates increased pressure on the bladder and, as such, is a trigger for bladder leakage, and bladder leaks can be the first sign of the presence of constipation. (Remember this fact; it will be repeated as it is often missed in client care.) Toileting avoidance due to fear of pain can develop into a chronic pain cycle with resistance to toileting, muscle tensing, and significant illness with potential megacolon. Interventions for care should ideally optimize nutrition and digestion, promote bladder and bowel functioning to "work" automatically, and for the child to have tools and habits to be the "boss" of their body.

MECHANICS OF PELVIC/VISCERAL FUNCTIONING

Understanding plumbing: control of urination

Central and peripheral nerves, and the bladder and pelvic muscles, ideally work in synchrony for function. Bladder filling, storage or holding, and emptying all involve relays that develop in infancy and childhood. Eventually, these processes become automatic. Behavioral habit training is the first branch of treatment, and it addresses education and attention focus. Toddlers typically learn to focus with prompting from parents and other care providers and respond to praise with repeated behavior patterns.

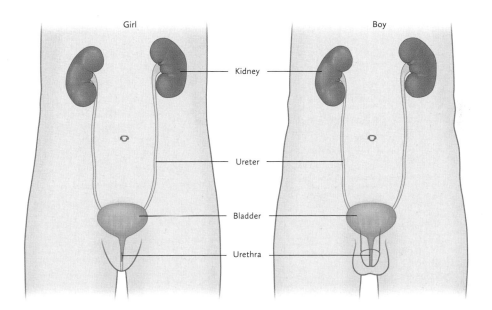

Figure 2.8 Kidneys and bladder.

For emptying urine, ideally, relaxed sitting (females) or standing (males) postures are used. The bladder contracts to empty, and pelvic muscles relax for ease of urination. This sounds simple, yet inadvertent tensing, clenching, and bearing down to speed emptying are often culprits in leakage (Figure 2.8). If too much urine is left in the bladder, as one leaves the toilet, post urination surprise leaks can occur. This is termed "post void micturition."

Understanding digestion and output

Digestion occurs in an amazing process from the mouth and through the entire gastrointestinal tract, with multiple nerve and sphincter (valve-like) regions that open and close. Many nerves are involved in the process, with signaling to the next region to prepare for action as needed, like a train calling ahead to stations in order to prepare for passengers. The vagus nerve is the master regulator for digestive functions, as well as facilitating relaxation and release of muscles (and their sphincters) for bladder and bowel emptying (Box 2.8). If an individual is under a high level of stress, the body may reduce blood flow to the gastrointestinal system and digestion may slow down, reducing the motility or movement along the "train tracks."

Box 2.8 The vagus nerve: relax, release, let go

The vagus nerve, cranial nerve 10, is recognized for "rest and digest" functions. It supplies parasympathetic input in regulating peristalsis, the wave-like contraction of the smooth muscle fibers that move solids and liquids along the system, such as swallowing and stomach motility, as well as bladder and bowel emptying. (The sympathetic system generally inhibits peristalsis, via limiting secretion and blood flow.) Pelvic rehabilitation ideally involves methods and programs to assist the enteric nervous system and vagus nerve towards optimized function. These methods will be profiled in future chapters.

PELVIC HEALTH CONDITIONS

Urinary incontinence

Urinary incontinence (UI), the involuntary loss of urine, is normal in infancy and up to ages 3 to 5 years in most cases. UI, also termed enuresis, may occur during the daytime, or at night, with bedwetting. Bedwetting is a challenge for parents and children (see Box 2.9). It is common in infants and young children, with dry nights developing between ages 3 and 5 years. Continence, "staying dry," is the goal for potty training. Continence may develop early, at age 3, but then a regression of function may occur with urinary incontinence occurring again at ages 4, 5, or later, in relation to environmental, medical, and/or behavioral factors.

other medical screening and intervention. However, a natural spontaneous acquisition of continence occurs between ages 5 and 9 years with annual improvement likely at 14% per year, and between ages 15 and 19 years, 16% improved per year (Forsythe and Redmond 1974).

Urinary problems in children can include UI, urinary hesitancy, weak stream, urinary withholding behavior, urinary retention, urinary tract infections, and vesicoureteral reflux (kidney and ureter dysfunction). Dysfunctional voiding symptoms can occur due to involuntary intermittent muscle contractions of the external urethral sphincter and pelvic floor muscle group observed during attempted voids and confirmed with urodynamic testing. Testing during bladder filling, holding, and emptying efforts may display a staccato pattern, and pre- and post-void volumes may show high post-void residual volume. Dysfunctional voiding patterns may be successfully treated with behavioral training, medical management, and rehabilitation care, including correction of dyssynergia (Zivkovic *et al.* 2012).

Constipation

Constipation is a condition that may include fewer than three stool outputs per week, straining or pain with defecation, hard or lumpy stools,

Box 2.9 Delays in maturation, and continence

A Canadian study of children with bedwetting (nocturnal enuresis) found that at 29 months of age 62.4% of children had bedwetting, diminished to 22.2% at 41 months, and the overall prevalence at 53 months was 9.7% (Touchette *et al.* 2005). In this study there was an association with premature birth, motor and speech delay, and hyperactivity and inattention in those with delayed attainment of continence. Incontinence may be a sign of a delay in central nervous system processing and warrant sensations of incomplete evacuation, or a sense of obstruction/blockage to emptying (Rome Foundation 2016) (Box 2.10).

Research demonstrates that identification and treatment of constipation in children produced subsequent improvement in reduced UI in 63–89 percent of children studied (Loening-Baucke 1997).

Fecal incontinence

Fecal incontinence (FI) is the involuntary loss of stool, termed feces or, in common vernacular, "poop." Fecal incontinence is common in infancy up to ages 3 to 5 years in typical development, and beyond that age becomes a concern. FI may range in its appearance from small balls to large firm masses, to softer matter and then liquid form, as displayed in the Bristol stool scale which identifies stool types #1–#7 (Figure 2.9).

In cases of constipation, firm stool may be present with softer stool leaking around it, creating soiling or smearing. Loss of loose stool in the case of constipation is termed encopresis. FI in children is typically related to constipation in 80 percent of cases, yet in 20 percent of cases "non-retentive" FI occurs, meaning that it is unrelated to any fecal retention/constipation (Koppen *et al.* 2016).

Medical management of encopresis involves multiple strategies. It can be confusing for parents to consider administering medicine to ease and increase stool output, yet the medications may make stool too loose and can also increase

stool leakage. In the case of retentive FI, the colon may lose its ability to contract to move the stool, which is a motility problem, as well as a child not sensing the "need to go."

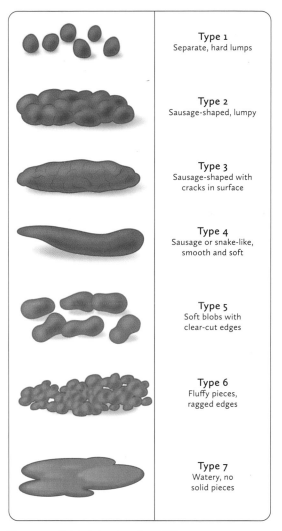

Figure 2.9 Bristol stool scale (BSS).

Enlarged colon, or megacolon

Over time with prolonged constipation, the colon can morph into a larger diameter shape, ranging from a few centimeters wide to over 5 cm or more. A child (or adult) may not have awareness of the enlarged colon. Health factors causing constipation, and possible techniques to retrain the colon, are listed below, as well as in Chapter 10 (Box 2.11).

Box 2.11 Enlarged colon, or megacolon

Severe constipation may require surgery, as in the case of megacolon. According to a study of children with irritable bowel disease (Benchimol *et al.* 2008), when the lumen of the large intestine becomes greater than or equal to 56 mm, toxic megacolon may be diagnosed, and approximately 70% of children may require a colectomy. Associated with toxic megacolon, these children may display dehydration, tachycardia, fever, electrolyte imbalances, and thickening of the intestinal walls. Medical intervention in the early stages of pediatric constipation is imperative in the prevention of megacolon.

Pelvic pain, continence issues, and trauma

Toddlers or children may have achieved continence and then begin schooling and encounter a teacher who does not, or cannot, allow on-demand toilet use. This can lead to a sense of dissociation from body signals (bladder or bowel filling) and a cessation of the normal response to use the toilet. A lack of privacy and bathroom antics from other children peering under stalls may also limit toilet use. An observed spider on a bathroom wall may create avoidance, or other stressors. Parents may need a private conference with a teacher to address the issues. A child may learn to "tune out and withhold," which then leads to accidents that may be associated with verbal or physical abuse from teachers or caregivers. Trauma may also occur with public shaming, such as wetting pants in front of class and being laughed at, thereby setting up an anxiety and fear in relation to bladder signals in the future.

Urinary urgency and frequency may develop in attempts to prevent recurrence.

Children may suffer with limited socialization and loss of play time with friends and anxiety due to their fear of accidents and the potential discovery of continence pads. Child sport participation may be curtailed or limited in relation to pelvic health concerns. Social rejection, bullying, and stigmatization may occur and consequently a child may withdraw from social activities and school participation. Negative interactions in medical evaluation and treatment may lead to a "white coat syndrome," with anxiety, fear, and avoidance regarding medical intervention, with a subsequent medical phobia. Finally, a consideration in pelvic health should be that continence problems in children may also be associated with sexual abuse, which providers have a mandate to report if this is suspected (De Bellis, Woolley, and Hooper 2013) (Box 2.12).

Box 2.12 Trauma sensitive therapy

Somatic experiencing may be transformational in a child who is traumatized by experiences related to their pelvic health condition. Body scanning, calming, therapeutic movement exploration, and guided visualization may be used by trauma sensitive therapists to facilitate a child's ability to release the mind, body, and spirit from trauma. A child needs to be able to recognize and respond to bodily signals, including pelvic sensations and functioning. If a "disconnect" and/or the presence of trauma is not identified in regard to sensory processing, therapies may offer tools for care that cannot be utilized due to the somato-emotional protective mechanisms in place. Yoga routines and Swiss ball programs can help a child to relax and release stress and trauma, as well as tune into body signals.

Pelvic floor muscle synergy and pelvic core mechanics

Toddlers learn to sit on a toilet and "let it go," to relax to allow bowel output and urination. Synergy between the abdominal wall and the pelvic floor muscles (PFM) involves a coordination between relaxing the PFM and firming the abdomen slightly for defecation. During defecation and generating intra-abdominal pressure, the external anal sphincter and levator ani muscles relax. Pressure is generated into the pelvic cavity to assist the rectum in elimination. For urination, the bladder muscle, the detrusor, contracts to squeeze urine out of the bladder into the urethra, and the pelvic floor muscles relax to allow urine outflow. Abdominal muscles may remain relaxed during urination. (In males, the bulbocavernosus muscle contracts to help squeeze urine out during urination.) In the case of normal trunk control for postural support, individuals easily sit on a toilet for elimination, or males, standing for urination.

Conservative care with nutrition, fluid and fiber management, and behavioral training are strategies that can produce positive results over time, yet require participation by teachers, parents, and ultimately a child internalizing positive health habits that become healthy routines.

Dyssynergia: clenching versus relaxing and "tight butts"

Pelvic floor dyssynergia is the inability to relax the pelvic floor muscles during attempted defecation or urination (Benninga *et al.* 2005) (Box 2.13). Unknowingly, individuals may actually be tightening muscles when they think they are relaxing. And individuals may bear down and release pelvic muscles when they think they are contracting and tightening the muscles. Dyssynergia is common in individuals with pelvic floor disorders. A coordination between muscle groups is required for urination and defecation.

Box 2.13 Physical therapy to train synergy

Pediatric pelvic physical therapy with exercise and biofeedback has been found to be of benefit in dyssynergic defecation. A retrospective study of 69 children receiving medical care found 76% demonstrating improvement, compared to 25% of patients receiving conservative treatment of medication alone. Patients with anxiety and low muscle tone had the best response rate (100%) (Zar-Kessler *et al.* 2019).

Fear of falling into the toilet: a cause for dyssynergia

Toddlers attempting training on tall toilets where their feet do not reach the ground may tense their trunk, pelvic, and leg muscles to avoid falling in the toilet and develop dyssynergic defecation and urination habits. Potty training on low toddler toilets and/or the use of footstools can help stabilize the body for bladder and bowel emptying. The "squatty potty" is a popular support stool for children or even adults, to assist in relaxation (Figures 2.10 and 2.11). And in regions where toilets are not available, individuals learn to squat and balance and relax their pelvic muscles to eliminate.

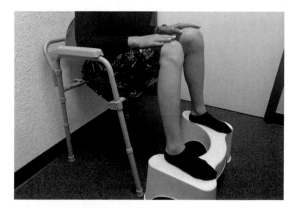

Figure 2.10 Squatty potty.

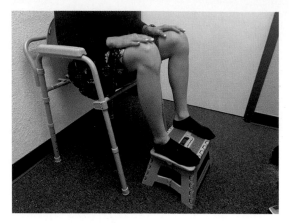

Figure 2.11 Footstool use.

Expectations for attainment of bladder and bowel control

The ability to achieve bladder and bowel control occurs in a range of two and three quarter years (33 months), up to 5 years old. Maturation of the nervous system, cognitive, sensory, and motor control, and parent training strategies are all important in toilet training. Developmental milestones may be delayed, with "red flags" including a lack of head control in supported sitting at 4 months, an inability to sit at 9 months, and an inability to walk independently at 18 months (Gerber, Wilks, and Erdie-Lalena 2010). Infants and children that have required surgeries may have missed developmental milestones and require transitions through developmental

"play" with postures and movement patterns for attainment of optimum functioning.

Requirements for bladder and bowel continence include functioning kidneys, ureters, bladder, and urethra, and a functioning gastrointestinal system, including absorption of nutrients and motility through the small intestine and colon to the rectum. The bladder and bowel need storage, as well as emptying capacities. Medical testing may be needed to clarify sources of pelvic symptoms; see Box 2.14.

> ## Box 2.14 Medical screening for pelvic problems
> Diagnostic testing with ultrasound, and urologic testing (cystoscopy, uroflowmetry) and gastroenterology testing (X-ray, ultrasound, and sitz markers showing timelines of marker placement along the digestive tract, and defecography), may identify organic structural causes that require medical attention and treatment (Raizada and Mittal 2008). However, most cases of UI and FI are functional, as there is no identified pathology, yet function is abnormal (Dohil *et al.* 1994). Functional bladder and bowel disorders respond best to behavioral intervention, utilizing conservative care practices as introduced here and outlined in further chapters.

GUT MICROBIOME

The infant gut microbiome (GM) from birth to age 3 years and beyond is an area of growing research interest. In relevance to pelvic health, the GM displays varied species depending on maternal health factors, birth type (surgical versus vaginal), feeding patterns (breast fed versus formula), and exposure to antibiotics and environmental influences. Pro-inflammatory microbes may have a larger presence in babies born by cesarean section, who are formula fed

(Yang *et al.* 2016). The GM influences stool type, the presence or absence of flatulence, homeostasis in the immune system, neurotransmitter production, and many other factors. Infants and children receiving surgeries and/or antibiotics may have a sequela of constipation, diarrhea, and other health problems in association with a low species GM. However, randomized controlled trials do not exist that provide guidelines for types of probiotics to assist pediatric pelvic health; more research is warranted (van Mill, Koppen, and Benninga 2019). Functional medicine providers may perform stool testing and supplementation with pre- and probiotic supplementation. See Chapters 10 and 14 regarding gut microbiome.

THE DEVELOPMENTAL SEQUENCE

Screening and therapeutic programming for the developmental sequence is a gold standard in pediatric therapy, with gross motor skills and cognitive skills as requirements for meeting pelvic health milestones for continence and independence. (Fine motor, speech, and activities of daily living are addressed by specialists as needed as well.)

Initially a baby has a predominance of flexor tone, and by three months begins to bring hands to midline, and to also open the arms to the side, and even lift the head in prone. Rolling begins to occur by four to five months, and by age six months, sitting. Extensor tone in the spine increases with prone positioning and a straight arm press up is achieved by five to six months. Trunk control with positioning on hands and knees and rocking at six months develops into crawling at nine months. Squatting with arm assistance, pulling up to kneeling (eight months), pulling up to standing (nine months), and cruising to step with support (9–12 months) are typical patterns. Gait with support at age 12 months, climbing stairs with support, and running at 24 months are typical gross motor timelines.

PELVIC MUSCLES AND THE CORE

Neuromuscular control systems and performance abilities are varied across individuals, and screening respiration, stability, and mobility patterns of the trunk, pelvis, and hip area are critical in pelvic screening and intervention. The pelvic muscle group is regarded as part of the "core" of the body, along with the transverse abdominis muscle group, the deep spine multifidus, and the respiratory diaphragm all working together for stability and mobility (Figure 2.12). Research studies identify automatic contractions between the pelvic floor muscles and transverse abdominis in response to anticipated exertion, and during activity (Park and Dongwook 2015). The diaphragm and its mobility in an up and down pattern is regarded as a pump or piston for health, for autonomic nervous system balance, digestive processes, and coordinated stability and mobility (Bordoni *et al.* 2018).

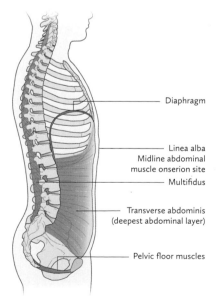

Figure 2.12 Lumbopelvic core.

THERAPY FOR PEDIATRIC PELVIC HEALTH

A multifaceted treatment approach is required, customized to each child and their family milieu, and recognizing barriers to rehabilitation. The child's health history of potential pelvic anomalies at birth, antibiotic use (gut microbiome disruption), surgery, cognitive status, gross and fine motor level skill, and somato-emotional state are all considered in planning care. Psychological stressors such as a recent move, loss of a family member, school change, or parental separation or divorce can also impact child health status and onset or aggravation of pelvic floor dysfunction.

The biopsychosocial model and pelvic health

The whole person view is considered with the biopsychosocial (BPS) model as outlined by the World Health Organization international classification functioning, disability, and health (Wade and Halligan 2017). The BPS model is useful in whole person care and identifies a health condition (such as pain or constipation), biological factors (body functions and structures/genetics), and individual activities (such as self-prompting to the toilet, and life as a student) and participation status (such as community outings or play with friends). The BPS model also considers environmental factors (such as bathroom stalls, tall toilets, no privacy) and personal factors (such as psychological and cognitive factors: anxiety, autism, OCD). Providers using the BPS model can include evidence-based medicine in a compassionate manner with recognition of all individual attributes and challenges (Rajindrajith, Devanarayana, and Benninga 2013; Scorza, Stevenson, and Canino 2013).

A framework for pediatric pelvic care will first address child psychosocial status, which may be indicated by body language, speech, and eye contact, as well as intake history. Pain, perceived lack of bodily control, and medical intervention such as enema therapy may have set the stage for fight or flight or freeze behavior, with sympathetic nervous system up-regulation. In the case of anxiety, fear, health care provider avoidance, and anger, trauma sensitive programming can help to promote trust and patient and parent program adherence. Pelvic health therapy has the potential to help a child feel comfortable in their body, confident in speaking up about the need for restroom use, and foster child-centered, empowered communication with holistic providers, and with medical care.

PEDIATRIC PELVIC PROGRAM OUTLINE

Pelvic therapy involves education, movement therapy, fluid and fiber management, nutrition adjustment, daily activity recommendations, encouraged toilet use after meals, and improved defecation and/or urination mechanics including posturing and muscle synergy. Movement therapy may be combined with bodywork/manual therapy for optimizing function. Teaching children to "say hello" to body areas can be helpful and add an element of play.

MANUAL THERAPY: SAYING HELLO TO THE BODY AND ITS PARTS

In application of manual therapy for pelvic health, hands-on care may be provided to the spine, abdomen, pelvis, hip, trunk, and other regions (Box 2.15). Treatment is performed ideally with parents or caregivers observing and receiving instruction in possible follow through with hands-on care at home if the parent is able and interested. A child can be directed to "say hello" to the area where the bladder sits, or the colon has its final "train tracks" in the left lower pelvis, and other hello cues. Laughter may accompany this education!

Surgical sites of scar tissue from procedures may be palpated by the therapist to assess superficial to deeper fascial systems in the musculoskeletal, neurological, visceral, and lymphatic regions, and to mobilize restrictions. Facilitation of full respiration may be attained with gentle work to the rib cage, diaphragm, and abdominal wall (Figures 2.13–2.15).

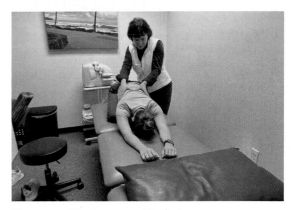

Figure 2.13 Diaphragm and lateral costal facilitation in child's pose.

Box 2.15 Compassion based manual therapy with client empowerment

Steps to provide manual therapy include:

1. Education of the client and family as to what will be done, and the rationale
2. Asking permission to provide hands-on care, as in "May I feel your belly to see how it is today?" or "May I place my hands on your back to help your breathing?" or "Would you like me to show mom or dad how to help your belly with a massage?"
3. Educating the client as to the option to say "no," "not today," or other statements to empower self-awareness, choice, and control
4. The therapist feeling energetically balanced and non-striving, having adequate time and attention for the client

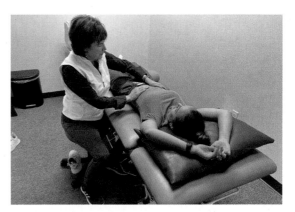

Figure 2.14 Abdominal wall/diaphragm facilitation, legs on bolster.

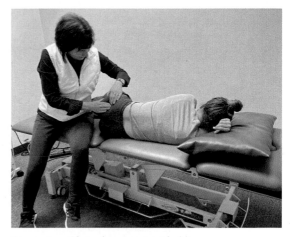

Figure 2.15 Gluteal massage, side lying.

Colon massage is very helpful in promoting awareness of body regions and body "signals" as well as restoring the motility function of the colon. (See Figure 10.2.)

Food sensitivities and allergies may be present, requiring analysis and nutrition training for parents and children. (Yet those in lower socioeconomic groups likely will not have access to this type of care.) Teaching and training in toilet mechanics is standard and can be accomplished with child friendly graphics and coloring books, parent and child education in the use of a footstool for stability, and the role of pelvic muscle relaxation required for emptying bladder and bowel. Sitting with knees open and relaxed diaphragm breathing is a starting point. Practice in gentle bearing down to assist bowel emptying requires abdominal wall tensing, and relaxing pelvic outlet muscles. Relaxed pelvic status for urination is trained, versus pushing urine out or rushing. Ultrasound and biofeedback may be used by medical providers to train function (Box 2.16).

Box 2.16 Real time ultrasound imaging (RUSI)

Medical providers can screen and train the effort for PFM relaxation, bearing down mechanics, as well as contraction/lift of the PFM. These mechanics may be screened with visual inspection, with digital palpation of the abdominal wall and external PFM, with real time ultrasound (RUSI), and/or with biofeedback (BFB) using electromyography sensors on either side of the external anal sphincter. RUSI and BFB guide accurate training of the PFM, including cues towards muscle strengthening for activities such as "stop a fart, stop your pee" as well as relaxation strategies and defecation mechanics. (BFB equipment allows the biologic signal of the nerve firing to be changed into a graphic representation on a computer screen.)

Graphics such as flowers, fractals, or spirals opening and closing can engender a peaceful sense during PFM BFB training.

Client self-care with parents' support

Tools for patient use include:

- daily tracking of supplements, fluid, fiber
- Bristol stool scale output tracking (#1–#7)
- episodes of urinary incontinence or fecal incontinence
- constipation: no output that day
- relaxed sitting on the toilet after meals
- colon massage
- exercise.

By utilizing a detective process, a tracker, the child and/or adult care provider can promote adherence to a program, and awareness of the triggers for the problems. A healthy habit tracker can be used to cue the child and the parents towards pelvic control and confidence, as well as optimizing hydration and nutrition.

For younger children, a reward system such as stickers, a toy box, verbal praise, and parent directed "special privileges" such as a park outing may help motivate towards compliance with pediatric pelvic rehabilitation. Children may choose a prompt they would prefer such as a chime sound on a computer or vibration on a watch to cue body scanning for bowel or bladder signals and for urinating every two hours if leaks are occurring from infrequent void attempts.

Therapeutic exercise can include aspects of the developmental sequence that address child specific limitations, such as reciprocal patterning with crawling, poor trunk stability, and altered respiratory dynamics. Stability ball exercises add an aspect of play that can be fun for the therapist and the child (Figures 2.16–2.21).

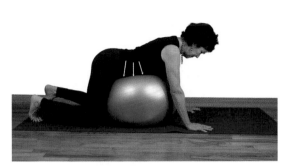

Figure 2.16 Quadruped on a ball.

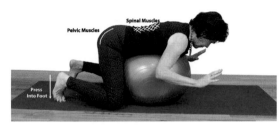

Figure 2.17 Rocking back.

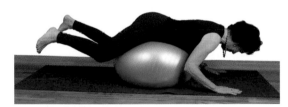

Figure 2.18 Rocking front.

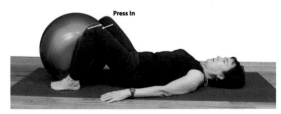

Figure 2.19 Ball squeeze.

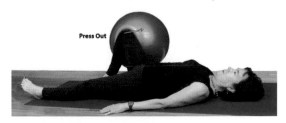

Figure 2.20 Ball push out.

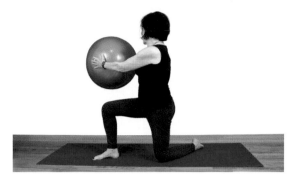

Figure 2.21 Half kneeling hold of ball.

Exercise strategies that are keys to focusing attention on breath and pelvic muscle control include primary movement patterns that are part of the typical developmental motor sequence. These exercises listed below require fundamental control of joint stability and mobility, and their skilled performance, or limitations, will guide programming. Children may enjoy these exercises and find them to be soothing routines, and they may be practiced as part of a family relax, rest, and stretch group exercise to engender a sense of wellbeing and play.

Yoga asanas (postures) are useful for promoting awareness of breath and relaxation versus tensing of the body, globally, as well as directing attention to the pelvic region. Lying down, face up (supine), initiate instruction and "play" with diaphragm breathing, rocking knees side to side, hip bridging, and pulling single, and then double knees to chest, with cues to notice hips, and easy breathing. Next, with both knees to chest, opening the knees and relaxing inner thighs and pelvic muscles, cuing to "relax the bottom." In quadruped, anterior–posterior rocking, to cat camel, to child's pose, to a press up. This may be followed by kneeling to squatting and standing. Crawling, bear crawls, catching and tossing balls, or squeezing a ball between the knees may be used for cuing muscle coordination. Pediatric pelvic health and dysfunction may benefit from multiple forms of treatment as portrayed in this chapter (Boxes 2.17 and 2.18).

Box 2.17 Pediatric pelvic therapy for constipation and encopresis

Jaquelyn received 12 physical therapy (PT) sessions over the course of 8 months, with once weekly for the first 6 weeks and tapering to once a month for the later visits. She used a tracking log and indicated Bristol stool type and bladder and bowel leaks. Her program included a strict, slow tapering of her laxative, and the addition of a few vegetable and fruit items to her diet, and increased hydration to 25–30 ounces per day. On advice, she stopped eating the "binding" foods of bananas and rice, and limited her bread intake. Manual therapy treated limitations in mobility of the rib, diaphragm, abdominal, gluteal, and colon areas, with education for parents to provide the similar massage if all parties were able and interested. Pelvic floor training for synergy used ultrasound and external biofeedback. Mat and stability ball exercises were instructed, emphasizing comfort, relaxation, and flow, and also light PFM tensing and relaxing. She enjoyed learning to use a stability ball for her pelvic health, and it felt somewhat similar to gymnastics she had begun prior to her pelvic health problems. She exhibited an improved affect as her pelvic health improved, with smiling and eye contact with her therapist during discussions and review of her monthly tracking log. She was able to return to dance and gymnastics class as well at the completion of the therapy.

Box 2.18 Medical management

Medical management requires adherence to behavioral interventions as listed above, as well as supplement use as needed, such as laxatives and stimulants and possibly suppositories and enemas. Emerging research points to the gut microbiome in pelvic health, yet this is not yet mainstream care. The MOP book (Hodges and Schlosberg 2018) discusses the "bottom up" approach to constipation with enema therapy, in addition to "top down" strategies that rely on fluid, fiber, and behavioral/nutrition management. Enemas may seem like drastic measures, but in the case of a chronically overstretched colon, signaling for a sense of fullness will not occur until the colon shrinks over the course of months and up to a year. Enemas may be traumatizing, and there are specialty seminars for pediatric pelvic health for providers needing introductory to advanced rehabilitation training and mentorship (Sandalcidi 2018).

In summary, pelvic health conditions in pediatrics are relatively common, and conservative care therapy can be composed of simple elements that create healthy habits, and allow the child to participate in family life, school, recreational, and community activities. Programs can be designed for fun and empowerment towards self-awareness and self-care. Child program cooperation, patience, and perseverance from parents, teachers, and all providers are required to overcome frustration and repeated challenges.

REFERENCES

Benchimol, E., Turner, D., Mann, E. H., Thomas, K. E., et al. (2008) "Inflammatory bowel disease; clinical and radiographic characteristics." *The American Journal of Gastroenterology 103*, 6, 1524–1531.

Benninga, M., David, C., Catto-Smith, A. G., Clayden, G., et al. (2005) "The Paris consensus on childhood constipation terminology (PAACT) group." *Journal of Pediatric Gastroenterology and Nutrition 40*, 3, 273–275.

Bordoni, B., Purgol, S., Bizzarri, A., Modica, M., et al. (2018) "The influence of breathing on the central nervous system." *Cureus 10*, 6, e2724.

Brantberg, A., Blass, H.-G. K., Haugen, S. E., Isaken, C. V., and Elk-Nes, S. H. (2006) "Imperforate anus; a relatively common anomaly rarely diagnosed prenatally." *Ultrasound in Obstetrics and Gynecology 28*, 7, 904–910.

Chase, J., Austin, P., Hoebeke, P., and McKenna, P. (2010) "The management of dysfunctional voiding in children: A report from the standardization committee of the international children's continence society." *Journal of Urology 183*, 1296-1302.

De Bellis, M. D., Woolley, D. P., and Hooper, S. R. (2013) "Neuropsychological findings in pediatric maltreatment: Relationship of PTSD, dissociative symptoms, and abuse/neglect indices to neurocognitive outcomes." *Child Maltreatment 18*, 171.

Dohil, R., Roberts, E., Jones, K. V., and Jenkins, H. R. (1994) "Constipation and reversible urinary tract abnormalities." *Archives of Disease in Childhood 70*, 56.

Forsythe, W. I. and Redmond, A. (1974) "Enuresis and spontaneous cure rate: Study of 1129 enuretis." *Archives of Disease in Childhood 49*, 4, 259-263.

Franco, I. (2011) "New ideas in the cause of bladder dysfunction in children." *Current Opinion in Urology 21*, 4, 334-338.

Gerber, R. J., Wilks, T., and Erdie-Lalena, C. (2010) "Developmental milestones: Motor development." *Pediatrics in Review 31*, 267-277.

Hodges, S. and Schlosberg, S. (2018) *The MOP Book: A Guide to the Only Proven Way to Stop Bedwetting and Accidents*. Bend, OR, USA: O'Regan Press.

Koppen, I. J. N., von Gontard, A., Chase, J., et al. (2016) "Management on functional nonretentive fecal incontinence in children: Recommendations from the Children's Continence Society." *Journal of Pediatric Urology 12*, 1, 56-64.

Loening-Baucke, V. (1997) "Urinary incontinence and urinary tract infection and their resolution with treatment of chronic constipation of childhood." *Pediatrics 100*, 228.

Park, H. and Dongwook, H. (2015) "The effect of the correlation between the contraction of the pelvic floor muscles and diaphragmatic motion during breathing." *Journal of Physical Therapy Science 27*, 2113-2115.

Pini-Prato, A., Mattioli, G., Giunta, C., Avanzini, S., et al. (2010) "Redo surgery in Hirschsprung disease; what did we learn? Unicentric experience on 70 patients." *Journal of Pediatric Surgery 45*, 4, 747-754.

Raizada, V. and Mittal, R. (2008) "Pelvic floor anatomy and applied physiology." *Gastroenterology Clinics North America 37*, 3, 493-509.

Rajindrajith, S., Devanarayana, N. M., and Benninga, M. A. (2013) "Review article: Faecal Incontinence in Children: Epidemiology, Pathophysiology, Clinical Evaluation and Management." *Alimentary Pharmacology and Therapeutics 37*, 37-48.

Rome Foundation (2016) "Rome IV diagnostic criteria for functional gastrointestinal disorders." Accessed 6/2/2022 at www.theromefoundation.org.

Sandalcidi, D. (2018) "Paediatric incontinence and pelvic floor dysfunction." *Journal of Pelvic, Obstetric and Gynecological Physiotherapy 122*, 5-8.

Sathyanarayana, S., Grady, R., Barrett, E. S., Redmond, B., et al. (2016) "First trimester phthalate exposure and male newborn genital anomalies." *Environmental Research 151*, 777-782.

Schultz-Lampel, D., Steuber, C., Hoyer, P. F., Bachmann, C. J., et al. (2011) "Urinary incontinence in children." *Deutsches Ärzteblatt International 108*, 37, 613-620.

Scorza, P., Stevenson, A., and Canino, G. (2013) "Validation of the World Health Organization disability assessment schedules for children. WHODAS-Child, in Rwanda." *PLoS One 8*, 3, e57725.

Solomon, B. D. (2011) "VACTERL/VATER Association." *Orphanet Journal of Rare Diseases 6*, 56.

Springer, A., van den Heijkant, M., and Baumann, S. (2016) "Worldwide prevalence of hypospadias." *Journal of Pediatric Urology 12*, 152.e1-7.

Thackery, E. and Harris, M. (2003) *Gale Encyclopedia of Mental Disorders (1st ed.)*. Detroit, MI: Gale.

Tjaden Butler, N. E. and Trainor, P. A. (2013) "The developmental etiology and pathogenesis of Hirschsprung disease." *Translational Research 162*, 1, 1-15.

Touchette, E., Petit, D., Paquet, J., Tremblay, R., et al. (2005) "Bed wetting and its association with developmental milestones in early childhood." *JAMA Pediatrics 159*, 12, 1129-1134.

TRAILS (2022) "5 Fs of Trauma Response." Accessed 10/10/22 at https://storage.trailstowellness.org/trails-2/resources/5-fs-of-trauma-response.pdf.

van Mill, M. J., Koppen, I. J. N., and Benninga, M. A. (2019) "Controversies in the management of functional constipation in children." *Current Gastroenterology Reports 21*, 6, 23.

von Gontard, A., Pirrung, M., Niemczyk, J., and Equit, M. (2015) "Incontinence in children with autism spectrum disorder." *Journal of Pediatric Urology 11*, 5, 264.e1-7.

Vuong, H. E. and Hsiao, E. Y. (2017) "Emerging roles for the gut microbiome in autism spectrum disorder." *Review, Society of Biological Society 81*, 411-423.

Wade, D. T. and Halligan, P. W. (2017) "The biopsychosocial model of illness; a model whose time has come." *Clinical Rehabilitation*, https://doi.org/10.1177/0269215517709890

Wang, Y. and Qian, H. (2021) "Phthalates and their impacts on human health." *Healthcare (Basel) 9*, 5, 603.

Wood, R. and Levitt, M. (2018) "Anorectal malformations." *Clinics in Colorectal Surgery 31*, 61-70.

Yang, I., Corwin, E. J., Brennan, P. A., Jordan, S., et al. (2016) "The infant gut microbiome; implications for infant health and neurocognitive development." *Nursing Research 65*, 1, 76-88.

Zar-Kessler, C., Kuo, B., Cole, E., Benedix, A., and Belkind-Gerso, J. (2019) "Benefit of pelvic floor physical therapy in pediatric patients with dyssynergic defecation constipation." *Digestive Disease 37*, 478-485.

Zink, S., Freitag, C. M., and von Gontard, A. (2018) "Behavioral comorbidity differs in subtypes of enuresis and urinary incontinence." *Journal of Urology 179*, 295-298.

Zivkovic, V., Lazovic, M., Vlalkovic, M., Slavkovic, A., et al. (2012) "Diaphragmatic breathing exercises and pelvic floor retraining in children with dysfunctional voiding." *European Journal of Physical Medicine and Rehabilitation Medicine 48*, 413-421.

FURTHER RESOURCES

Bodywork definition, https://en.wikipedia.org/wiki/Bodywork_(alternative_medicine)

The Environmental Working Group, www.ewg.org/consumer-guides

Kids Bowel and Bladder, https://kidsbowelbladder.com

CHAPTER 3

Pelvic Health in Teens and Young Adults

Part I of this chapter introduces pelvic health challenges and related musculoskeletal conditions that may occur in teens and young adults. Part II presents systems for screening movement and injuries, and then, progressive therapeutic exercise strategies for health and healing.

Movement therapists and bodyworkers may be the first holistic health resources that teens are exposed to, and this care can support mind–body–spirit health that is a vibrant taproot for fruitful development into adulthood. Some teens may pursue careers in the healing arts and sciences in response to their injuries and their care received.

PART I PELVIC HEALTH CHALLENGES AND RELATED MUSCULOSKELETAL CONDITIONS

During the lifespan from preteen to young adult, there are many influences on pelvic function. Teens undergo rapid musculoskeletal maturation, ideally with neuromuscular control developing towards stability, strength, coordination, agility, flexibility, and ease with walking and running. Athletic participation may begin or expand from childhood sports, as well as hiking, dance, or other types of exercise, ideally helping to strengthen growing bones and muscles, and overall physical fitness (Box 3.1). Musculoskeletal growth spurts are remarkable, as teens mature towards their adult height. However, rapid growth in teens may cause vulnerability towards injury, such as growth plates in bones.

Endocrine changes, genetics, and environmental influences combine to produce sexual characteristic maturation and body type profile. Body types may tend towards leaner, "ectomorphic" type, rounder, "endomorphic" type, or muscular, "mesomorphic" type, yet most body types are a combination of these profiles.

> ### Box 3.1 Appropriate exercise intensity
> Teens should not strength train with resistance at a maximum level because their skeletal "growth plates" are not yet mature, and at risk for fracture. The maturation of the lumbar, pelvic, and hip bones spans from ages 9 to 20, with females maturing a few years earlier than males. In the pelvic region, secondary (final) ossification occurs at the femur, acetabulum, ilium, ischium, and pubis as chondrocytes mature into osteoblasts, to mature ossification (Verbruggen and Nowlan 2017).

During teen development, gender identity may shift from female or male identity and affiliations, towards identification as non-binary, lesbian, gay, bisexual, transgender, or queer (LGBTQ+). Non-binary and LGBTQ+ identities in youth and teens may involve challenges for psychological, social, and cultural wellbeing, and also entail medical intervention for hormonal and surgical procedures. Providers working with the LGBTQ+ population should be capable of respect, recognition of individual expression, and provide a client-centered approach to health and wellness in any intervention or refer to another provider.

FEMALES

Health conditions in the teen life phase include premenstrual syndrome, premenstrual dysphoric disorder, dysmenorrhea, endometriosis, thyroid disorders, and polycystic ovarian syndrome. Sexually active teens may experience dyspareunia (pain with sex), vaginismus (vaginal spasm), urinary tract infection, or sexually transmitted disease. All of these conditions can be associated with pelvic floor muscle (PFM) spasm, altered respiratory patterns, and possibly the development of chronic pelvic pain.

Females in general suffer more pain than males, with research summarizing, "It is becoming very evident that gender differences in pain and its relief arise from an interaction of genetic, anatomical, physiological, neuronal, hormonal, psychological and social factors which modulate pain differently in the sexes" (Pieretti *et al.* 2016).

Premenstrual syndrome (PMS) may include symptoms of bloating, weight gain, mood changes, nausea, and other symptoms. Lifestyle practices that help with stress management and reducing inflammation in the body are found to be helpful for PMS. Meditation, exercise, nutrition, and yoga practices are correlated with reduced PMS symptoms (Hashim *et al.* 2018; Viswanthan and Pinto 2015; Wilson 2022). PMS may be screened with the PMS assessment form, which may also be used to track the results of treatments for research (Guthrie 2022).

As PMS symptom severity increases, it may become a disabling cluster of symptoms that is more serious, as in premenstrual dysphoric disorder (PMDD) (see Box 3.2 and Table 3.1). Due to alterations in hormone levels, neurotransmitters, and significant mood alterations based on physiologic processes, PMDD may require medical screening and pharmaceutical intervention in addition to standard therapies for PMS.

Box 3.2 PMS and PMDD

PMS and PMDD both include cyclical symptoms that occur before menses, and medical screening is used to differentiate between the two. PMS is reported to occur in 80% of women, with a range of severity, and PMDD in 5% of women. The number of symptoms and their severity help differentiate between the conditions and require tracking over a few months of the menstrual cycle. A useful tracker is the Daily Record of Severity of Problems (DRSP) (Endicott, Nee, and Harrison 2007). Risk factors for PMS and PMDD are multifactorial, and treatment may include behavioral therapy, hormone and/or antidepressant medication, lifestyle modifications, and chasteberry and calcium supplements (Hofmeister and Bodden 2016; Lustyk *et al.* 2009; Pearlstein and Steiner 2012; Robinson and Ismail 2015).

Table 3.1 PMS and PMDD symptoms

Symptom types	PMS	PMDD
Sleep	Variable	Possible insomnia or hypersomnia
Somatic symptoms	Breast tenderness, headaches, muscle and joint pains, swelling, bloating, weight gain One or two of these symptoms	A few of these symptoms
Affective symptoms	Anxiety, depressed mood, irritability, feelings of overwhelm, concentration difficulties, emotional lability, loss of interest in activity participation, low energy levels, food cravings, over-eating Only a few of these symptoms	A multitude of these symptoms
Functional level at home, community, work	Mild to moderate impairment with the need to limit or stop home, community, and/or work participation during the premenstrual phase	Moderate to severe impairment in home, community, and/or work participation during the premenstrual phase

(Endicott et al. 2006; Hofmeister and Bodden 2012; Pearlstein and Steiner 2012; Robinson and Ismail 2015)

Dysmenorrhea

Dysmenorrhea, or painful menstruation, occurs in a wide range of females, with incidence rates from 16 percent to 91 percent (Ju, Jones, and Mishra 2014). Dysmenorrhea can include premenstrual symptoms as well as symptoms during menses. Typical symptoms include pain, cramping, nausea, headache, diarrhea, and vomiting. Severe disabling pain is found in 2 percent to 29 percent of women, with activity limitations such as bed rest required, and missing school, work, and other functional roles (see Box 3.3).

Risk factors for dysmenorrhea may include a positive family history of dysmenorrhea, younger age, insufficient exercise, a poor diet, and exposure to life and work stress as precipitating factors. Obesity is an associated risk factor in some but not all research studies. There is a protective effect from regular physical exercise, self-care, nutrition awareness, parturition, and oral contraceptive use (Bavil *et al.* 2016). Dysmenorrhea is caused by uterine contractility in response to prostaglandin hypersecretion. Dysmenorrhea may be an isolated medical occurrence, or also occur in association with two medical conditions, endometriosis and adenomyosis (Bernardi *et al.* 2017).

> **Box 3.3 Symptom tracking, and considering if care is needed**
>
> Do we take cyclical pain complaints seriously, and consider hormone, neurovascular, and endocrine fluctuations in an individual, or write pain off due to "emotional instability"? Teaching teens to track their mood, pain, and menses over a few months can provide insight and patterns in relation to the menstrual cycle, as well as assist therapists with providing care. Validating symptoms and offering programs for wellness can lessen symptom burden.

Menstrual cycle trackers in the form of electronic applications (apps) are widespread in use and may help individuals to identify symptoms and decrease the stigma associated with menstruation. (Symptom burden may be shared with an individual's health care provider to help with screening and optimizing treatment.) The apps may also be used to track fertility, and as birth control, yet they may not always be accurate and may result in unwanted pregnancies (Earle *et al.* 2019).

Research validates beneficial self-care skills to help with dysmenorrhea, including the use of acupressure, nutrition, the use of heat, and aerobic and/or more gentle and sustainable exercise such as yoga and Pilates (Armour *et al.* 2019). Exercise is one of the key foundations that may lighten the burden of dysmenorrhea, with sample exercises below (Figures 3.1–3.9).

Gentle exercise for PMS and dysmenorrhea, moving in a flow:

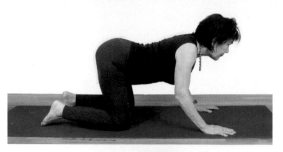

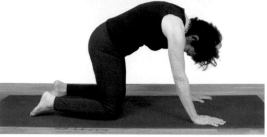

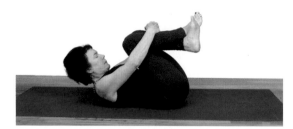

Figure 3.1 Knees to chest, supine.

Figure 3.4 Cat camel.

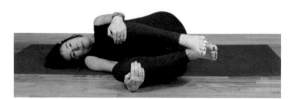

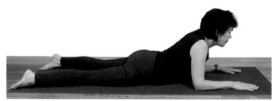

Figure 3.2 Rocking supine, right and left.

Figure 3.5 Sphinx (partial press up).

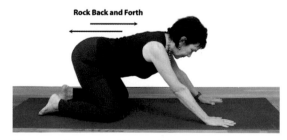

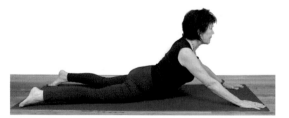

Figure 3.3 Posterior glide, rocking in quadruped.

Figure 3.6 Press up.

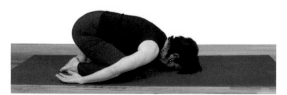

Figure 3.7 Child's pose.

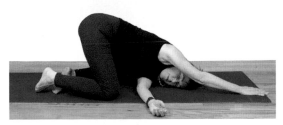

Figure 3.8 Thread the needle.

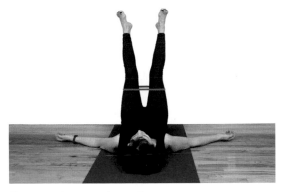

Figure 3.9 Legs up the wall.

Exercise is promoted for improved health and reduced pain and other symptoms related to PMS and dysmenorrhea (Office on Women's Health 2021).

Endometriosis and polycystic ovarian syndrome

Endometriosis and polycystic ovarian syndrome (PCOS) conditions are typically not diagnosed until after years of suffering.

Endometriosis is a systemic inflammatory health condition that characteristically includes endometrial (uterine) tissue occurring outside the uterine lining, and dysmenorrhea and infertility are often present (see Box 3.4). This occurs in 10 percent to 15 percent of females in their reproductive years (Agarwal *et al.* 2019; Asghari *et al.* 2018). Endometriosis is present in 30 percent to 45 percent of women with infertility. Sadly, it takes an average of 12 years for women with endometriosis to receive a diagnosis, and pain presentation may be misleading with abdominal, pelvic, bladder, bowel, and even radiating leg pain being present.

> **Box 3.4 Endometriosis**
> Genetics, epigenetics, oxidative stress, inflammatory cytokines, and hormonal influences are all involved in endometriosis disease initiation and progression. Historically, women have received birth control, pain medications, and surgery for endometriosis. Laparoscopic surgery or hysterectomy for endometriosis is common, yet tissue removal does not eradicate the symptoms in all, with a recurrence rate of 3.3–62% (Rizk *et al.* 2013; Soliman *et al.* 2017). The failure of sole surgical treatment points to the need to consider systemic influences that are pro-inflammatory.

The role of oxidative stress, as well as the potential for an anti-inflammatory lifestyle, is being studied in endometriosis, with recent research stating, "Overall, the available literature focuses on the efficacy of antioxidant therapy in the treatment and mitigation of endometriosis" (Vitale *et al.* 2018). Pelvic physical therapy, nutrition, lifestyle coaching, mindfulness, yoga, increasing physical activity, and endometrial excision surgery may dial down the inflammatory processes and provide pain reduction, or even total relief in some cases (Orbuch and Stein 2019).

PCOS is the most common endocrine disorder in women of reproductive age, occurring in 8 percent to 13 percent of women (Teede *et al.* 2018), and undiagnosed in up to 50 percent of females (see Box 3.5). Multiple studies confirm the benefit of lifestyle modification and exercise in PCOS (Harrison *et al.* 2011; Ibanez *et al.* 2017; Woodward *et al.* 2020) in reducing hyperinsulinemia (high blood sugar) and improving insulin sensitivity. However, a recent research review indicates, "45 percent of women with PCOS have reported that they have never been provided information about lifestyle management. This highlights a significant gap in knowledge and is reflective of the lack of evidence-based guidance for lifestyle modification" (Aly and Decherney 2021).

Box 3.5 PCOS
There are four phenotypes of PCOS, with possible anovulation, hyperandrogenism, enlarged ovaries with cysts, and infertility. Symptoms may include pelvic pain, weight gain, acne, male pattern hair growth, acanthosis nigrans (skin changes), and depression. Long-term sequelae may include infertility, diabetes, high cholesterol, and cardiovascular disease.

MALES

Teen males may develop swelling of the testes or have an exacerbation of swelling that was present in childhood, and this is typically diagnosed as a hydrocele.

Hydroceles form from a failure of the patent process vaginalis (embryologic) tissue to close at the inguinal ring. In children this condition may be closed at the inguinal ring with surgery (groin region), but in males over 10–12 years old a scrotal approach may be used (Koutsoumis, Patoulias, and Kaselas 2014).

Testicular swelling may occur from a dilation of the veins that drain the testicle, with the condition termed varicocele (see Box 3.6). Varicoceles occur most often in the left testicle, and occur in <1 percent pre-puberty, and are common in 5–30 percent of adolescent males. The varicocele may be asymptomatic, but it can be associated with future hypogonadism, infertility, and pelvic pain (Chung and Lee 2018).

Box 3.6 Varicocele treatments
Surgical techniques for varicocele in adolescents may be reserved for cases that progress in size and show a reduced blood flow on ultrasound. Improved testicular symmetry is gained postoperatively, yet some males not receiving surgery may spontaneously normalize volume during adolescent growth, termed "catch-up growth." For males beyond adolescence that are seeking fertility treatment and present with a varicocele, semen analysis is used pre and postoperatively, and demonstrates improved testicular function in spermatogenesis (Chung and Lee 2018).

FEMALES AND MALES

Adolescent females and males may develop abdominal and pelvic pain, which may stem from conditions discussed previously in this chapter, or other medical conditions requiring care (see Box 3.7). Females with significant dysmenorrhea may also have endometriosis, with bladder and bowel pain, and be at risk for chronic pelvic pain. Adolescent males can develop prostatitis-like pain, with symptoms including abdominal and pelvic pain, painful urination and ejaculation, and the risk of developing chronic pelvic pain. A Canadian study found adolescent males reported mild pelvic pain at an incidence rate of 8.3 percent, and moderate to severe symptoms in 3 percent, and the condition was associated with depression, catastrophizing, and reduced quality of life (Tripp *et al.* 2009).

Box 3.7 Medical screening, antibiotics, and the gut

Pelvic pain, abdominal and/or pelvic regions swelling, dermatological changes, vaginal or penile discharge, or bladder or bowel dysfunction require medical screening and testing. Ruling out infection, such as sexually transmitted disease, versus cancer conditions, appendicitis, physical and/or sexual abuse, and other conditions is required. With recurrent infections, or suspected infections, individuals may receive a single dose or repetitive antibiotic use, with changes in the gut microbiome (GM). The GM is typically less diverse in association with antibiotic use, demonstrating low diversity of species. Low species diversity in the GM may lead to health risks in neuroendocrine functioning, metabolic signaling, mood, immune system function, and disease risk versus resilience (Jasarevic, Morrison, and Bale 2016). These authors state, "mounting evidence suggests that microbial communities in the gut may be capable of altering the individual at a phenotypic level, including hormone-driven metabolic and behavioral phenotypes." Specialty testing of stool biome, and/or supplementation with probiotics and optimizing nutrition, may help rebalance the GM, although socioeconomic disparities exist in health literacy and the availability of wellness care (see Chapter 14).

CONNECTIVE TISSUE VARIATIONS

Genetics have great influence on connective tissue flexibility. Generalized joint laxity (GJL) is a condition where joints have greater than average range of motion, or laxity, due to connective tissue consistency. GJL is also termed generalized joint hypermobility. GJL occurs in 10–20 percent of the population, and it is not always associated with pain, but it does increase potential risk for injury such as anterior cruciate ligament (ACL) tears in the knee (Steinberg *et al.* 2021; Tingle *et al.* 2018).

Screening for GJL is based on the Beighton scale, which views the full end-range of motion at specific joints. Scoring >5/9 on this scale is considered positive for hypermobility (Beighton, Solomon, and Soskolne 1973; Grahame 1990). (See Table 3.2.)

More complex connective tissue disorders fall under the heading of joint hypermobility syndromes (JHS), such as Ehlers-Danlos syndrome. Variants of JHS may include arteriovascular dysfunction, and associated tendencies towards increased pain perception, autonomic dysfunction, and depression. JHS may include musculoskeletal disorders such as reduced muscle strength, and a tendency towards dislocation injuries, sports injuries, pelvic floor dysfunction, hemorrhoids, varicose veins, and abdominal hernias (Salnikova, Khadzhieva, and Kolobkov 2016).

ORTHOPEDIC CONSIDERATIONS

Injuries that involve the low back, the pelvis, and the hip and leg can occur in daily teen and young adult life. The back, hip, and pelvis are an integrated system for stability and mobility, and the region is termed as a whole the lumbo–pelvic–hip (LPH) complex. Also, conditions of the toes, foot, ankle, and knee may cause compensatory changes at the LPH as well. Health care providers interfacing with this population, as well as parents, coaches, and movement therapists, ideally can consider the "kinematic chain" as connected from the foot to the top of the head.

Injuries to the LPH and lower extremity can occur with or aggravate pelvic pain due to the cumulative responses in the neurological and myofascial system to protect injured areas. The body tends to "hug" an area with muscle spasm and shortening in order to protect it when injured (see Box 3.8). An accumulation of injuries and conditions may change myofascial structure and function, and this has been defined as somatic dysfunction in the field of osteopathy (Chaitow and Lovegrove Jones 2012; Freyer 2016). Somatic dysfunction may solely involve myofascial structures, or there may be associated neurological and visceral disorders as well.

Individuals presenting for pelvic therapy treatment as young adults, and into their elder years, may have histories of LPH injuries as well as their presenting pelvic health condition (see Box 3.9).

> ### Box 3.9 Catastrophic thinking and mind, body, spirit support
> Teens may develop "catastrophic thinking" in relation to orthopedic and/or pelvic health conditions that manifest at this delicate, sometimes tumultuous phase of life. First experiences of pain, and adults in their social milieu that may have chronic pain, can deepen worry and anxiety, and lead to despair and depression. Pain problems that limit or stop athletic and/or social participation may add fuel to the fire. Compassionate care providers can use storytelling, including tales of resiliency, to encourage adaptability, growth, confidence, and resourcefulness. Movement therapies that are pain-free and safe can be a respite at this time, as well as start a new path for fitness, self-confidence, and self-esteem.

> ### Box 3.8 Visual screening, and intuition with therapy
> Movement therapists and bodyworkers can optimally recognize palpable changes in the myofascial system "feel," as well as possible visible signs of tension or laxity in body surface contours, posture asymmetries, and altered movement patterns. Often, prior injuries may not be remembered and reported to providers, but be "found" by therapists and released in structures in holistic treatment.

SPECIFIC ORTHOPEDIC CONDITIONS

Orthopedic conditions that may occur involving the LPH and lower extremity are common in teens and include overuse symptoms with tendonitis, sprains, strains, as well as fractures and other serious orthopedic conditions, as listed in Boxes 3.10–3.12. The conditions listed focus on orthopedic youth presentation, yet also may occur with advancement in fitness and sport into the twenties and beyond.

> ### Box 3.10 Red flags!
> Pain which persists should receive medical attention for screening and ruling out infections, fractures, tumors, or other serious conditions.

Box 3.11 Patient case

Lucy played soccer from ages 12 to 27, and noted a sense of discomfort, pain, and tightness in her hips and spine in the later years of play. At age 23 she fractured her right big toe during a soccer game and walked in a cast boot for 8 weeks. It healed but she occasionally had episodes of toe pain with walking, and a limp. At age 24 she developed multiple bladder infections and began to experience bladder pain, with urgency and frequency of urination, and a condition termed "bladder pain syndrome." In addition to the bladder pain, following months of recreational road bike riding in her later twenties, she developed pelvic nerve pain, diagnosed as pudendal neuralgia. Her bladder symptoms and her pudendal neuralgia began to impact her quality of life in her late twenties, with limited sitting tolerance, pain with sex, and limited fitness due to pain flares with activity.

Physical therapy (PT), orthopedic and pelvic screening, and evaluation in her early thirties identified limited motion in her trunk, lumbar spine, hip joints, sacrum, ankle, and foot. (She had a medical referral for pelvic pain.) Lucy had tenderness and pain in her abdomen, pelvic floor muscles (PFM), adductors, and hamstrings. In particular, abdominal wall tightness, upper chest respiration pattern, and a short, tight pelvic floor were found, with no mobility of pelvic muscles on palpation (see Chapter 4 regarding PFM tightness). Her gait demonstrated limitations in stride length, push off, and trunk rotation, and a shorter stride on her right leg versus her left.

The therapy she received over the course of a year included standard pelvic therapy for the short pelvic floor, pudendal nerve region Botox treatment by her gynecologist, and treatment to her LPH and lower extremity. Myofascial treatment and movement therapy provided the mainstay of her recovery. Specifically, joint and soft tissue mobilization and therapeutic exercise helped her walk with a smoother, longer stride. Mobilization for all the diaphragms (pelvic, respiratory diaphragm, and thoracic inlet) and thoracic and lumbar spine rotation helped with movement flow. Medical therapeutic yoga, behavioral therapy, massage therapy, medication management, and a switch to hiking, surfing, dance, and yoga (and stopping long bike rides) allowed her to progress to a pain-free status.

Box 3.12 Sports and injury profiles

A large European review found the highest incidence of injury in teen sports occurred with soccer (31.1%), followed by handball (8.89%), sports associated with school athletics (8.77%), skiing (5.95%), and biking (5.71%). In the lower extremity, the knee and the ankle joints were injured at the rate of 29.79% and 24.02%, respectively. Males were injured at twice the rate of girls, presumably due to more aggressive play and contact in sport, in addition to larger body mass (Habelt et al. 2011).

Dance injuries are common, and a 29-year review of dance research found that injuries may occur at the following rate: ankle/foot: 14–54%, knee injuries: 16.2%, hip: 13.1%, and spine: 7–62% (Rinonapoli et al. 2020). Injury profiles included acute, traumatic injuries as well as overuse, microtrauma injuries.

KINEMATIC CHAIN

We all have a kinematic chain of linked myofascial, joint, and bone structures. These are interlinked structures from the toes, foot, ankle, knee, hip to pelvis, spine, and the trunk and upper body. Conditions such as strains, sprains, or fractures can potentially influence structures and functions near and far, above and below. With consideration of biotensegrity, and awareness of compressive and tensile forces throughout the body, stability and movement-mobility can occur with ease, or with dysfunction along the lower extremity "chain" with effects at the pelvic region (see Figure 3.10 and Box 3.13).

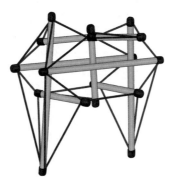

Figure 3.10 Human body biotensegrity model.

Box 3.13 Biotensegrity

Biotensegrity is becoming increasingly recognized as a more thorough explanation of the mechanics of motion: it examines the basic physics of natural forms through geometry and shows how even the most complicated organism can be better understood through the simplest of models. Tensegrity demonstrates the natural balance of forces, the dynamic tension network, and an integrated movement system that is applicable to all living things. The term tensegrity is a contraction of the words "tension" and "integrity" and was coined by the architect Buckminster Fuller.

(Scarr 2014)

Orthopedic conditions are listed per region, below, with readers advised to consult references and further resources as needed per your area of interest and level of specialization. Consider that the severity of an injury is manifest in altered gait and performance, as well as potential pain, including pain at rest. Conservative care with rehabilitation, bracing, therapeutic modalities, limiting or stopping performance, and/or surgery may be required for these conditions (see Box 3.14).

Toes, foot, ankle

- Sprains, strains, anterior and posterior impingement syndromes.
- Calcaneal bone osteochondrosis (a breakdown of cartilage and bone), also known as Sever-Blanke disease, may be associated with a tendinopathy of the Achilles insertion at the calcaneus, and pain is produced primarily during jumping (Rinonapoli *et al.* 2020).

Knee

- Patellofemoral pain may occur with conditions: patellar tendonitis, dislocation, bursitis, subluxation, rupture, and apophysitis of the tibial tubercle (bony overgrowth of the quad insertion site on the tibia) (Osgood-Schlatter disease).
- Patellofemoral pain is most common in ages 39–50, yet this occurs in over 13 percent of individuals aged 10–19 (Glaviano *et al.* 2015).
- Meniscus and anterior or posterior cruciate ligament tears.

Hip

- Iliotibial band syndrome, snapping hip syndrome, piriformis syndrome, and femoral-acetabular impingement (FAI) (Hart *et al.* 2009).
- Hip dysplasia: congenital alterations in the congruency and alignment of the ball (femoral head) and socket (acetabulum).
- Slipped capital femoral epiphysis (SCFE), a condition where the head of the femur slips backwards, resulting in stiffness, pain, and varying degrees of instability (Peck, Voss, and Voss 2017).
- Dysplasia and SCFE may lead to ligament and cartilage tears, and bony changes requiring surgery to continue performance, as profiled in a study of ballet dancers and gymnasts (Weber *et al.* 2014).
- Legg-Calve-Perthes disease: an avascular necrosis of the femoral head and adjacent structures (Mazloumi, Ebrahimzadeh, and Kachooei 2014). This may require surgical fixation.

Box 3.14 Critical rest and recovery

Rest is not a "four letter word" and yet it may be treated with disdain, fear, or avoidance for many reasons. Sever-Blanke, tibial tubercle apophysitis, and slipped capital femoral epiphysis are examples of forces exceeding compressive and tensile integrity. Genetics, overtraining, and/or incomplete bone maturation may underlie these conditions, and yet teens may continue on in pain, perhaps due to love of the sport, or parental encouragement, parental or peer pressure, or other factors. A therapist's professional advice may not match teen and parent goals, and this may create a sense of moral and ethical conflict for a health care provider in a circumstance where one sees a client's condition worsening and others are nonchalant regarding long-term effects, focusing on immediate performance goals.

Pelvis

Pelvic pain can occur in various locations, from the pubic symphysis, hip joint, sacroiliac joint, coccyx, spine, and multiple muscle groups. Pelvic pain can also be due to hernias, abdominal/pelvic visceral pathology such as ulcerative colitis, overactive bladder, PCOS, oncology conditions, and irritation of nerves in the region. Pain generators may be bone, muscle, organ, or nerve, or a combination of these factors (Phillip 2016; see Box 3.15).

Box 3.15 Red flags for teens needing medical screening

Pelvic region pain suddenly occurring in relation to a fall, motor vehicle accident, or athletic maneuver will demonstrate range of motion limitations and exacerbation with specific maneuvers on testing and demonstrate gait limitations if a fracture or significant tissue strain is present. Due to rapid healing in youth, mild injuries recover rapidly, yet persistent pain resulting in impairment requires screening and treatment. Pain elicited with mechanical testing leads to identification of joint and muscle irritation, whereas cyclical pain related to menstrual cycles, digestion, or sexual function leads to consideration of visceral drivers in pain.

Spine

- Strains and sprains
- Spondylolysis, a lowering of disc height, typically asymptomatic
- Spondylolisthesis, an anterior slippage of a vertebral segment, and this

condition may be asymptomatic or present with low back pain and lower extremity pain and require treatment (Foreman *et al.* 2013).

Research identifies varied incidence rates of spondylolisthesis in sport, with up to 47 percent of high level participants in gymnastics, diving, rowing, and weight lifting having the condition (Cavalier *et al.* 2006; Harvey *et al.* 1998). If the vertebral slippage is significant, surgery may be required to stabilize the segments, as in a case profiling a 15-year-old lacrosse player and skateboarder (Kolber and Hanney 2017), yet many individuals are symptom free.

CONSIDERATIONS IN TEEN SPORT AND HEALTH

Single sport participation is increasingly popular in youth and adolescence, yet health risks are well documented including physical injury and psychological distress (Stop Sports Injuries 2022). According to Smucny *et al.* (2015), vulnerability to injury is profiled in light of adolescent growth spurts, non-closure of bony and cartilaginous growth plates, high training volume, and inadequate rest. Emotional distress may arise from social isolation, overscheduling, lack of autonomy, self-esteem, and identity related solely to sports performance. Overall, athletes perform better and sustain sport participation when cross training and rest are scheduled. Athletes should not train for more hours per week than their age, and they should be given at least one day a week off for full rest.

Low energy availability and thinness

Teens may develop insufficient caloric intake in relation to the relative energy demands of sport, with a sequelae of negative health consequences. Relative energy deficiency in sport (RED-S) was historically addressed as the female athletic triad

(see Box 3.16). Current perspectives recognize female and male athletes with insufficient caloric intake, limited to absent menses (amenorrhea) and low bone mineral density, with risk for stress fractures. Parent, trainer, and coach education, as well as education for athletes on nutritional requirement in sport, is advised to prevent and/or intervene in this condition (Logue *et al.* 2020; Melin *et al.* 2015).

Box 3.16 RED-S

Awareness of RED-S is optimally considered in all athletes, as RED-S includes risks for injury and changes in the hypothalamus pituitary axis functioning, with potential reproductive health impairment and other problems. Obsessive compulsive behavior trends, anxiety, perfectionism, and high training loads are associated with some individuals with RED-S. Recent guidelines advise screening resting metabolic rate and providing questionnaires that screen the desire for thinness and symptoms related to low energy availability (Logue *et al.* 2020; Melin *et al.* 2015).

Wellness in pelvic health, and movement performance in the teen life phase, is represented by ease of functioning. Mild pelvic health conditions are common, such as PMS in the female reproductive cycle, or strains and sprains to the LPH and leg. However, some conditions such as endometriosis or RED-S may have related neuro-endocrine changes that have systemic effects, as well as associated psychological distress. Awareness of teen health concerns and challenges can help care providers to have an "antenna up" to consider if the teen needs specialty health care.

▢ PART II STABILITY, MOBILITY, SCREENING, AND TREATMENT

This section discusses movement control, screening methods, and treatment progressions. These paradigms are further addressed in other chapters.

The inclusion of the following information will provide readers as to the "big picture" that is often missed in beginners providing pelvic health programs. How the body moves as a whole can promote health or lead to pelvic pain and/or other symptoms of PFD.

CONCEPTS IN PELVIC JOINT AND MUSCLE FUNCTIONS

Pelvic stability and mobility

Optimum pelvic function requires adequate articular interface, such as the interlocking facet joints between the sacrum and ilium (SI), and dense ligaments around the SI, lumbosacral, and hip region. Stability of the pelvic ring also requires adequate muscle tone and activation to meet demands for motion, with a firing of the transverse abdominis, the pelvic floor muscles, and the spinal multifidi working as the core units, with outer superficial muscles activating in synchrony. The transverse abdominis, pelvic floor muscles, and the deep lumbar multifidus may not fire as needed for specific tasks as desired. For gentle activities such as walking or for more demanding fitness endeavors, this may lead to pain, and/or PFD such as urinary incontinence.

Sacrum motion in relation to ilium motion is a "locking" process in standing where the sacral base (top) moves anterior, termed nutation, and the sacral apex and ilia (most inferior section, laterally) move posterior, and the SI bony anatomy and ligaments lock the bones in place during weightbearing. In standing, the sacrum is nutated relative to the ileum. In non-weightbearing the sacrum can move posterior relative to the ilium, termed counternutation. Flexed sitting with pressure on the coccyx is a position of counternutation, which is also a position of a SI joint that is "unlocked." Injuries disrupting ligamentous support, and/or hypermobility syndromes, may allow excess bony SI motion, and the "force" system of muscles and myofascial slings must work harder to support stability and controlled mobility (see Box 3.17).

In addition to SI dynamics, the pelvic floor, lumbar spine, abdomen, and trunk require adequate ligamentous and myofascial support for stability and mobility. Local and far-reaching myofascial slings are involved in human performance, such as the latissimus dorsi (lats) and its connection into the transverse abdominis and thoracodorsal fascia into the lumbar and pelvic regions.

Active motion, passive mobility tests, and palpation of muscle groups are used to determine if the lumbar, pelvic, or hip regions are unstable or unlocking.

Activities of daily living (ADL)

Basic functional movement testing includes ADL, such as the performance of sit to stand, gait, bending and reaching tasks, squatting, and stair climbing. Basic ADL require adequate stability, mobility, balance, and neurological control. Bladder, bowel, or pelvic pain symptoms should not be present with resting or dynamic movement patterns.

Box 3.17 Optimal rehabilitation: screening and testing first

A form of simplistic therapeutic intervention is to "treat" (i.e. massage, soft tissue mobilization, stretch) an area of pain without considering why the pain is there. Heartfelt providers can want to "fix" a pain site but not yet have the skills to discern linkages in dysfunctional patterns from an integrative viewpoint. However, the healing arts take years of study and practice to develop expertise. Screening tests can identify limitations in stability or mobility, what, and why, in motor control problems. Over time, experts can find the problem links and fine tune therapeutic methods for healing.

Movement control

There are multiple rehabilitation formats to assess movement control. A holistic view is to consider the biotensegrity model when viewing form and function. Foundational studies to adequately evaluate and treat problems involving movement control include human anatomy and physiology, kinesiology, biomechanics, and pathology.

Viewing alignment, stability, and mobility, providers can find patterns that are creating pain and/or loss of function. All rehabilitation formats utilize education seminars with lab skills requiring in-person practice to refine provider screening and treatment formats.

Therapeutic rehabilitation programs

Below is a list of rehabilitation programs which may be studied via textbooks, webinars, and free online introductory and even advanced YouTube videos. The beauty of these skilled rehabilitation programs is that they analyze structure and function to decipher the neuromuscular and biomechanical reasons for pain and function loss versus solely treating symptoms.

- Developmental neuromuscular system (DNS) (Frank, Kobesova, and Kolar 2013; Kobesova *et al.* 2020)
- Functional movement assessment (FMA) in medical therapeutic yoga (Garner 2016)
- Movement system impairments (MSI) (Sahrmann 2002; Sahrmann, Azevedo, and Van Dillen 2017)
- Integrated systems model (ISM) (Lee 2022; Lee and Lee 2020).

These programs are utilized by providers treating LPH pain and dysfunction, as well as other conditions. These programs may also help reduce PFD such as bladder, bowel, or sexual health challenges, with improved intra-abdominal and trunk pressure system regulation and pelvic muscle control. Providers may use one system for therapy or use a combination of these approaches for rehabilitation. Verbal cuing, manual contacts and mobilization, positioning, and therapeutic exercises are used to develop integrated kinetic chain function by each of the approaches listed above.

Sahrmann *et al.* (2017) discuss "signs" which may occur before symptoms, which may be altered joint mechanics, limitations in range of motion or strength, inability to hold postures, or the specific onset of pain in certain positions. In the hip a "sign" may be instability in single limb stance, with rotation of the femur, and anterior groin pain may occur as a "symptom" (Box 3.18).

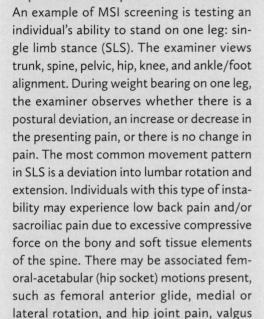

Box 3.18 Movement system impairment example

An example of MSI screening is testing an individual's ability to stand on one leg: single limb stance (SLS). The examiner views trunk, spine, pelvic, hip, knee, and ankle/foot alignment. During weight bearing on one leg, the examiner observes whether there is a postural deviation, an increase or decrease in the presenting pain, or there is no change in pain. The most common movement pattern in SLS is a deviation into lumbar rotation and extension. Individuals with this type of instability may experience low back pain and/or sacroiliac pain due to excessive compressive force on the bony and soft tissue elements of the spine. There may be associated femoral-acetabular (hip socket) motions present, such as femoral anterior glide, medial or lateral rotation, and hip joint pain, valgus knee inclination, ankle–foot pronation, or other deviations. Cuing, manual therapy, and therapeutic exercise can be utilized in progressive rehabilitation treatment to optimize function and reduce pain.

A stabilization series exercise program can target the body region and "impairment." An impairment in single limb stance would be, for example, pain that develops with an attempted "tree pose" in yoga, or pain that occurs with running which requires more single limb control than walking (see Box 3.19). A condition such as single limb stance and concomitant lumbar extension and rotation would likely train the spine, abdominal wall, thorax, pelvic floor, hip, knee, ankle, and foot.

Box 3.19 Progressive stabilization exercises

The following stabilization exercises may appear robotic, especially at the beginner level, and yet they are the patterns that infants and toddlers display as repetitive patterns in the developmental sequence; the exercises scaffold in levels of difficulty that produce the ability to roll, crawl, climb, walk, run, pivot, and play! Consider that a teen (or adult) may have missed a toddler stability-to-mobility phase or has limited motor programming and kinesthetic sense, and optimally they can improve their foundations for motor control with the series listed.

The following exercise sequences could be used in rehabilitation (Figures 3.11–3.34). This is not a cookbook for any one program, it uses the developmental sequencing model as applied to human stability, mobility, and performance. Endurance is built over time with increased challenges holding static postures, and increased repetitions with specific mobility patterns that show performance deficits with screening. With expertise, providers train clients in progressive work on the weak links. Through neuromuscular re-education, the entire system can perform better for the desired goals of treatment.

Stabilization/developmental series exercise program
FOUNDATIONS FOR STABILITY AND MOBILITY
Photo sequence, Level 1:

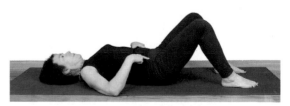

Figure 3.11 Neutral spine, supine.

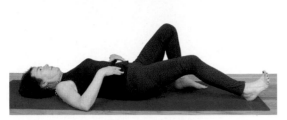

Figure 3.12 Heel slide.

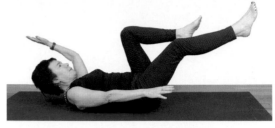

Figure 3.17 Alternate upper extremity and lower extremity flexion and extension.

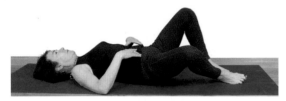

Figure 3.13 Knee drop out.

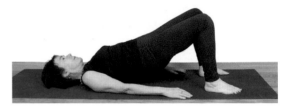

Figure 3.18 Hip bridge.

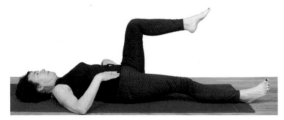

Figure 3.14 Single knee to 90/90.

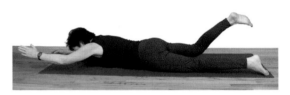

Figure 3.19 Prone arm and leg up.

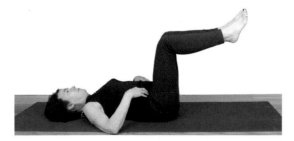

Figure 3.15 LE 90/90 tabletop.

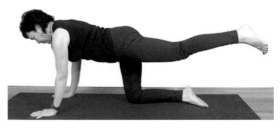

Figure 3.20 Quadruped single limb extension.

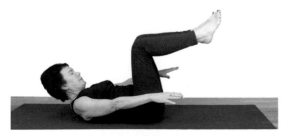

Figure 3.16 Head lift and tabletop and arms flexed.

Level 2:

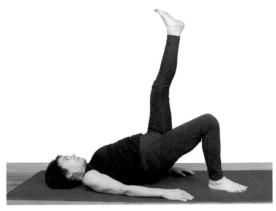

Figure 3.21 Single limb bridge.

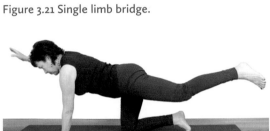

Figure 3.22 Quadruped alternate extremity raise.

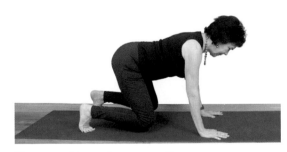

Figure 3.23 Down dog preparation.

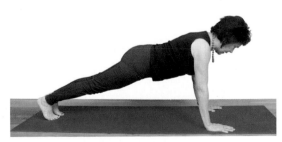

Figure 3.24 Plank on knees to full plank.

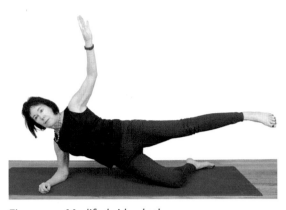

Figure 3.25 Modified side plank.

Level 3:

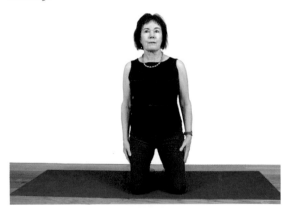

Figure 3.26 Kneel.

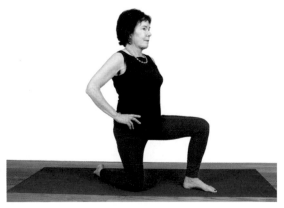

Figure 3.27 Half kneel.

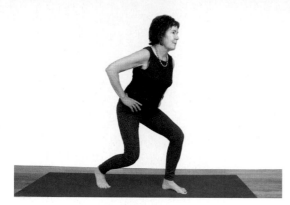

Figure 3.28 Kneel to stand.

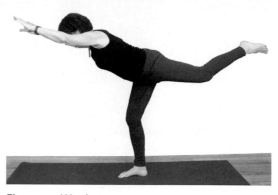

Figure 3.31 Warrior 3.

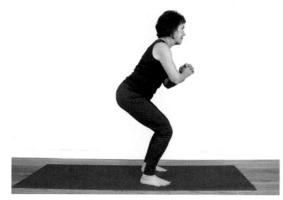

Figure 3.29 Squat.

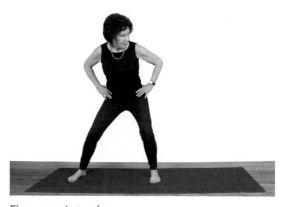

Figure 3.32 Lateral steps.

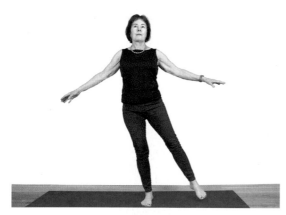

Figure 3.30 Single limb balance.

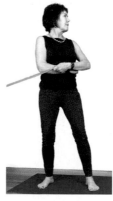

Figure 3.33 Resisted rotations.

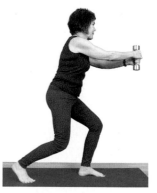

Figure 3.34 Matrix series, with drivers.

Movement screening: quick tests

BEIGHTON SCALE

A simple connective tissue screen may be performed with the Beighton hypermobility scale. If hypermobility is present, and injuries are occurring due to lack of support and stability for joints, then bracing, increased stability training, and even changing fitness activities may be indicated.

Table 3.2 Beighton scale criteria

Joint criteria	Hypermobility	Right/Left	Point value
Fifth finger extension	Beyond 90 degrees	+ +	1 + 1
Thumb abduction apposition to forearm	Contact of thumb to forearm	+ +	1 + 1
Elbow hyper extension	Beyond 10 degrees	+ +	1 + 1
Knee hyper extension	Beyond 10 degrees	+ +	1 + 1
Spinal flexion	Palms contact floor	+	1
			Total: 9

(Beighton, Solomon, and Soskolne 1973)

Observing gait and other movements can identify problems that can be helped with bodywork and movement therapy.

When screening for joint laxity, posture holds, and movement patterns, providers are looking at how the myofascial system functions, and what may be causing pain or loss of performance (see Box 3.20).

CONSIDERATIONS IN SCREENING

- Is stability and control present?
- Is balance control present?
- Is there a wobble or pivot point?
- Are certain parts moving a lot, and others appear tight or stiff?
- Is pain produced during the test?
- If pain is produced, is it from myofascial stretching, or from joint compression, or both?
- Screening tests are a starting point for providing therapeutic movement programs, which may be simple or complex depending on the needs of the individual being tested.

Box 3.20 Lumbar, pelvic, and hip weakness and pain

Janelle began to have anterior hip pain and mild low back pain in high school. She participated in a recreational dance group, and also practiced running and gym workouts with machines and free weights. In college she was screened for her LPH function, and deficits were noted in her stabilization testing. She was unable to maintain single leg stance (SLS) without a pelvic drop on the unsupported side. She exhibited lumbar extension and rotation in SLS. With manual muscle testing she demonstrated gluteus maximus, medius, and hip external rotation weakness. She was unable to hold a plank pose without an increased lordosis (low back arch), and hip bridging on one leg demonstrated a pelvic drop on the unsupported side. She had anterior hip pain with hip flexion, adduction, and internal rotation pain. She was prescribed an LPH stabilization program, focusing on the gluteus maximus, medius, and hip external rotator group, and multifidus and transverse abdominis training for functional position holds. She received manual therapy for five sessions, emphasizing facilitation of the LPH and core muscles. After 10 weeks of performing the LPH stabilization program 4–5 times a week, her movement testing indicated stability in poses, including SLS, and a pain-free status regarding her hip and spine.

YOGA AND PILATES

Yoga and Pilates represent mind–body exercise formats which include strengthening, stretching, and attention to respiration, and are robust platforms for lifelong fitness and wellness. (Readers can recognize yoga and Pilates poses as presented in the stabilization series.) Yoga and Pilates programs are excellent adaptable fitness formats for teens. Stability and also flow of movements in these programs can soothe stress and enhance wellbeing, vital for health and self-care, and provide fitness foundations for teens and through the lifespan.

SUMMARY

The teen years are regarded as a phase of mind, body, and spirit maturation, with the potential onset of sex-specific pelvic health conditions which may not be diagnosed until an older age. Fitness and sport participation in youth ideally does not include injuries that are permanent in the LPH region, or the associated kinetic chain into the lower limb. Injuries may create impairments that contribute to challenges that linger across the lifespan.

Great joy may be experienced in teen competence and skill acquisition in sport and recreational activity, as well as empowerment towards self-care. Therapists ideally can screen stability, mobility, gait, and other functional tasks in clients presenting with pelvic health conditions and optimize treatment with a view towards fluidity of motion for all stages of life.

REFERENCES

Agarwal, S. K., Chapron, C., Giudice, L. C., Laufer, M. R., et al. (2019) "Clinical diagnosis of endometriosis: A call to action." American Journal of Obstetrics and Gynecology 220, 4, 354.e1–354.e12.

Aly, J. M. and Decherney, A. H. (2021) "Lifestyle modifications in PCOS." Clinical Obstetrics and Gynecology 64, 1, 83–89.

Armour, M., Smith, C., Steel, K., and Macmillan, F. (2019) "The effectiveness of self-care and lifestyle interventions in primary dysmenorrhea; a systematic review." BMC Complementary and Alternative Medicine 19, 1, 22.

Asghari, S., Valizadeh, A., Aghebati-Maleki, L., Nouri, M., and Yousefi, M. (2018) "Endometriosis: Perspective, lights, and shadows of etiology. Review." Biome Pharmacotherapy 106, 163–174.

Bavil, D. A., Dolation, M., Mahmoodi, Z., and Baghban, A. A. (2016) "Comparison of lifestyles of young women with and without primary dysmenorrhea." Electronic Physician 8, 3, 2107–2114.

Beighton, P., Solomon, L., and Soskolne, C. L. (1973) "Articular mobility in an African population." Annals of Rheumatic Diseases 32, 413.

Bernardi, M., Lazzeri, L., Perelli, F., Reis, F. M., and Petraglia, F. (2017) "Dysmenorrhea and related disorders." Europe PMC 6, 1645.

Cavalier, R., Herman, M. J., Cheung, E. V., and Pizzutillo, P. D. (2006) "Spondylosis and spondylolisthesis in children and adolescents: Diagnosis, natural history and management." Journal of the American Academy of Orthopedic Surgeons 14, 7, 417–424.

Chaitow, L. and Lovegrove-Jones, R. (2012) Chronic Pelvic Pain and Dysfunction. Edinburgh: Churchill Livingstone.

Chung, J. M. and Lee, S. D. (2018) "Current issues in adolescent varicocele: Pediatric urological perspectives." The World Journal of Men's Health 36, 2, 123–131.

Earle, S., Marston, H., Hadley, R., and Banks, D. (2019) "Use of menstruation and fertility app trackers: A scoping review of the evidence." British Medical Journal Sexual and Reproductive Health 47, 2.

Endicott, J., Nee, J., and Harrison, W. (2006) "Daily record of severity of problems (DRSP): Reliability and validity." Archives of Women's Mental Health 9, 1, 41–49.

Foreman, P., Griessenauer, C. J., Watanabe, K., Conklin, M., et al. (2013) "L5 spondylolysis/spondylolisthesis: A comprehensive review with an anatomic focus." Child's Nervous System 29, 209–216.

Frank, C., Kobesova, A., and Kolar, P. (2013) "Clinical commentary, dynamic neuromuscular stabilization and sports rehabilitation." *International Journal of Sports Physical Therapy 8*, 1, 62–73.

Freyer, G. (2016) "Somatic dysfunction;an osteopathic conundrum." *International Journal of Osteopathic Medicine 22*, 52–63.

Garner, G. (2016) *Medical Therapeutic Yoga*. London: Handspring Publishing.

Glaviano, N. R., Kew, M., Hart, J. M., and Saliba, S. (2015) "Demographic and epidemiological trends in patellofemoral pain." *International Journal of Sports Physical Therapy 10*, 3.

Grahame, R. (1990) "The hypermobility syndrome." *Annals of Rheumatological Disease 49*, 3, 199–200.

Guthrie, A. (2022) *Premenstrual assessment form*. Accessed 2/9/2022 at https://wholehealthtoronto.com/wp-content/uploads/2014/05/PremenstrualAssessment-Form.pdf.

Habelt, S., Hasler, C. C., Steinbruck, K., and Majewski, M. (2011) "Sports injuries in adolescents." *Orthopedic Reviews 3*, 2, 18.

Harrison, C. L., Lombard, C. B., Moran, L. J., and Teede, H. J. (2011) "Exercise therapy in polycystic ovary syndrome: A systematic review." *Human Reproduction Update 17*, 2, 171–183.

Hart, E. S., Metkar, U. S., Rebello, G. N., and Grottkau, B. E. (2009) "Femoral acetabular impingement in adolescents and young adults." *Orthopedic Nursing 28*, 3, 117–124.

Harvey, C. J., Richenberg, J. L., Saifuddin, A., and Wolman, R. L. (1998) "The radiological investigation of lumbar spondylolysis." *Clinical Radiology 53*, 723–728.

Hashim, M. S., Obaideen, A. A., Jahrami, H. A., *et al.* (2018) "Premenstrual syndrome is associated with dietary and lifestyle behaviors among university students: A cross-sectional study from Sharjah, UAE." *Nutrients 11*, 8, 1939.

Hofmeister, S. and Bodden, S. (2016) "Premenstrual syndrome and premenstrual dysphoric disorder." *American Family Physician 94*, 3, 236–240.

Ibanez, L., Oberfeld, S. E., Witchel, S. F., Auchus, R. J., *et al.* (2017) "An international consortium update: Pathophysiology, diagnosis, and treatment of polycystic ovarian syndrome in adolescence." *Hormone Research in Pediatrics 88*, 6, 371–395.

Jasarevic, E., Morrison, K. E., and Bale, T. L. (2016) "Sex differences in the gut microbiome-brain axis across the lifespan." *Philosophical Transactions of the Royal Society B 371*, 1688, 20150122.

Ju, H., Jones, M., and Mishra, G. (2014) "The prevalence and risk factors for dysmenorrhea." *Epidemiological Reviews 36*, 104–113.

Kobesova, A., Davidek, P., Morris, C., Andel, R., *et al.* (2020) "Functional postural-stabilization tests according to dynamic neuromuscular stabilization approach: Proposal of novel examination protocol." *Journal of Bodywork and Movement Therapies 24*, 84–95.

Kolber, M. J. and Hanney, W. J. (2017) "A grade iv isthmic spondylolisthesis." *Journal of Orthopedic and Sports Physical Therapy 47*, 12, 971.

Koutsoumis, G., Patoulias, I., and Kaselas, C. (2014) "Primary new onset hydroceles presenting in late childhood and pre-adolescent patients resemble the adult type hydrocele pathology." *Journal of Pediatric Surgery 49*, 1656–1658.

Lee, D. (2022) The Integrated Systems Model (ISM). Accessed 1/24/2022 at https://learnwithdianelee.com/the-integrated-systems-model.

Lee, D. and Lee, L. J. (2020) *The Pelvic Girdle: An Integration of Clinical Expertise and Research*. Edinburgh: Churchill Livingstone.

Logue, D. M., Madigan, S. M., Melin, A., Delahunt, E., *et al.* (2020) "Low energy availability in athletes 2020: An updated narrative review of prevalence, risk, within-day energy balance, knowledge, and impact on sports performance. Review." *Nutrition 12*, 3, 835.

Lustyk, M. K., Gerrish, W. G., Shaver, S., and Keys, S. L. (2009) "Cognitive behavioral therapy for premenstrual syndrome and premenstrual dysphoric disorder: A systematic review." *Archives of Women's Mental Health 12*, 2, 85–96.

Mazloumi, S., Ebrahimzadeh, M., and Kachooei, A. (2014) "Evolution in diagnosis and treatment of Legg-Calve-Perthes disease." *Archives of Bone Joint Surgery 2*, 22, 86–92.

Melin, A., Tornberg, A. B., Skouby, S., Moller, S. S., *et al.* (2015) "Energy availability and the female athletic triad in elite endurance athletes." *Scandinavian Medicine and Science in Sports 25*, 610–622.

Office on Women's Health (OASH) (2021) "Premenstual syndrome (PMS)." Accessed 9/21/2022 at www.womenshealth.gov/menstrual-cycle/premenstrual-syndrome.

Orbuch, I. K. and Stein, A. (2019) *Beating Endo: How to Reclaim Your Life From Endometriosis*. New York: Harper Wave.

Pearlstein, T. and Steiner, M. (2012) "Premenstrual dysphoric disorder, burden of illness and treatment update." *Focus: The Journal of Lifelong Learning in Psychiatry 10*, 1.

Peck, D. M., Voss, L. M., and Voss, T. T. (2017) "Slipped capital femoral epiphysis; diagnosis and management." *American Family Physician 15*, 95, 12.

Pieretti, S., Di Giannuario, A., Di Giovannandrea, R., Marzoli, F., *et al.* (2016) "Gender differences in pain and its relief." *Annali dell'Istituto superiore di sanità 52*, 2, 184–189.

Phillip, P. A. (2016) *Pelvic Pain and Dysfunction*. New York: Thieme.

Rinonapoli, G., Graziani, M., Ceccarini, P., Razanno, C., *et al.* (2020) "Dance, epidemiology of injuries connected with dance; a critical review on epidemiology." *Medicinski glasnik (Zenica) 17*, 2, 256–264.

Rizk, B., Fischer, A. S., Lofty, H. A., Turki, R., *et al.* (2013) "Recurrence of endometriosis after hysterectomy: Facts, views, and visions." *Obgyn 6*, 4, 219–227.

Robinson, L. L. and Ismail, K. M. (2015) "Clinical epidemiology of premenstrual disorder: Informing optimized patient outcomes." *International Journal of Women's Health 7*, 811–818.

Sahrmann, S. (2002) *Diagnosis and Treatment of Movement Impairment Syndromes*. St Louis, MO: Mosby.

Sahrmann, S., Azevedo, D. C., and Van Dillen, L. (2017) "Diagnosis and treatment of movement impairment syndromes, masterclass." *Brazilian Journal of Physical Therapy 21*, 6, 391–399.

Salnikova, L. E., Khadzhieva, M. B., and Kolobkov, D. S. (2016) "Biological findings from the PheWas catalog: Focus on connective tissue related disorders (pelvic floor dysfunction, abdominal hernia, varicose veins, and hemorrhoids)." *Human Genetics 135*, 7, 779–795.

Scarr, G. (2014) *Biotensegrity: The Structural Basis of Life.* Edinburgh: Handspring Publishing.

Smucny, M., Parikh, S. N., and Pandya, N. K. (2015) "Consequences of single sport participation in the pediatric and adolescent athlete." *Orthopedic Clinics of North America 46*, 249–258.

Soliman, A. M., Du, E. X., Yang, H., Wu, E. Q., and Haley, J. C. (2017) "Retreatment rates among endometriosis patients undergoing hysterectomy or laparoscopy." *Journal of Women's Health 26*, 6.

Steinberg, N., Tenenbaum, S., Zeev, A., Pantanowitz, M., *et al.* (2021) "Generalized joint hypermobility, scoliosis, patellofemoral pain, and physical abilities in young dancers." *BMC Musculoskeletal Disorders 22*, 1, 1–11.

Stop Sports Injuries (2022) *Best Practices in Youth Sports Injury Reduction and Prevention.* Accessed 6/7/2022 at https://www.ncys.org/safety/stop-sports-injuries.

Teede, H. J., Misso, M. L., Costello, M. F., Dokras, A., *et al.* (2018) "Recommendations from the international evidence-based guideline for the assessment and management of polycystic ovarian syndrome." *Human Reproduction 33*, 9, 1602–1618.

Tingle, A., Bennett, O., Wallis, A., and Palmer, S. (2018) *Physical Therapy Reviews.* Abingdon: Taylor and Francis.

Tripp, D. A., Nickel, C., Ross, S., Mullins, C., and Stechyson, N. (2009) "Prevalence, symptom impact and predictors of chronic prostatitis-like symptoms in Canadian males age 16–19." *BJUI International 103*, 8, 1080–1084.

Verbruggen, S. W. and Nowlan, N. C. (2017) "Ontogeny of the human pelvis." *The Anatomical Record 300*, 4, 643–652.

Viswanthan, P. and Pinto, N. (2015) "The effects of classical music based chakra meditation on the symptoms of premenstrual syndrome." *International Journal of Indian Psychology 2*, 3, 133–141

Vitale, S. G., Capriglione, S., Peterlunger, I., La Rosa, V. L., *et al.* (2018) "The role of oxidative stress and membrane transport systems during endometriosis: A fresh look at a busy corner." *Hindawi Oxidative Medicine and Cellular Longevity 7924021.*

Weber, A. E., Bedi, A., Larson, C. M., *et al.* (2014) "The hyperflexible hip: Managing hip pain in the dancer and gymnast." *Sage Journals 7*, 4.

Wilson, D. (2022) *St. John's Wort.* Accessed 2/9/2022 at https://www.healthline.com/health/pms-supplements#st.-john's-wort.

Woodward, A., Broom, D., Dalton, C., Metwally, M., and Klonizakis, M. (2020) "Supervised exercise training and increased physical activity to reduce cardiovascular disease risk in women with polycystic ovarian syndrome: Study protocol for a randomized controlled feasibility trial." *Trials 20*, 1, 1–8.

CHAPTER 4

Pelvic Pain

This chapter will delve into the varied conditions of pelvic pain that are common, how it may feel in the somatic experience of the individual, and insights into therapeutic options for pain care. Manual myofascial and visceral techniques and movement therapy will be profiled, with client cases that illustrate rehabilitation strategies from simple problems to more complex presentations.

Considerations in pelvic pain rehabilitation include:

- What is the root cause of the pain, or are there multiple causes or drivers?
- Is medical screening and intervention needed (see red flags below) or are symptoms mild and appear likely to respond to conservative care such as lifestyle education, manual therapy, and exercise?
- What is the client's mindset regarding their expectations, and their goals—what do they hope to achieve with care?
- Can the client sleep, sit, walk, and perform basics of life, or are they homebound with their condition?
- Is psychological, mind–body support indicated, as in anxiety, depression, insomnia, or anger?
- Are there signs of emotional, physical, or sexual trauma, and trauma-sensitive care indicated?
- Is the provider confident that they can provide care, or can they add teamwork with acupuncture, massage, chiropractic, nutrition, gut microbiome, sleep therapy, fitness trainers, or other professionals?

Pelvic pain is what prompts an individual to seek medical care. It is a phenomenon that may occur as a temporary experience, or it may entail a chronic health condition. Pelvic pain may limit movement, breath, and functioning, with each person having unique reactions to pain (Box 4.1). Therapeutic treatment for pain can help restore breath, function, mobility, and even vitality in the best results from care.

> ### Box 4.1 Client body language and therapy options
>
> Consider an individual's body language in care. Confident individuals who move with ease and face a therapist, and even lean towards them, are typically ready to engage in treatment. Body movements observed can provide clues into overall "Gestalt" of an individual and their soma. Those that are flexed, bent, and turned away from a therapist with arms and legs crossed may need gentleness and patience. Factors such as predominant upper chest respiration and frequent sighing can benefit, when ready, from lengthening, opening the limbs to the sides, and restoration

of full breath. Jittery, jumpy individuals that stand at attention, talk, and move fast, and thrust themselves into movement, may benefit from grounding, flowing, closing, bending, and centering programs. Offering the right amount of movement at the best time for a client requires sensitivity and patience.

Pelvic pain may require medical screening by medical specialists. Individuals need to be referred to medical screening with "red flags" as listed in Box 4.2 and Table 4.1.

Box 4.2 Red flags for pelvic pain 👓

Abdominal and pelvic pain may be due to appendicitis, infection, inflammation such as pelvic inflammatory disease, diverticulitis, hernia, ruptured ovarian cyst, ectopic pregnancy, placental abruption, cystitis, pyelonephritis, ureterolithiasis, ovarian vein thrombosis, endometriosis, or other conditions such as vascular or cancer related conditions. Medical screening requires a complete medical history, abdominal and pelvic evaluation, and possible ultrasound, radiology, and lab tests performed by a health care provider (Kruszka and Kruszka 2010).

Table 4.1 Red flags

Pain intensity	Pain location	Swelling	Other symptoms	Medical history	Sensory and/or motor changes
Increasing over time to moderate, to severe. Pain does not improve with rest or changing positions.	Localized or spreading. Abdominal tenderness. Possible radiating pain from the abdomen, spine, from pelvis into hips and thighs.	Mild to moderate swelling, abdomen, groin, legs. Bloated or distended abdomen, perineum.	Sweating or chills, cramping, nausea or vomiting, fever, loss of appetite, constipation, diarrhea, weight loss, increasing fatigue. Bladder: increased urgency, frequency, urine loss or retention. Blood in the urine. Irritable bowel symptoms. Blood in the stool.	History of cancer, or trauma, or recent infection. Immune suppression.	Saddle (perineal) numbness. Progressive sensory and motor loss in the legs.

(Funston et al. 2018; Gerwin and Kruszka 2010; Leerar et al. 2007; Motamed et al. 2012)

A limited number of interventions may help rehabilitate a simple, non-complicated pelvic pain condition. For example, pelvic pain localized to the coccyx from repeated falls during snowboarding, ice skating, or trips and falls may benefit from pelvic myofascial treatment in just a few sessions (see Boxes 4.3 and 4.4). Many individuals with pelvic pain have overactive pelvic floor muscles, and benefit from conservative care (Morrison 2016).

Box 4.3 Coccyx pain 💜

Andre was a beginning snowboarder, age 22, who fell onto his tailbone (coccyx) multiple times in his first few days of practice. As he practiced more, he fell less often, but noted increasing difficulty sitting, and an ache in his coccyx. He presented to physical therapy (PT) within two months of his pain onset. He scored his pain at level 4/10 coccyx pain on a visual analog scale, where 10 = maximum pain (Gallagher *et al.* 2002). His chief problems were limited sitting of 30–45 minutes, pain moving from sit to stand, pain with stair climbing, and with running. Key findings on his evaluation were shallow respiration, with low diaphragm, rib, and abdominal wall mobility, and myofascial pain. His low back, iliopsoas, gluteals, hamstring, and pelvic floor muscles had limited myofascial mobility, with tenderness and trigger points throughout. His coccyx and anococcygeal ligament were tender on external palpation. Pain occurred with mobility testing externally, with the coccyx unable to comfortably extend from a flexed position. Andre received diaphragm, rib, pelvic floor, iliopsoas, gluteal, and hamstring muscle myofascial treatment and respiratory and flexibility exercises, including yoga (also see Andre in Boxes 4.13 and 4.17).

Box 4.4 Causes of coccyx pain

Coccyx alignment may be excessively flexed, tucked under, or excessively straight, yet alignment variances do not necessarily cause symptoms. Other factors may cause coccyx region pain, such as levator ani spasm, or anococcygeal ligament strains or stretch from vaginal childbirth. Excessive squat workouts may also cause coccyx pain.

CHRONIC PELVIC PAIN

If persistent beyond three months, pain problems may be labeled as chronic. In chronic pelvic pain (CPP), there may be a continuous presentation, over 24 hours, or most of a day or night. Or CPP may have a cyclic presentation such as that occurring in females with menstruation (dysmenorrhea) or pain with sex (dyspareunia) (see Boxes 4.5 and 4.6).

Box 4.5 Incidence rates of CPP

A systematic review of CPP (Latthe *et al.* 2006) found prevalence rates ranged from 16.8% to 81% (dysmenorrhea), 8% to 21.8% (dyspareunia), and 2.1% to 24% (non-cyclical pain). In male chronic pelvic pain related to the prostate or bladder, prevalence rates are between 2% and 16% according to an expert consensus (Krieger, Nyberg, and Nickel 1999).

Box 4.6 Emotional and sensory reactions to chronic pain

Privacy, fear, and "being tough and carrying on" may lead to denial and dismissal of pelvic pain, of bodily symptoms, and somato-emotionally "shutting off" the area. Hence the "layers of the onion" as seen in global body tension. There is often tactile defensiveness, self-isolation, guarding, and armoring up of the myofascial body. Those that provide movement training may not be a threat, yet any provider that uses touch, palpation, and hands-on care may open the layers hiding the pain and walk in the pain trenches with the individual requesting care. Providers may not be equipped for the depth of emotion stirred up during treatment sessions, and how to validate and confirm symptoms, yet to also steer the client gently towards resiliency and healing. Some clients may release myofascial tension easily. An individual may feel profound interconnections in their health history and realize somato-emotional aspects of pain. Each journey is different for the care provider and care recipient.

Cross talk among systems

CPP is a complex syndrome. It may include pathologic changes in the central and peripheral nervous system processing, the pelvic organs (viscera) functioning, and dysfunction in the associated muscular and fascial system. Visceral dysfunction, such as bladder and urethra pain from a urinary tract infection, may lead to organ "cross talk" where associated structures such as the bowel and/or pelvic muscles may begin to transmit pain signals via facilitated neural pathways (Woolf 2014). CPP may involve multiple body systems, such as relays between myofascial, visceral, and nervous systems (Box 4.7).

> ## Box 4.7 Chronic primary pelvic pain syndrome (CPPPS)
>
> The European Association of Urology (EAU) uses the term chronic primary pelvic pain syndrome (CPPPS) to delineate a syndrome where there is no detected infection or other cause for the pain. Associated health conditions with CPPPS may be chronic fatigue syndrome, fibromyalgia syndrome, Sjögren's syndrome, or other complex health challenges. Additional aspects such as negative cognitive, emotional, behavioral, and functional aspects in the patient's life should be recognized. In addition to pain, there may be symptoms of urinary tract, sexual, bowel, or gynecological dysfunction (Engeler *et al.* 2012).

Co-morbidities presenting with pelvic pain may involve physiological problems in body systems such as cardiovascular, gastrointestinal, gynecologic, endocrine, urologic, lymphatic, metabolic, myofascial, neural, and orthopedic dysfunction. Individuals with obesity may have systemic inflammation, as well as disrupted sleep, depression, and osteoarthritis in the hip and knee (Box 4.8). Adipose tissue is regarded as a metabolically active system that is pro-inflammatory (Okifuji and Hare 2015).

Pelvic pain may disrupt a client's ability to function in their emotional, social, and physical roles. Loss of participation in family and work life, hobbies, community, and recreation activity limitations are common in CPP. Factors such as negative affect (mood), fatigue, high pain ratings, and social function limitations were found to correlate with the level of patient overall dysfunction in a large research study of 613 women with CPP (Fenton *et al.* 2015).

> ## Box 4.8 Inflammation and obesity
>
> Obesity is defined as a body mass index of >30kg/m². Obese individuals demonstrate elevated serum markers of inflammatory substances such as C reactive protein (CRP), interleukin-6, and an accumulation of macrophages. There is also an increase in inflammatory markers post-operatively, as well as a greater tendency for degenerative disc disease, low back pain, and osteoarthritis (Okifuji and Hare 2015).

Neuroplasticity

Depression can aggravate pain, and pain can lead to a depressed state; in chronic pain states and with depression, similar structural central nervous system brain changes are observed. Changes in anatomical structures demonstrate the principle of neuroplasticity. Chronic pain causes an enlargement of nerve centers processing pain, and shrinkage of nerve structures associated with pain inhibition and multimodal sensory and motor processing (Doan, Manders, and Wag 2015). Positive changes in neural processing may occur with healing therapies (Brumange *et al.* 2019; Zeidan *et al.* 2012).

Pain and "danger"

Pain typically alerts us of a danger, a need to pay attention to an area, and to protect it. Yet pain signals, their processing in the body, and the perception of pain is not localized to singular neural tissues, or groups of neurons. There is typically an associated threat or danger level, as well as somato-emotional processing in the experience of pain.

Pain perception can be understood by considering the context of the pain in an individual's life (Box 4.9). Rehabilitation can use storytelling and patient resource books, such as *Explain Pain* (Moseley and Butler 2015). Training in a consideration of thoughts about pain can help shift perception towards non-aggravating statements such as "I am sore but safe, I am getting stronger, I am releasing discomfort" (Butler and Moseley 2014).

Box 4.9 Pain, distress, and resilience

Pain can irritate, pain can annoy, distress, and traumatize, pain can wall us in, pain can trap us, isolate us. Yet pain can teach us to let go, to reach out, to connect, to show vulnerability and ask for and receive help.

Hope

One of the biggest keys to healing is a client's ability for hope, ability for resiliency, and to be able to visualize a future positive health status. Research for individuals with fibromyalgia received treatment where they visualized their "best possible self," practiced guided imagery, and showed significant improvement (Molinari *et al.* 2018). Considering this and other research, providers can help the mind, and perceptions and thoughts about pain as key tap roots for healing (see Boxes 4.10 and 4.11).

Box 4.10 Storytelling for teaching

Storytelling by providers can offer alternative scenarios for individuals feeling stuck in the mud, in the trenches of pain. By describing similar client cases and illustrating examples of improved function, a sense of hope may emerge. Offering a team of providers and options for care can empower decision making skills.

Box 4.11 Biopsychosocial (BPS) model

Interventions for CPP optimally include a whole person view of function and health. In the BPS model a health condition is considered a biological, social, or psychological problem, with associated alterations in function, termed "impairments." Impairments may include limitations in function in home, work, community, and recreation participation. Genetics, health history, physical environment, and biological functioning are considered, versus a sole diagnosis. Feeling safe, loved, nourished, and cared for by family and community helps develop stability and a sense of belonging, as well as healthy boundaries and self-care. With the BPS, care providers can discern multiple causes for pain, as well as potential assets towards healing (Fenton *et al.* 2015).

ADVERSE CHILDHOOD EXPERIENCES: ACE SCORE

The social, psychological, and physical environment in early life has been identified as a factor in future health or illness. Early childhood experience with exposure to stress and trauma can set up an individual for health challenges throughout their life, including increased propensity towards experiencing pain. ACE can be scored from 0 to 10, and correlate with health status, and risk of disease over a lifetime (Hughes *et al.* 2017; Metzler *et al.* 2017; Ramiro, Madrid, and Brown 2010; Zarse *et al.* 2019). Clients can be guided with therapy to help recognize experiences and patterns that have contributed to their ill health over time, including the ACE score (Box 4.12).

Providing peace, centering, and grounding in therapy with options for ongoing self-care, even self-love and empowerment, can wash over prior negative influences and promote healing.

Maureen Mason

tobacco, and illicit drug use, and increased likelihood of pain, health risk behavior, and disease are seen in those with higher ACE scores (Metzler *et al.* 2017; Zarse *et al.* 2019) (Box 4.13).

Box 4.12 ACE

For full terminology see the ACE questionnaire (Felitti *et al.* 1998).

Before age 18:

1. Exposure to verbal abuse or threats (put downs, insults, humiliation, threatened with harm)
2. Physical abuse (pushed, grabbed, slapped, items thrown)
3. Sexual abuse (touching, fondling, penetration)
4. Feeling unloved, lack of family bonds
5. Insufficient food, hygiene, medical care, or parents with alcohol or drug abuse unable to care for you
6. Loss of biological parent through divorce, abandonment, or other reason
7. Observation of mother or stepmother often receiving physical abuse
8. Have a household member that was a problem drinker or alcoholic or used street drugs
9. Have a household member depressed or mentally ill or attempt suicide
10. Have a household member go to prison.

Box 4.13 Patient case: Andre, ACE score

Andre, a snowboarder, had a very low ACE score: 1/10. His parents divorced when he was 16, and he rarely saw his dad ("abandonment or loss of a parent"), yet was close with his mom and siblings. He was confident, relaxed, and expressed a strong family connection. He recovered with bodywork and movement therapy with a few sessions.

Unrecognized or unresolved emotional, physical, or sexual trauma can contribute to chronic health conditions, which may manifest with exacerbated pelvic floor dysfunction.

Therapists providing trauma-sensitive care and resiliency training can address how trauma "lives in the body" (Levine and Phillips 2012) (Box 4.14).

Box 4.14 Soothing the senses, reducing pain

Therapists can consider and support all aspects of life, of being, that promote wellness in our clients. Humming, dancing, singing, creating art, and walks in nature can be rich positive sensory experiences that calm the nervous system and enhance comfort and joy in life. The greater the abundance of positive sensory experience with sight, sound, scent, touch, and taste, the more the nervous system is bathed in uplifting somatic experiences. Teaching clients options for a "shift" from negative self-talk and stressors to soothing oneself with comfort and enjoyable sensory experiences can provide a breakthrough in the treatment of chronic pain.

Most adults score one or more on the ACE scale, yet a score of four or higher is associated with long-term health consequences and challenges that may involve social, psychological, and physical functioning. Poor self-care, propensity for alcohol,

PELVIC FLOOR DYSFUNCTION (PFD)

PFD is an umbrella term for pelvic health problems, which may include pelvic pain, and limitations with functions and symptoms pertaining to the bladder, bowel, pelvic organ prolapse (POP), and/or sexual activities.

PAIN SCREENING

Screening for pain includes specific questions regarding the exact location of pain, the duration of pain (constant or intermittent), the nature of pain (sharp, dull, aching, burning, stinging, tingling, radiating), and aggravating or relieving methods (rest, exertion, supplements, medications, specific postures or stretches). Answers to these questions help a provider see the 24-hour experience and life impact of pain.

MYOFASCIAL PELVIC PAIN

Individuals with pelvic pain may have myofascial system problems, with multiple tender and trigger points (Box 4.15). Pain may be localized in tender points or referred from one region to another, as in the case of trigger points.

Structurally, the pelvic fascia courses in layers from external skin and muscles into internal visceral structures, nerves, and the vascular and lymphatic system. Tautness of tissue may compress myofascial, neurovascular, and lymphatic structures, leading to varied presentations of pain and possible swelling. Conversely, weakness and laxity in certain areas (such as a torn knee ligament) may lead to tightness and guarding, spasm, and pain in other areas such as the hamstrings, hip flexors and pelvic floor muscles, and low back to help provide stability.

> **Box 4.15 Pain terminology** ᴏᴏ
>
> Tender point: A discrete area of soft tissue that is tender to palpatory pressure (<4 kg) yet otherwise cannot be distinguished from other tissue (Gerwin 2001; Wolfe *et al.* 2013).
>
> Trigger point: An area that may be taut or a hyperirritable nodule, is painful and may be hypersensitive, may refer pain, and may have associated muscle weakness, restricted motion, and possible autonomic and trophic changes (Gautschi 2012; Killens 2018).
>
> Myofascial pain syndrome (MPS): Regional pain that originates in myofascial trigger points which are found in skeletal muscle and characterized by hyperirritable spots or nodules. MPS may be localized or associated with satellite trigger points (Desai, Saini, and Saini 2013; Saxena *et al.* 2015, Simons, Travell, and Simons 1999).

FIGHT OR FLIGHT "WIND UP" IN THE PELVIS, AND POSSIBLE "NUMBING"

Heightened nervous system activity in fight, flight, or freeze often shows up in the pelvis; this is often manifested in the clenching of muscles. An ongoing heightened state of nervous system arousal can persist post-infection, injury, or after exposure to trauma, be it emotional, physical, sexual, or a combination. Non-restorative sleep, those with high ACE scores, and those suffering unrecognized losses such as bereavement may be wound up and not able to participate in therapy due to cognitive and somato-emotional barriers. Sympathetic overdrive and/or trauma may manifest in not recognizing or feeling sensations in the body, feeling numb, and demonstrating poor self-care, including limited participation in therapy.

PAIN REFERRAL ZONES

Pain may be referred into local or distant areas with myofascial palpation, stretch, or compression, as in a "referred pain pattern." Sensitized nerves may be present in MPS, aggravating pain symptoms, and creating local and referred pain in the distribution of the nerve.

In Figure 4.1 we see individual spinal nerve levels which supply specific regions. We also see the same areas with overlapping innervations from peripheral nerves that represent a few combined root levels.

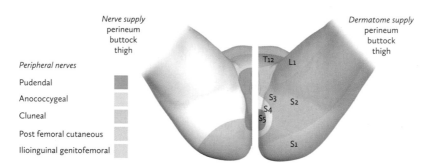

Figure 4.1 Nerve supply to perineum, buttocks, and thighs.

The iliohypogastric, ilioinguinal, and genitofemoral nerves supply sensation and motor innervation to the lower abdomen and upper pelvis, genital region, and hip. The iliohypogastric nerve derives from T12 and L1, the ilioinguinal nerve from L1, and the genitofemoral nerve from L1 and L2. There are multiple sites for potential compression and injury to these nerves, including contusions with sports or trauma, surgeries such as tummy tucks (abdominoplasty), and hernia repairs with mesh.

The lateral femoral cutaneous nerve is sensory to the lateral thigh and skin of the upper buttock. This nerve derives from L2 to L3, and it may be compressed by tight belts or other factors, causing numbness in the outer thigh, termed "meralgia paresthetica."

The obturator nerve is sensory and motor, and it derives from L2 to L4, and supplies the skin of the anterior and medial thigh, and the adductor muscles. The obturator nerve passes through the obturator foramen along with the obturator artery and vein.

Cluneal nerves and sacral nerves supply the

skin of the buttocks and the pelvic area outside the region of the pudendal nerve. Additional sensation is provided via the segmental branches of the lumbosacral plexus, L1 to S5.

Nerve branches from the lumbar and sacral spine innervate the deepest pelvic structures, including L5–S1 to obturator internus, L5–S2 piriformis, and the nerve to the levator ani S2–S5. The pudendal nerve emanates from S2-4 and is sensory and motor to the pelvic floor (Figure 1.15).

Sensitized nerves and neuralgias

If a neural system is placed in a position of stretch and a referral of symptoms occurs in the nerve distribution, this is termed a "sensitized nerve" (Box 4.16). With greater inflammation there may be sharp stabbing pain present. In the case of an inflamed nerve, limited motion, extreme muscle guarding, and intense pain with stretch may indicate a neuralgia, or a localized nerve root as in radiculopathy. Associated weakness, numbness, and protective regional muscle spasm may occur with neuralgia and this type of pain is typically not appropriate for manual or exercise therapy and may be aggravated by well-intentioned movement and bodywork.

> **Box 4.16 Pudendal nerve**   👓
> The pudendal nerve can be irritated with prolonged sitting, bike riding, high intensity squat training, as well as due to individual propensity to myofascial tightness (see Figure 1.15). The pudendal is sensory, motor, and autonomic to the urogenital triangle, and external anal triangle. If irritated or "sensitized" it may manifest symptoms in the clitoral area, penile tip or shaft, pain in the perineum, and/or pain in the anal triangle. Symptoms may be mild, or symptoms may be significant and severely limit sitting, sexual function, cause possible pain with urinary and bowel function, and the ability to simply rest. Rare cases may need injections and/or surgery, yet typically ceasing perpetuating factors and restoring myofascial mobility can help its healing (Hibner *et al.* 2010).

Respiration

Respiratory function is often impaired in CPP conditions, with shallow respiration and limited rib, sternal, and diaphragm mobility. The diaphragm and its connections with muscular, visceral, vascular, and lymphatic structures is of utmost importance. Chronic stress and/or injuries, as well as exercise habits, can lead to a shortening of myofascial structures in the trunk and abdomen, and impaired diaphragm, posterior-lateral, and basal rib regions.

HANDS-ON HEALING WORK: MANUAL THERAPY

As a foundation, providers with a good sense of self-care will ground themselves and work with manual therapy assessment and treatment with a sense of curiosity and discovery (Box 4.17). Hands-on care can start with "listening" to sense the overall soma and any pulls or tensions into certain zones. A hand placed flat on the abdomen at the umbilicus may feel "pulled" towards a hernia scar, or deep into the pelvis at a viscera, or up to the diaphragm.

Manual techniques for myofascial assessment and pain reduction are numerous and may include:

- a neutral, gentle palpation of the skin, with fingertips, or the entire hand, or two hands, and then

- a deeper depth of palpation into the myofascial system.

When sensing a myofascial restriction, a sense of pull into a diagonal, or deeper zone, or other discovery, the use of further myofascial mobility testing can be helpful, such as moving towards or around a restriction in a clock pattern, or a star pattern (Killens 2018). Myofascial mobility work can entail multiple techniques such as:

- holding, gliding, moving into "ease" towards the restriction, with one or two hands
- stacking, or guiding associated layers with lateral bending and/or rotational component.

And then when the time feels right, the manual therapist may perform:

- a sustained holding with pressure, a stretch, distraction, unwinding, or other technique to guide the myofascial region into elongation, into mobility, towards lengthening
- sweeping strokes of broad expanses of the myofascia, from effleurage into deeper kneading as in petrissage
- strumming, lifting, and "skin rolling" where the myofascial structures are lifted and stroked through like a rolling wave across several centimeters
- oscillating or jiggling the region to encourage mobility
- active release therapy which strokes through distinct anatomical layers and engages client contraction and/or relaxation-stretch of the muscles during treatment (Spina 2007).

Research on the efficacy of manual therapy and other interventions for pelvic pain identifies health care provider attributes and interactions that are associated with client improvement, as listed (Bishop, Bialosky, and Alappatu 2020) (Boxes 4.18–4.20):

- forming a sense of a "therapeutic alliance" with the client needing care
- provider skill, with expertise from advanced studies and experience
- a sense of confidence and self-efficacy by providers
- the use of positive language regarding potential benefits of care
- shared decision making in consideration of preferences for types of care.

Box 4.17 Patient case: Andre's therapy

Andre, the snowboarder with coccyx pain, benefitted from:

- myofascial release to areas of tenderness, trigger points, and pain, including sustained pressure on tender and trigger points, skin rolling, and petrissage
- multiplanar leg, hip, trunk, spine stretches, and targeted "unwinding" hamstring, gluteal, adductor, iliopsoas, and abdominal muscles
- respiratory training in coordination with PFM relaxation techniques
- yoga asana as pictured in Figures 4.2–4.13 (a partial list), with an initial small range of motion eventually expanded as he became comfortable, stable, and pain-free.

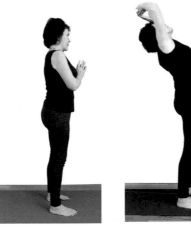

Figure 4.2 Mountain.   Figure 4.3 Back bow.

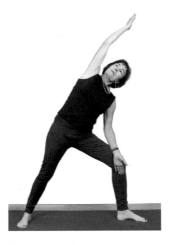

Figure 4.6 Triangle pose.

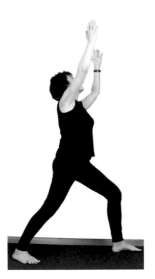

Figure 4.4 Warrior I.

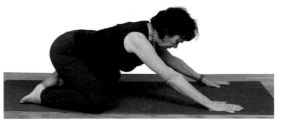

Figure 4.7 Quadruped rocking with PFM relaxation.

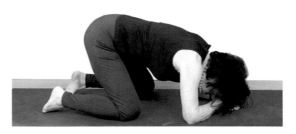

Figure 4.8 Modified child's pose or puppy pose.

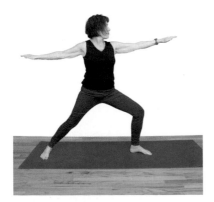

Figure 4.5 Warrior II.

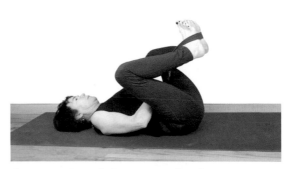

Figure 4.9 Happy baby supported with strap.

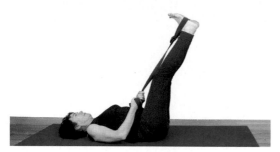

Figure 4.10 Hamstring stretching supported with strap.

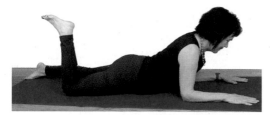

Figure 4.11 Partial press up (sphinx) and knee flexion.

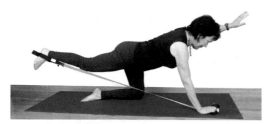

Figure 4.12 Superman facilitated with handibands (Hauptmann 2022).

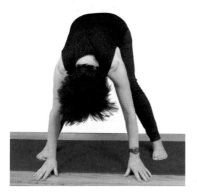

Figure 4.13 Wide forward bend.

These poses were held with a minimum of three breaths per pose with the incorporation of mindfulness and intention setting for a sense of lightness and flow in his body. He performed the program 4–5 times per week.

Box 4.18 Manual therapy for pain reduction

A systematic review (Wasserman *et al.* 2018) found decreased pain with manual therapy to the abdomen in the post-surgical time frame, with soft tissue mobilization (STM) for surgical abdominal adhesions reducing pain and increasing function. STM was also found to be helpful for treating chronic abdominal symptoms.

Complex pain

Box 4.19 Myofascial and nerve pain

Suzanna, age 26, attended PT for right-sided sacroiliac, hip, and pelvic pain. She worked as an accountant and sat for more than ten hours a day. She stood at attention and had a stiff, firm feel to her gluteals, lumbar muscles, hamstrings, and iliotibial band. Her spinal and hip motions were limited, along with tight hip flexors and a straight leg raise on the right side limited to 50 degrees. Her psoas muscles were tight bilaterally with hip extension to 5 degrees. Manual therapy assessment revealed low back, sacroiliac joint, and hip greater trochanter pain with abundant tender and trigger points. She had a loss of myofascial mobility in all areas of pain, and significant tightness in the hamstring muscles, the biceps femoris, and semitendinosus. Additionally, the pudendal nerve, and specifically the perineal branch, showed nerve sensitization with palpation externally at its exit from the ischial spine region, with referred pain into the labia and clitoral region. Her obturator internus muscle, palpated internally, was found to recreate her right hip pain (see Figure 4.18).

She benefitted from several sessions of manual therapy emphasizing myofascial mobilization for the abdomen, spine, hips, external and internal pelvic floor muscles, and hamstrings. She received rib mobilization and respiratory and lumbopelvic hip stretches, and added yoga stretches and intermittent walks into her workday. Switching to a standing desk and practicing pelvic floor relaxation throughout the day helped reduce her pudendal pain.

> **Box 4.20 Balancing the body**
> Manual therapy and movement practices can help restore symmetry, balance, and flow to the body.

VISCERAL MANUAL WORK

The deepest level of manual therapy involves organ specific assessment and treatment, as in visceral mobility work (Barral 2006; Horton 2015; Wetzler 2009). This therapy relies on a generous dedication to study in all aspects of anatomy, while developing palpatory skills that provide a platform for a total body screen, as well as local regional assessments (Boxe 4.23).

Visceral functioning relies upon optimum glides of organs in relation to the skeletal frame, as well as organ to organ mobility, which is the organs' "physiologic" range of motion. This also involves a therapeutic approach towards organ motility, or overall function. Detective work in evaluation and treatment can lead to a discovery of stiffness or lack of mobility in a region, such as the alignment and mobility of the uterus in the bowl of the pelvis. An example of the role of the viscera in pain production is in the case below (Box 4.21).

- Pain localized to cesarean scar and right sacroiliac joint
- Palpation identifies tender, stiff, and painful cesarean scar
- Uterus situated in a side bend and inferior positioning towards the right on organ specific mobility testing
- Limited superior glide, side bend, and rotational mobility of the bladder and uterus
- SI region pain reproduced on myofascial visceral testing anteriorly
- Therapeutic myofascial cesarean scar and visceral treatment towards symmetry and mobility
- Resolution of pain with manual therapy and a therapeutic exercise program

Organ specific and myofascial mobilizations can be outstanding in relieving postpartum pain of this nature.

> **Box 4.21 Postpartum pain: Sheila**
>
> - Six months postpartum: pelvic pain, worse with menses, physical exertion with reaching, bending, standing, and lifting her infant

Although the world is full of suffering, it is full also of the overcoming of it.

(Helen Keller)

Box 4.22 Exercise for healing

Exercise instruction that follows manual therapy can empower the individual with self-care and opportunities for somatic experiencing. Movement can allow discovery and a sense of freedom in the body and help relieve stress. Healing exercise strategies involve inviting individuals to:

- move in any direction that is comfortable
- use their intuition to decide how much to move
- practice ease, non-striving, comfort, and non-violence to self
- notice their breath, breathe comfortably
- explore physical sensations, such as gravity, pressure, stretch, a sense of air on skin which is not covered by clothing
- use routines that feel good
- notice warmth as muscles increase activity
- notice fatigue, and changes in muscle activation with exertion
- choose to work into fatigue to build stamina, endurance, and power.

Manual therapy directly to the pelvic muscles and viscera is a specialty, with a brief portrayal of the process as follows, with accompanying photos on a medical model of the pelvic structures (Figures 4.14–4.20) and pelvic manual therapy equipment (Figures 4.21–4.24).

Box 4.23 Direct pelvic treatment

Depending upon licensure, specialty training, and clinical practice act, following history and pelvic function screening, examination and testing may proceed. This is assessment of the sensory, motor, myofascial, and reflex testing of external, and possibly internal, PFM pelvic floor structures (Van Delft, Thakar, and Sultan 2015).

THE SHORT, TIGHT PELVIC FLOOR

Myofascial assessment of the pelvic floor may identify taut, hypomobile, stiff tissues. In some individuals, a "short pelvic floor" is present, in which case the PFM can neither contract and lift, or relax, bulge, and descend. It was originally described by Fitzgerald and Kotarinos (2003) who advise a multimodal approach to intervention due to the complex nature of the condition. Manual therapy with a variety of techniques as listed prior can help a short PFM group develop flexibility, and this may also reduce associated PFD.

PFM mapping: digital examination sites and/or myofascial release sites

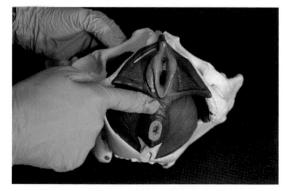

Figure 4.14 External view of urogenital triangle, anal triangle, and perineal body (inferior view of female pelvic anatomy).

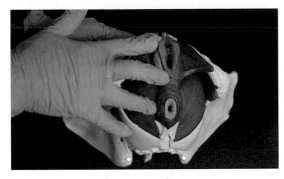

Figure 4.15 Perineal nerve supply zone.

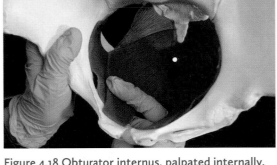

Figure 4.18 Obturator internus, palpated internally.

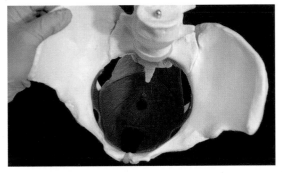

Figure 4.16 Levator ani viewed from above.

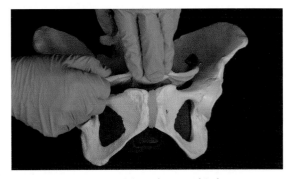

Figure 4.19 Uterus position above pubic bone.

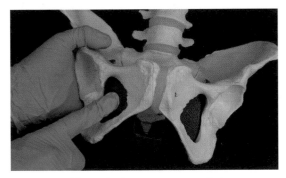

Figure 4.17 Obturator internus, external view.

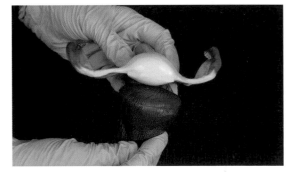

Figure 4.20 Uterus position above bladder.

Many terms are utilized to describe myofascial pain in the pelvic area, with trends in medical diagnoses over time favoring certain "diagnoses," for example:

- Pelvic floor tension myalgia
- Non-relaxing pelvic floor muscles
- Levator ani syndrome
- Vaginismus
- Pelvic and perineal pain.

Once an individual learns about their PFM and identifies triggers or habits that exacerbate their condition, they can steer towards practices that prevent symptoms, and also find relief with the self-care practices as well as direct exercise and manual therapy (Boxes 4.22 and 4.24).

Box 4.24 Suzanna's therapy: ♥
myofascial and nerve pain treatment
Suzanna, presented earlier, benefitted from several months of myofascial mobilization for the abdomen, spine, hips, external and internal pelvic floor muscles, and hamstrings. She received rib mobilization and respiratory and lumbopelvic hip stretches, and added yoga stretches and intermittent walks into her workday.

She received pudendal nerve anatomy education, as well as potential aggravating factors such as bike riding, sitting on rigid surfaces, and performing intense squats. The use of pudendal decompression pillows and options to create a padded seat with a folded jacket for outings was provided.

training and pleasure (see Chapter 13). There is potential for harm in incorrect pelvic equipment use, in causing increased pain, or even retention, tearing, and fistulas, therefore individuals ideally should consult a medical pelvic specialist for pain care and training and safety guidelines as needed.

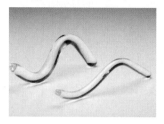

4.21 Clear serenity wand.

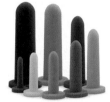

Figure 4.22 Intimate Rose dilator set.

Specialized pelvic health equipment may be used for external and internal mapping, self-care, and myofascial release tools (Figures 4.21–4.24). Pelvic health equipment, or tools, can also provide feedback via pressure, stretch, and movement, regarding correct performance of PFM contraction, lift, descent, and bulge-relax, all of which can help with awareness, embodiment, and myofascial pain reduction (Box 4.25).

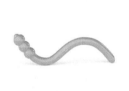

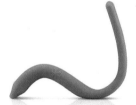

Figure 4.23 TheraWand LA, posterior view.

Figure 4.24 Intimate Rose vibrating wand.

Myofascial assessment and treatment

Myofascial treatment is one of the safest interventions for clients with pain. Yet it is important to recognize body language and signs that indicate a need for "hands-off care." In the most private region of the body—the pelvis—shame and fear may be present, along with anxiety about new procedures, and a heightened fear-avoidance and tactile defensiveness reaction with palpation. Provider sensitivity is needed to prevent harm and empower clients.

Box 4.25 Precautions with
equipment
Many individuals may simply regard the items pictured as "sex toys," yet in the case of pelvic pain they may be painful to use and may represent a threat or danger to those with a history of trauma. The term "toy" may be associated with child behavior and stigma and be unacceptable per religious and/or cultural training. At the other end of the spectrum, this equipment may be used for sexual health

Nervous system down training

Screening the habitual respiratory pattern can be a way into the body for care, and a teachable tool for wind-down of sympathetic towards parasympathetic. In the absence of pelvic floor mobility and a lack of synchrony between the diaphragm and pelvic core, exercise and manual therapy may have limited results. Somatic experiencing, dance, yoga, Pilates, qigong, tai chi, personal training, and aerobic exercise are formats that can help re-set the nervous system.

YOGA AND PILATES

Yoga and Pilates are mind–body exercise formats that help in pain rehabilitation (Box 4.26). Writings by Patanjali outline the eight-fold path, recognized as the limbs of yoga (Miller 1995). The first four limbs are yama, niyama, asana, and pranayama, which "concentrate on refining our personalities, gaining mastery over the body, and developing an energetic awareness of ourselves" (Carrico 2021). The other four limbs are the deeper meditative spiritual practices of pratyahara, dharana, dhyana, and samadhi.

> **Box 4.26 Yoga benefits, and precautions**
>
> Yoga has great potential for health benefits. Research validates the health benefits of yoga on statistically reducing pelvic pain and benefits towards reducing anxiety and depression (Cramer *et al.* 2018; Nag and Kodali 2013; Saxena *et al.* 2017), which make it a valuable mind–body method for intervention. However, a large review found a lifetime prevalence of injuries at 21.3–61.8%, typically non-permanent sprains and strains (Cramer, Ostermann, and Dobos 2018). Instructor training in safety and injury prevention is important.

Medical therapeutic yoga (MTY) is a resource which offers healing mind–body–spirit programming (Garner 2016). Modifications are used for conditions such as spondylolisthesis, pubic or pelvic girdle pain, femoral acetabular impingement, pudendal sensitization, or other conditions. Pranayama and meditation practice guidelines are important aspects of MTY.

Restorative yoga postures (asanas) may be used to calm, center, and often reduce pelvic pain. Positions can be held in a time frame that feels best, from 30 seconds to a few minutes or longer, and also using pillows, bolsters, blocks, and straps.

Pranayama practice includes awareness of breath and controlling the rate and depth of respiration. Depending on what is needed by an individual, such as relaxation and calming, or charging up and energizing, instructions can vary (Garner 2016).

- Deep relaxation "diaphragm" breathing
- Transverse abdominal engagement for stability and postural control, during diaphragm and lateral costal breathing
- Ujaii breathing, victorious warrior breath
- Alternate nostril breathing (Figures 4.25 and 4.26)

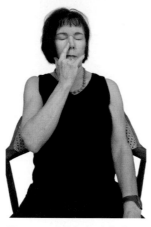

Figure 4.25 Exhale, inhale left nostril.

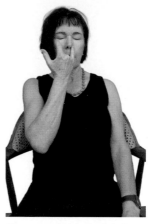

Figure 4.26 Exhale, inhale right nostril.

MEDITATION (SEE CHAPTER 12)

Pilates is a popular mind–body workout format which may be performed as mat exercise or with the reformer, the Wunda chair, and other equipment (Pilates and Miller 1998; Wood 2018). Pilates concepts of breathing, concentration, control, centering, precision, fluidity, stamina, and relaxation combine to create a mind–body experience with improved health measures based on studies (Fleming and Herring 2018; Lin *et al.* 2016). Pilates exercises are low impact and can help individuals find self-care formats (Hauptmann 2022) as well as enjoyable classes for wellness (see Figures 4.27–4.33).

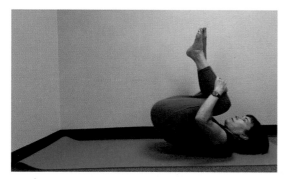

Figure 4.27 Rolling like a ball.

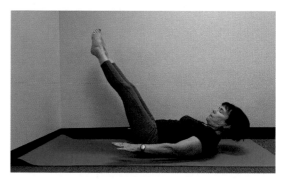

Figure 4.28 The hundred.

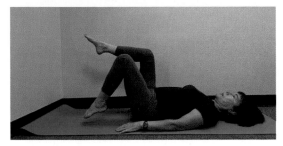

Figure 4.29 Toe taps.

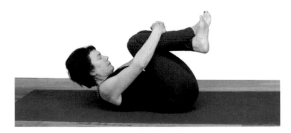

Figure 4.30 Swimmer.

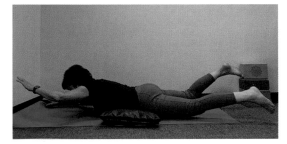

Figure 4.31 Double knee to chest.

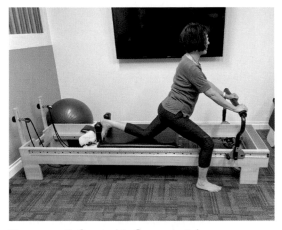

Figure 4.32 Reformer hip flexor stretch.

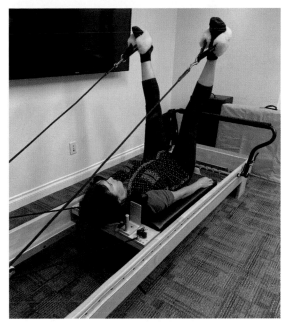

Figure 4.33 Reformer legs in straps.

Instructors may cue pelvic relaxation, and/or tightening the pelvic region, in yoga (Sweta *et al.* 2021) or Pilates. "Mula bandha," cues a contraction of the anterior PFM, and "ashwini mudra," the posterior muscles (Box 4.27). However, repeated tightening of the PFM is not functional and susceptible individuals who have a tendency to pelvic clenching may even develop nerve sensitization in the pelvic region, such as pudendal neuralgia (Yildirim and Goksenoglu 2019).

> Box 4.27 Mula bandha: 🦋
> engage, and release
> Light contractions for awareness and core control, followed by PFM relaxation, is likely the best applications of mula and ashwini cuing.

SUMMARY

Pain is part of the experience of being human, and pelvic pain has many causes, and many presentations, with a different journey for each person. With emerging models of neuroplasticity and understanding the vast potential benefits of mind–body approaches, resilience can be celebrated in stories about the healing of chronic pain. Remarkably, over time, transformations can happen for some, but not for everyone, and this is an enigma in complex pain.

Care providers are advised to build and work with a team. Lightening or softening the burden of pain is an act of compassionate care and skill. Holistic approaches can engage the mind, body, and spirit in treatment, promoting positive sensory input, which can promote gratitude, wellness, enhanced health, and reduced pain.

REFERENCES

Barral, J. P. (2006) *Urogenital Manipulation*. Seattle, WA: Eastland Press.

Bishop, M. D., Bialosky, J. E., and Alappatu, M. J. (2020) "Riding a tiger; maximizing effects of manual therapies for pelvic pain." *Journal of Women's Health Physical Therapy 44*, 1, 32–38.

Brumange, S., Diers, M., Dannels, L., Moseley, G. L., *et al.* (2019) "Neuroplasticity of sensorimotor control in low back pain." *Journal of Orthopedic and Sports Physical Therapy 49*, 6, 402–414.

Butler, D. S. and Moseley, G. L. (2014) *Explain Pain* preconference seminar at the combined sections meeting. American Physical Therapy Association, Las Vegas, NV, USA, 2014.

Carrico, M. (2021) "Get to Know the 8 Limbs of Yoga." *Yoga Journal Online*. Accessed 6/7/2022 at https://www.yogajournal.com/yoga-101/philosophy/8-limbs-of-yoga/eight-limbs-of-yoga.

Cramer, H., Lauche, R., Anheyer, D., Pilkington, K., *et al.* (2018) "Yoga for anxiety; a systematic review and meta-analysis of randomized controlled trials." *Depression and Anxiety 35*, 9, 830–843.

Cramer, H., Ostermann, T., and Dobos, G. (2018) "Injuries and other adverse events associated with yoga practice: A systematic review of epidemiological studies." *Journal of Science and Medicine in Sport 21*, 2, 147–154.

Desai, M. J., Saini, V., and Saini, S. (2013) "Myofascial pain syndrome: A treatment review." *Pain Therapy 2*, 1, 21–36.

Doan, L., Manders, T., and Wag, J. (2015) "Neuroplasticity underlying the comorbidities of pain and depression." *Neural Plasticity*, APA PsychNet article 504691, https://doi.org/10.1155/2015/504691.

Engeler, D., Baranowski, A. P., Elneil, S., Hughes, J., *et al.* (2012) "Guidelines on chronic pelvic pain." *European Association of Urology 57*, 1, 35–48.

Felitti, V. J., Anda, R. F., Nordenberg, D., Williamson, D. F., *et al.* (1998) "Relationship of childhood abuse and household dysfunction to many of the leading causes of death in adults. The adverse childhood experiences (ACE) study." *American Journal of Preventative Medicine 14*, 4, 245–258.

Fenton, B. W., Grey, S. F., Tossone, K., McCarrol, M., and Von Gruenigen, E. V. (2015) "Classifying patients with chronic pelvic pain into levels of biopsychosocial dysfunction using latent class modeling of patient reported outcomes." *Pain Research and Treatments*, Article ID 940675.

Fitzgerald, M. P. and Kotarinos, R. (2003) "Rehabilitation of the short pelvic floor." *International Urogynecological Journal 14*, 261–268.

Fleming, K. M. and Herring, M. P. (2018) "The effects of Pilates on mental health outcomes: A meta-analysis of controlled trials." *Complementary Therapies in Medicine 37*, 80–95.

Funston, G., O'Flynn, H., Ryan, N. A. J., Hamilton, W., and Crosbie, E. J. (2018) "Recognizing gynecological cancer in primary care: Risk factors, red flags, and referrals." *Advances in Therapy 35*, 590.

Gallagher, E., Bijur, P. E., Latimer, C., and Silver, W. (2002) "Reliability and validity of a visual analog scale for acute abdominal pain in the ED." *American Journal of Emergency Medicine 20*, 4, 287–290.

Garner, G. (2016) *Medical Therapeutic Yoga*. Edinburgh: Handspring Publishing.

Gautschi, R. U. (2012) "Trigger points as a fascia-related disorder." In R. Schleip, T. W. Findley, L. Chaitow, and P. A. Huijing (eds) *Fascia, The Tensional Network of the Human Body*. Edinburgh: Churchill Livingstone.

Gerwin, P. S. and Kruszka, S. J. (2010) "Evaluation of acute pelvic pain in women." *American Family Physician 82*, 2, 141–147.

Gerwin, R. D. (2021) "Classification, epidemiology, and natural history of myofascial pain syndrome." *Current Pain Headache Reports 5*, 5, 412–420.

Hauptmann, M. (2022) Hooked On Pilates®. Accessed 9/21/22 at hookedonpilates.com.

Hibner, M., Desai, N., Robertson, L. J. and Nour, M. (2010) "Pudendal neuralgia." *Journal of Minimally Invasive Gynecology 17*, 2, 148–153.

Horton, R. (2015) "Clinical review: The anatomy, biological plausibility and efficacy of visceral mobilization in the treatment of pelvic floor dysfunction." *Journal of Pelvic, Obstetric and Gynaecological Physiotherapy 117*, 5–18.

Hughes, K., Bellis, M., Hardcastle, K. A., Sethi, D., *et al.* (2017) "The effect of multiple adverse childhood experiences on health: A systematic review and meta-analysis." *The Lancet Public Health 2*, 8, e356–e366.

Killens, D. (2018) *Mobilizing the Myofascial System*. Edinburgh: Handspring Publishing.

Krieger, J. N., Nyberg, L., and Nickel, J. C. Jr. (1999) NIH consensus definition and classification of prostatitis. *Journal of the American Medical Association 282*, 3, 236–237.

Kruszka, P. S. and Kruszka, S. J. (2010) "Evaluation of acute pelvic pain in women." *American Family Physician 82*, 2, 141–147.

Latthe, P., Latthe, M., Say, L., Gulmezoglu, M., and Kahn, K. S. (2006) "WHO systematic review of prevalence of chronic pelvic pain: A neglected reproductive health morbidity." *BMC 6*, 177.

Leerar, P., Boissonnault, W., Domholdt, E., and Roddey, T. (2007) "Documentation of red flags by physical therapists for patients with low back pain." *Journal of Manual and Manipulative Therapy 15*, 1, 42–49.

Levine, P. A. and Phillips, M. (2012) *Freedom from Pain: Discover Your Body's Power to Overcome Physical Pain*. Boulder, CO: Sounds True Inc.

Lin, H. T., Hung, W. C., Hung, J. L., Wu, P. S., *et al.* (2016) "Effects of Pilates on patients with chronic non-specific low back pain: A systematic review." *Journal of Physical Therapy Science 28*, 10, 2961–2969.

Metzler, M., Merrick, M. T., Klevens, J., Ports, K. A., and Ford, D. C. (2017) "Adverse childhood experiences and life opportunities: Shifting the narrative." *Children and Youth Services Review 72*, 141–149.

Miller, B. S. (1995) *Yoga, Discipline of Freedom: The Yoga Sutras Attributed to Patanjali*. New York: Bantam Books.

Molinari, G., Garcia-Palacios, A., Enrique, A., *et al.* (2018) "The power of visualization: Back to the future for pain management in fibromyalgia syndrome." *Pain Med 19*, 7, 1451–1468.

Morrison, P. (2016) "Musculoskeletal conditions related to pelvic floor muscle overactivity." In Padoa, A. and Rosenbaum, T. Y. *The Overactive Pelvic Floor*. New York: Springer.

Moseley, G. L. and Butler, D. S. (2015) "Fifteen years of explaining pain: The past, present and future." *Journal of Pain 16*, 9, 807–813.

Motamed, F., Mohsenipour, R., Seifirad, S., Yusefi, A., *et al.* (2012) "Red flags of recurrent abdominal pain in children: Study on 100 subjects." *Iran Journal of Pediatrics 22*, 4, 457–462.

Nag, U. and Kodali, M. (2013) "Meditation and yoga as alternative therapy for primary dysmenorrhea." *International Journal of Medical & Pharmaceutical Sciences 3*, 7, 39–44.

Okifuji, A. and Hare, B. D. (2015) "The association between chronic pain and obesity." *Journal of Pain Research 8*, 399–408.

Pilates, J. H. and Miller, W. J. (1998) *Pilates' Return to Life Through Contrology*. Idaho: Presentation Dynamics.

Ramiro, L. S., Madrid, B. J., and Brown, D. W. (2010) "Adverse childhood experiences (ACE) and health-risk behaviors among adults in a developing country setting." *Child Abuse and Neglect 34*, 842–855.

Saxena, A., Chansoria, M., Tomar, G., and Kumar, A. (2015) "Myofascial pain syndrome: An overview." *Journal of Pain and Palliative Care Pharmacotherapy 29*, 16–21.

Saxena, R., Gupta, M., Shankar, N., Jain, S., and Saxena, A. (2017) "Effects of yogic intervention on pain scores and quality of life in females with chronic pelvic pain." *International Journal of Yoga 10*, 1, 9–15.

Simons, J., Travell, D., and Simons, L. (1999) *Myofascial Pain and Dysfunction: The Trigger Point Manual*. Philadelphia: Lippincott Williams & Wilkins.

Spina, A. A. (2007) "External coxA saltans (snapping hip) treated with active release techniques®: A case report." *Journal of Canadian Chiropractic Association 51*, 1, 23–29.

Sweta, K. M., Godbole, A., Prajapati, S., and Awasthi, H. H. (2021) "Assessment of the effect of mulabandha yoga therapy in healthy women, stigmatized for pelvic floor dysfunctions: A randomized controlled trial." *Journal of Ayurvedic and Integrative Medicine 12*, 3, 514–520.

Van Delft, K., Thakar, R., and Sultan, A. H. (2015) "Pelvic floor muscle contractility: Digital assessment versus transperineal ultrasound." *Ultrasound in Obstetrics and Gynecology 45*, 2, 217–222.

Wasserman, J. B., Copeland, M., Upp, M., and Abraham, K. (2018) "The effect of soft tissue mobilization techniques on adhesion-related pain in the abdomen: A systematic review." *Journal of Bodywork and Movement Therapies 23*, 2, 262–269.

Wetzler, G. (2009) Gynecologic Visceral Manipulation Seminar, 10.8.2009–10.11.2009, sponsored by the Section on Women's Health of the American Physical Therapy Association. Pomona, CA.

Wolfe, F., Brähler, E., Hinz, A., and Häuser, W. (2013) "Fibromyalgia prevalence, somatic symptom reporting, and the dimensionality of polysymptomatic distress; results from a survey of the general population, randomized controlled trial." *Arthritis Care Research 65*, 5, 777–785.

Wood, S. (2018) *Pilates for Rehabilitation: Recover from Injury and Optimize Function*. Windsor, ON, Canada: Human Kinetics.

Woolf, C. J. (2014) "What to call the amplification of nociceptive signals in the central nervous system that contribute to widespread pain?" *Pain 155*, 1911–1912.

Yildirim, M. A. and Goksenoglu, G. (2019) "A rare and late presentation of pudendal neuralgia in a patient with fibromyalgia after Pilates exercises." *Turkish Journal of Physical Medicine and Rehabilitation 65*, 1, 80–83.

Zarse, E. M., Neff, M. R., Yoder, R., Hulvershorn, L., *et al.* (2019) "The adverse childhood experiences questionnaire: Two decades of research on childhood trauma as a primary cause of adult mental illness, addiction, and medical diseases." *Cogent Medicine 6*, 1, 1581447.

Zeidan, E., Grant, J. A., Brown, C. A., McHaffie, J. G., and Coghill, R. C. (2012) "Mindfulness meditation-related pain relief: Evidence for unique brain mechanisms in the regulation of pain." *Neuroscience Letters 520*, 2, 165–173.

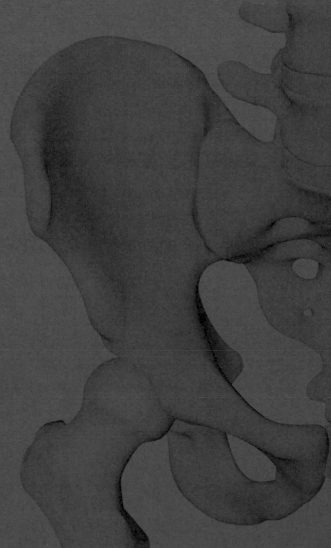

PERINATAL CHANGES, CHALLENGES, AND RESILIENCE IN PELVIC HEALTH

CHAPTER 5

Pregnancy, Birth, and Early Postpartum: Profiles in Resilience

J. MICHELLE MARTIN AND MAUREEN MASON

Pregnancy is a wonderful journey. It is the process of creating a new human being. Spiritually, it is profound in the creation of a new life, life that is both an intimate part of the mother, yet totally separate, with a genetic mix of ancestors across generations that may trace back thousands of years to mitochondrial DNA (23andMe 2021) (Box 5.1).

> Box 5.1 Parents: journeys of love 🦋
> For birth parents, experiencing the dichotomy of creating an infant who is from ovum and sperm, yet a totally separate being that will ideally grow to independence, is a dance that is carried throughout parenthood. Parenthood may also occur via in vitro fertilization, surrogacy, or adoption and they are all journeys of love and require a dance between nurturing, protecting, dependency, and independence.

Pregnancy is characterized by many changes, both during and after, for ten months and beyond. This chapter follows the journey into three distinct sections: pregnancy, birth, and postpartum. It will detail unique pelvic health medical features pertaining to each phase, and movement therapy and bodywork therapy to assist each phase. This chapter will also present socioeconomic and historical profiles that help us understand modern perinatal health care and challenges, and prompt readers to improve perinatal care.

PREGNANCY

Pregnancy begins or is counted from the first date of the last menstrual cycle. Typically, pregnancy is segmented into trimesters, 13-week intervals, with each interval presenting its own symptoms, changes, and potential concerns. The journey is unique to each pregnant individual, and for each pregnancy (Box 5.2): easy, uncomplicated, full of the joy of new life, or with a bit of distress, and even unexpected challenges.

First trimester

This is typically the time most individuals discover that they are pregnant—often due to a missed period (Box 5.3). Typical symptoms present at this time may include:

- nausea and vomiting due to changes in hormone levels, including increased levels of human chorionic gonadotropin (hCG)
- potentially decreased appetite due to nausea
- increased sensitivity to odors, likely a protective biologic function
- fatigue, which may be due to increasing levels of progesterone
- enlarged, tender breasts
- changes in mood/emotional changes.

Second trimester

The second trimester is special for many reasons. It is the period of time when fetal movements are first felt. It is the time when some women find out the sex of the fetus, if ultrasound screening is available. It is the time when many start to feel as though they are finally pregnant as they are now experiencing abdominal growth and those around them become aware of their joyous surprise. Yet this time may also be filled with more challenges (Box 5.4). As the body continues to accommodate the growing fetus, the mom may experience some of the symptoms listed below, yet each pregnancy is unique.

1. Decreased digestion, due in part to progesterone. This can also be responsible for constipation, hemorrhoids, and pelvic discomfort.
2. Musculoskeletal changes with all the muscles of the "canister" of the trunk (diaphragm, abdominals, quadratus lumborum, spinal muscles, pelvic floor muscles) stretching. Balance challenges with a higher center of gravity, and increased weight. These can result in the onset of back pain, hip pain, round ligament pain, as well as pelvic girdle pain (primarily sacroiliac joint pain and pubic symphysis dysfunction).
3. Neurological symptoms may occur; many pregnant individuals might report pain along the sciatic nerve distribution at the buttock and/or posterior thigh or leg, or at the antero-lateral thigh consistent with lateral femoral cutaneous nerve involvement (meralgia paresthetica). Other areas of nerve irritation may occur as well, such as the upper extremity symptoms of numbness, burning, and pain.
4. Increased sense of heaviness or pressure at the lower abdomen and perineum

may occur as weight gain continues, and as the fetus continues to develop.

5. Bladder urgency from weight gain and direct pressure, as the uterus sits upon and hugs the bladder.

6. Swelling at the extremities, as pelvic pressure may hinder circulation, yet overall blood volume increases to support growth and cushion the baby.

7. Skin changes such as stretch marks, linea nigra (a central "stripe" on the abdomen), and skin dryness.

8. Hot flashes and increased sweating, related to increased metabolic rate and hormone changes.

weight gain and fatigue. All potential symptoms described in the second trimester may increase in intensity in the last three months of pregnancy. It is difficult to stoop to don socks and tie shoes, due to abdominal girth. Moms may often feel out of breath, and there is an increased rate of respiration due to a lower excursion ability for the diaphragm. Braxton Hicks contractions occur; the uterus involuntarily contracts at times, as preparation for its performance during vaginal birth; these contractions may be tolerated with ease or feel uncomfortable (Box 5.6). Pain may also occur from stretch of structures such as the Ligament of Cleyet, which spans from the cecum and appendix to the fallopian tube and uterus (Burch 2003; Wetzler 2010; Figure 5.1 and Box 5.5).

> ### Box 5.4 Bodywork with doulas
> According to the recipient of bodywork in her middle trimester, having a doula perform a small jiggling of the myofascial trunk and pelvis, with small oscillations, felt soothing and relaxing and allowed the body to feel a sense of ease with pregnancy. The pregnant woman was in side-lying position, and a doula led therapists in an introductory workshop in Spinning Babies (spinningbabies.com 2022), where a scarf was looped loosely around the lower pelvis, and helped provide oscillations around the trunk in a very small range of motion. Spinning Babies providers may be doulas, midwives, or nurse providers who offer support online, as well as in-person care. Considerations of daily routines, movement therapy, the use of gravity in varied positions, and comfort and ease are supported for an optimized journey through the perinatal time.

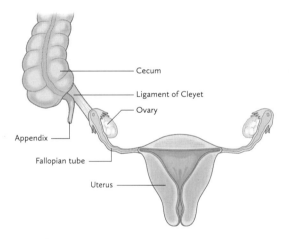

Figure 5.1 Second trimester view of cecum, Ligament of Cleyet, and uterus.

> ### Box 5.5 Manual therapy intervention
> Myofascial care and visceral mobilization may provide pain relief for stretch related pains from the round ligament, Ligament of Cleyet, and other structures. This work requires multiple levels of client screening, evaluation, and therapeutic intervention as provided by advanced providers.

Third trimester

Going into the third trimester, growth of the abdomen is more apparent, and some pregnant individuals tend to "slow down" due to the increased

There are postures that may be comforting to mothers in this phase, as noted here, and provide rest as a preparation for caring for an infant soon (Figures 5.2 and 5.3).

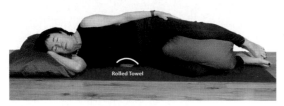

Figure 5.2 Third trimester restorative yoga with side-lying head, waist, and lower extremity support pillows.

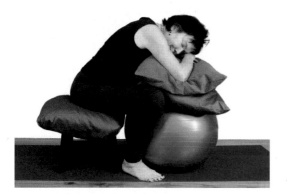

Figure 5.3 Third trimester modified child's pose: pregnant female seated on stool leaning over ball (also a laboring pose).

Box 5.6 Preemies: infant and parents need help

Once a fetus reaches 27 weeks' gestational age, they are termed "viable," meaning if a situation arose where they were to be born prematurely, there is a good chance that they would survive. A preemie birth may be accompanied by great community support, yet also be a time of anxiety, stress, and sleep deprivation for parents while an infant is in neonatal intensive care. This may be traumatic for parents, who are then taxed with caring for a newborn who needs special care after discharge.

Understanding the biopsychosocial aspects of pregnancy

Providers optimally can view a pregnant person from a biopsychosocial model, considering factors beyond the physical, and physiological. Psychological factors such as anxiety levels and coping skills play a role in the health of a pregnancy (Rizzardo *et al.* 1985). A pregnant person's emotional levels can impact anxiety, mood, appetite, and even physical activity or the desire to engage in any activity. Socioeconomic status also plays a role in maternal health as living conditions and financial means can dictate a person's access to care, maternal health education, and other resources, not only for pregnancy but beyond.

The intersection of race and pregnancy

Currently within the US there have been significant disparities regarding health care for minorities and other marginalized populations. This is a worldwide phenomenon as well. Many pregnant individuals lack access to care, including prenatal services, maternal fetal medicine specialists, or may be limited based on proximity. Furthermore, stresses outside of the environment, such as medical or health related factors can add insult to injury.

According to research by Margaret Buhrer (Buhrer 2016), "a lack of proper sex education, and the lack of access to affordable or free birth control, is a part of a cycle of events that directly prevents marginalized groups from improving their socioeconomic status." As such, these events play a role in maternal outcomes well before an individual has even conceived. Additionally, these same issues impact not only pregnant individuals but families in general, from premature births to maternal/obstetric mortality, which is 3–5 times higher in Black birthing individuals than their white counterparts. The perpetuation of these same issues leads to the generational concerns within specific communities regarding birth outcomes.

According to Howell *et al.* (2016), the site of birth plays a critical role in birth disparities: "The black–white maternal mortality disparity is the largest disparity among all conventional population perinatal health measures." And the authors further state, "for every maternal death, 100 women experience severe maternal morbidity, a life-threatening diagnosis, or undergo a life-saving procedure during their delivery hospitalization. Like maternal mortality, severe maternal morbidity is more common among Black than white women." This research found that white birthing individuals were more likely than their Black counterparts to deliver in facilities, more specifically hospitals with lower morbidity rates (65 percent white versus 23 percent of Black deliveries). Furthermore, the research indicated that the location of birthing facility or delivery may contribute as much as 47.7 percent of the racial disparity in severe maternal morbidity rates in New York City (Boxes 5.7 and 5.8).

Box 5.7 Medical screening: pre- eclampsia and eclampsia
Women with limited access to care and low socioeconomic status are more likely to suffer from pre-eclampsia or eclampsia. Pre-eclampsia is a sudden rise in blood pressure in a pregnant individual with no prior hypertension history, and this usually begins around the 20th week of pregnancy. Blood pressure readings at or above 140/90 mmHg, protein in the urine, and swelling are signs of pre-eclampsia, and blood pressure monitoring during pregnancy and urinalysis is critical to check for this. If untreated, maternal and fetal health are at risk, and the progression to eclampsia involves seizures and coma, and possible fetal and maternal mortality (Duley 2009).

Box 5.8 Medical ethics, historical use and abuse
The fields of obstetrics and gynecology owe a debt to enslaved women who became experimental subjects in the development of surgical techniques. Many of the fields' most pioneering surgical techniques were developed on the bodies of enslaved women who were experimented on until they either were cured or died. Owens and Fett (2019) discuss historical facts regarding race, medical experimentation, and injustice in the legacies of slaves and surgeries, stating, "The deep roots of these patterns of disparity in maternal and infant health lie with the commodification of enslaved Black women's childbearing and physicians' investment in serving the interests of slave owners." The slaveholding surgeon François Marie Prevost pioneered cesarean section surgeries on American enslaved women's bodies through repeated experimentation. James Marion Sims, another famed 19th-century gynecologist, created the surgical technique that repaired obstetrical fistula by experimenting on a group of Alabama enslaved women (Owens and Fett 2019).

Many maternal deaths are preventable. Providers of health care to people in the perinatal journey can help optimize health and health care service and help mend the sad socioeconomic injustice that is prevalent today (Box 5.9).

Box 5.9 The intersection of sexuality and pregnancy
One of the important considerations that we need to be aware of is the fact that not every pregnant individual identifies as female, as in the case of trans men. There is an increased incidence of non-binary individuals who are

giving birth, along with trans male individuals who have made the decision to expand their family and become pregnant. Unfortunately, due to lack of education, provider biases and lack of access to care exist. According to the study "Transgender Men Who Experienced Pregnancy After Female-to-Male Gender Transitioning," some trans male individuals have gender dysphoria due to their changing body appearance—weight gain, enlarged breasts, growing abdomens. Care must be taken to ensure that these individuals are able to receive the appropriate care that they need to ensure a healthy and happy physiologic and emotional pregnancy, birth, and postpartum period.

Profiles: Musculoskeletal concerns during pregnancy

The physiology of pregnancy and related musculoskeletal changes is a complex and remarkable process. Ideally, the pregnant person's body displays resilience in structure and function. Health and wellness care providers can step in to help birthing persons address musculoskeletal concerns and facilitate an "easier" and tolerable if not pain-free prenatal experience.

Cantu and Grodin (2001) discuss connective tissue continuity throughout the body in their text *Myofascial Manipulation*. The authors describe a continuous tension which is exhibited by connective tissue within our bodies, involving interconnections throughout muscles, tendons, ligaments, and fascia. There is a balance at play in tension and mobility in a normally functioning body. We need to consider the extensive physical changes that will occur will impact all connective tissue structures.

Many individuals during pregnancy will experience low back pain, sacroiliac joint pain, occasional sciatica, round ligament pain, pubic symphysis dysfunction, and hip pain (Box 5.10). Increased weight gain along with the weight and

pressure of the growing fetus inside the pelvic and abdominal cavities contribute to postural shifts and potential biomechanical compensations, leading to pain.

Apart from pelvic related discomforts, many pregnant individuals may experience carpal tunnel syndrome (Bahrami *et al.* 2005), diastasis rectus abdominis (Mota *et al.* 2018), and neurological complaints (Ferraz *et al.* 2017) including the upper and lower extremities.

Box 5.10 Patient case: Sarah ♥

Sarah was a 29-year-old female, currently in her third pregnancy, which she stated was different from her other two. She reported that she started having a significant amount of low back pain but also pain at the front of the pelvis, which she described as a sharp but intermittent discomfort. She reported difficulty with turning in bed, and walking, especially up the stairs, and noticed that when she carried her toddler.

On examination, she was shown to have both sacroiliac (SI) joint pain as well as pubic symphysis dysfunction. Her treatment included activity modification, use of an SI belt, manual therapy for SI alignment correction, and therapeutic exercise. She was instructed in SI belt application to add stability, including application while lying down, and positioning to avoid excess hip compression that could cause meralgia paresthetica (lateral femoral cutaneous nerve irritation). Activity modification education included pacing work/rest, by taking more breaks throughout the day, avoiding a staggered stance, optional weight shifting to one side when standing for long periods, carrying the toddler evenly using a baby carrier whenever possible, and learning how to transfer from sitting to standing or turn in bed with spine and pelvic symmetry. Training was provided in strengthening exercises to stabilize the low back and hips to decrease back pain (Figures 5.4 and 5.5). Overall, she noted decreased symptoms after the initial session with report of full resolution by session number six.

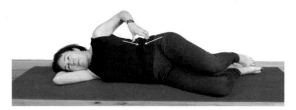

Figure 5.6a Hip hike, quadratus lumborum.

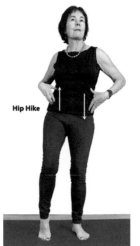

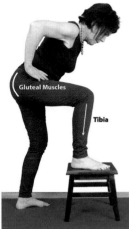

Figure 5.4 Contract–relax for quadratus lumborum.

Figure 5.5 Contract–relax for correction of an anterior rotation.

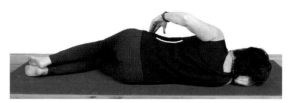

Figure 5.6b Hip depress downward, quadratus lumborum stretch.

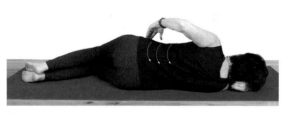

Figure 5.7 Lumbar rotations: multifidus.

Exercise during pregnancy

During pregnancy, there are many physiological changes that an individual may experience, as described. One of the greatest recommendations for pregnant persons is exercise! Once upon a time, exercise during pregnancy was a big "no-no" (Perales, Artal, and Lucia 2017). However, in recent years, persons have been recommended to exercise during pregnancy even if they had not done so previously.

For women with back, leg, and pelvic discomfort, if they are unable to tolerate weight-bearing fitness activities, they may perform exercise in side-lying position for core training and stretching, as illustrated below (Figures 5.6–5.14).

These are side-lying examples for pregnant individuals with pelvic discomfort, MM gentle series. Note the lumbopelvic core strengthening followed by relaxation-stretch.

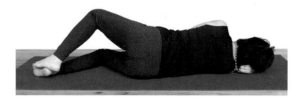

Figure 5.8 Clam.

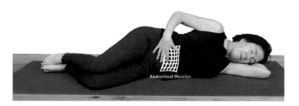

Figure 5.9 Transverse abdominis (TRA) contract.

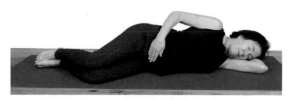

Figure 5.10 Diaphragm breathing.

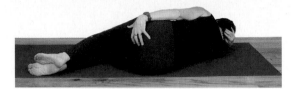

Figure 5.11 Pelvic floor muscles (PFM) contract 10%/relax.

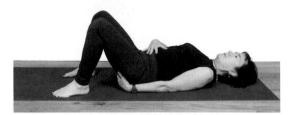

Figure 5.12 Transverse abdominis (TRA) and pelvic floor muscles (PFM).

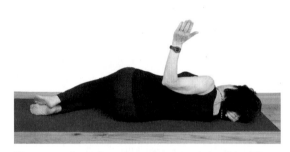

Figure 5.13 Scapular spine retract and shoulder ER.

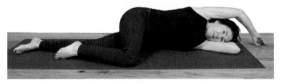

Figure 5.14 Piriformis stretch and arm reach into abduction; lateral costal respiration.

Exercise has many benefits that include increasing the chance for an uncomplicated delivery (Poyatos-León *et al.* 2015). According to the American College of Obstetricians and Gynecologists (ACOG), "a healthy woman with a normal pregnancy may continue regular exercise or begin a new program."

Screening the pregnant client for fitness programs

In consideration of exercise during pregnancy, providers and trainers need to identify how to competently assess individuals for activity. It is easy to say "go forth and exercise" but providers need to make sure that they are safe, especially if embarking on this type of activity for the first time. Examples of such tools being used to adequately assess pregnant individuals are:

1. The Physical Activity Readiness Questionnaire (PAR-Q). The PAR-Q is a series of questions to assess readiness for exercise but more importantly to determine if a medical follow-up is needed prior to exercising.
2. The Physical Activity Readiness Medical Examination (PARmed-X), www.eparmedx.com. The PARmed-X is a questionnaire usually conducted by medical professionals and involves a checklist of medical issues that will warrant supervision and/or special consideration and management. Collaborations between medical clinicians and fitness professionals is important to ensure adequate management of the pregnant individual.

A thorough functional assessment and evaluation by a skilled fitness professional may include physical therapists, strength and conditioning coaches, and personal trainers that all have experience working with the pregnant and postpartum populations. Functional movements such as moving from supine to side-lying to sitting and sitting to standing may be difficult. Pushing, pulling, reaching, and squatting are an important part of everyday life. Care providers for pregnant individuals need to be able to assess quality of movement and range of motion within functional tasks as listed. A skilled professional can identify when stability exercises are needed, such as with complaints of pelvic girdle pain;

when scaling may be necessary, such as later in pregnancy when they may need to be modified to accommodate the growing abdomen; and also, how to maintain fitness level throughout the pregnancy. Mobility programs such as Spinning Babies may be referred as teamcare.

BIRTH PREPARATION

The birthing process is an amazing one, and preparation for the birthing individual is ideal. Preparation may take a variety of forms, from general childbirth education and the physiologic changes that occur during pregnancy and delivery as well as more targeted birth preparation including breathing, pelvic floor relaxation, hypnotherapy, and other strategies to better manage anxieties and fears, as well as to better prepare families for the process (Odent 2019). Pelvic floor physical therapists, doulas, and midwives are equipped to render education and practical strategies for pregnancy and birth, along with emotional support.

The goal for any pregnancy and delivery is a healthy birthing person and baby(ies), and to that end, focusing on a physiologic birth process is key. Simply put, it is the process of allowing labor to take its natural course without intervention, allowing both the birthing person and baby to partake in the "magical" dance that will ultimately result in the birth of the baby.

Ensuring a healthy pregnancy, minimizing stress, and allowing for appropriate mobility are all things that help moms to be physically equipped and ready to handle the birthing process. Also of importance is ensuring a healthy prenatal environment, including adequate support and low stress, as well as intrapartum or labor support. Encouraging upright positions and general mobility has been shown to decrease labor and need for intervention, decrease cesarean rates, decrease pain, increase patients' overall satisfaction, and increase likelihood of achieving a physiologic birth relative to those who remain semi-recumbent (Ondeck 2019).

A useful resource during this time is a birth doula. While there are several specialties within the spectrum of being a doula, including birth, postpartum, cesarean birth, and even death doulas, a birth doula is an individual, usually a lay person but not necessarily, who supports a birthing person throughout their pregnancy and, more specifically throughout the birthing process, being an advocate and ally to ensure that they will achieve as close to a physiologic birth as possible and in particular that they achieve as close to the birth experience they desire as possible.

Research indicates that in general those who utilized a doula not only had better birth outcomes, but that they were four times less likely to have a low birth weight baby and two times less likely to experience a birth complication involving either themselves or their baby (Gruber, Cupito, and Dobson 2013). An article from Doulas of North America (DONA) International, the leading educator of doulas throughout the world, indicated that having a doula during birth has been shown to reduce the likelihood of a cesarean birth anywhere from 28 percent to 56 percent (www.dona.org). Additionally, those in marginalized communities who tend to be at risk of poor birth outcomes have shown better outcomes as the use of a doula appears to help disrupt "the pervasive influence of social determinants as predisposing factors for health during pregnancy and childbirth" (Kozhimannil et al. 2016).

In consideration of the birthing process, not only does the pregnant person have a job but so does the baby. The baby moves through different postures in utero, and ideally is positioned well for birth. At 32–36 weeks, the baby takes on a "head down" position otherwise known as a cephalic position, where they are positioned with the head down and chin tucked ready to enter into the pelvis and facing the spine. This is an ideal position and also referred to as occiput (back of the baby's head) anterior. At other times, the baby might be positioned head down but facing mom's abdomen and this is referred to as occiput posterior or "sunny-side up." Babies may also be positioned breech or transverse, with the former being where the buttocks are ahead and the latter where the baby is lying across the abdomen. Breech births may proceed spontaneously with good outcomes when moms are able to move in the upright position, as recorded in birth videos (Reitter, Halliday, and Walker 2020), yet there is often a need for assistance in turning a baby (version) and/or cesarean delivery.

As the baby prepares to exit the body, there are a few movements that need to occur. As the baby's head engages in the pelvis, they begin to tuck the head a little more as they continue to descend. The baby then starts to rotate to accommodate the changes of the pelvis as they continue to traverse the pelvis. Once the baby has come to the most distal part of the pelvis, the head extends, and the baby begins to rotate from face down about 90 degrees to allow for clearance of the coccyx, then comes expulsion and out comes the baby! While the baby is performing this marathon style feat, the laboring individual's body is working as well. The pelvis moves to accommodate the baby's movements, first with sacral extension/posterior pelvic tilt to create increased room for the baby's head into the pelvis. Then, as the baby moves down, the sacrum has to flex or move into an anterior pelvic tilt and the coccyx moves out of the way. This is clearly an indication that birth is definitely not a passive act, and everyone has to play their part, parent and baby alike!

Regarding birth preparation, providers need to make sure that the birthing individual is able to make informed decisions—they need all of the information to make the best decisions for themselves and their families. It is imperative, when pregnant individuals are educated, that they not only know about physiologic birth and the uncomplicated birth process but that they also know of options for managing pain. Moms should be educated regarding potential complications and when a cesarean may be necessary. Additionally, education regarding postpartum physiologic changes in pelvic function, sleep disruption, mood changes, and breastfeeding support should be offered.

Our society has trended towards either being pro-epidural or pro-natural birth. For many individuals however, length of labor, pain tolerance, position of the baby, and/or potential labor complications may warrant pain medication being utilized. Pain relief options may include an epidural, intravenous pain medications, or even nitrous oxide gas. It is important that individuals find out from their birth facility what is available (for example, nitrous oxide is not available at all facilities) and from medical providers when the appropriate time would be for those to be administered.

Regarding the need for a cesarean birth, this can range from failure to progress or dilate, to fetal or maternal distress. There are times when cesarean birth is planned, such as conditions where a placental abnormality occurs (placenta accrete). However, there may be times when an individual might find themselves needing an emergency cesarean such as when they experience a prolapsed umbilical cord. In either case, education prior to birth is key, so that these individuals and families are prepared mentally and emotionally, and expectations are set early.

PELVIC FLOOR INJURIES: OASIS INJURIES

Sometimes the best plans may not always go smoothly and there are times when there are injuries that occur as a result of the birthing process. Here we cover some of the aspects of pelvic floor injuries that may occur with birth, such as obstetric anal sphincter injuries (OASIS).

The deep pelvic floor muscles are collectively referred to as the levator ani muscles and are at risk of distension from prolonged labor or even the risk of avulsion/separation (Caudwell-Hall *et al.* 2017). According to this research, disruption of the deepest pelvic muscle group, the levator ani, may occur from the use of forceps, a prolonged second stage, and perineal tearing. OASIS injuries are associated with the pelvic floor disruptions of urinary incontinence, bowel incontinence, pain, and prolapse.

Perineal tearing, also known as perineal lacerations, refers to the tears that occur in the area of the perineum during the delivery process. There are four grades or degrees of tears (Harvey *et al.* 2015), as listed in Table 5.1.

Table 5.1 Perineal injuries with vaginal birth

Grade of injury	Anatomical location of pelvic floor injuries with childbirth	Medical care	Health impact
Grade 1	The skin of the perineum and no other structures (underlying fascia and muscles intact)	Typically not required, self-healing	None, or minimal increased risk for PFD
Grade 2	The perineal muscles, from superficial, to potentially deep perineal muscles of the urogenital triangle	Sutures	Minimal to moderate increased risk for PFD
Grade 3a, 3b, 3c	Tearing of the posterior structures of external anal sphincter complex, with possible internal sphincter injury, as well as the perineal muscles, fascia, and skin	Surgical repair	Moderate to significant increased risk for PFD
Grade 4	Tearing of anal epithelium, external anal sphincter muscle into the rectal mucosa and internal sphincter, as well as the perineal muscles and fascia	Surgical repair	Significant risk for PFD

(Bidwell et al. 2018; Harvey et al. 2015; Meister et al. 2016)

The latter two types of tears often result in fecal incontinence as well as a longer course of healing in the postpartum period, as well as possible surgical repair by a specialist. Some physicians still practice the use of an episiotomy, an intentional cut to the perineum believed to allow for an easier and less complicated delivery as well as decreasing perineal trauma. However, research has repeatedly refuted the necessity of episiotomies stating that they offer no protection to the perineum as previously assumed (Vale de Castro Monteiro *et al.* 2016).

In 2017, a Cochrane review regarding perineal trauma (Aasheim *et al.* 2017) involving data from over 20 clinical research papers with over 15,000 participants was indicative of the following:

1. Warm compresses did not have a clear impact on the incidence of an intact perineum; those who utilized it appeared to have fewer third and fourth degree tears.
2. The incidence of intact perineum was increased in the perineal massage group and there were fewer third or fourth degree tears.

While the above techniques appeared to decrease third and fourth degree tears, there was inconsistency regarding outcomes and there was insufficient evidence to show if other techniques improved outcomes.

BIRTH TRAUMA AND RESILIENCY

Birth trauma and resiliency is of extreme importance. A review and meta-analysis of 59 studies of the prevalence of PTSD during pregnancy and postpartum showed that 4 percent of women develop PTSD after birth (Dikmen-Yildiz, Ayers, and Phillips 2017b). The study also went on to add:

> key vulnerability factors were depression in pregnancy, fear of childbirth, poor health or complications in pregnancy, a history of PTSD, or counselling for pregnancy or birth-related factors. The strongest risk factors during birth were a negative subjective birth experience, having an operative birth (i.e. assisted vaginal or caesarean section), lack of support during birth, and dissociation. (Dikmen-Yildiz, Ayers, and Phillips 2017b)

It should be noted that the outcome of a birth is not determined by the perspective of the clinical professionals but by that of the birthing individual. While most physicians may be of the opinion that a vaginal/non-operative delivery is a successful delivery, for a birthing individual, there is much more to be considered, including how they felt, how they were treated, whether they felt secure, and whether they felt involved or included in decision making processes. Not only do physical considerations need to be made, but emotional safety is of the utmost importance when working with the birthing individual (Boxes 5.11 and 5.12).

In order to truly be resilient, one needs a supportive structure or community. Many birthing individuals are transplants to their respective locations, meaning that they are not originally from that place and relocated for reasons that might have included work, personal choice, or possibly even family. We cannot take for granted that everyone has a supportive network, and it is imperative that as clinicians

and birthing professionals we encourage them to build their network early and to be aware of the resources available to them. Research has shown that women who are deemed resilient typically reported having more social support, increased satisfaction with their health care professionals, less depression, less fear of the childbirth experience, and fewer traumas since birth (Dikmen-Yildiz, Ayers, and Phillips 2017a).

Box 5.11 Perinatal depression 👓

Depression occurs in 25% of women in the perinatal time frame. In clinical evaluation, a two week period during which five of nine symptoms occur is necessary for diagnosis. These symptoms may include loss of energy, lack of interest or pleasure, weight loss, depressed mood, sleep disturbance (insomnia or hypersomnia), agitation or retardation, frequent thoughts of death or suicide, feelings of worthlessness or guilt, and diminished concentration or indecisiveness.

Risk factors for perinatal depression include status as a single mother, unwanted or unplanned pregnancy, general life stress, and social stress as well as domestic violence, lack of social support, and low socioeconomic status. Prior history of miscarriage or still birth is associated with perinatal depression (Stuart-Parrigon and Stuart 2014).

Postpartum depression occurs in 10–15% of women and is distinct from "baby blues" which are categorized as transient, mild symptoms of insomnia, irritability, anxiety, mood lability, and tearfulness. Maternal psychosis, also termed puerperal psychosis, is rare, seen in 1/500 to 1/1000 deliveries, and is associated with maternal suicide and infanticide. Rapid onset of behavior change may be seen in this condition. Hospitalization, medication management, and counseling support are vital (Sharma and Sharma 2012). Providers may use the Edinburgh depression scale to screen individuals in the perinatal time frame. The Edinburgh depression scale has been validated for its psychometric properties to detect women at risk for depressive symptoms, or to detect major depression (Berginck *et al.* 2011).

Box 5.12 Patient case: Martina, ♥
depression awareness and medical care
Martina's tears rolled down her cheeks during her massage therapy to help with back pain. At three months postpartum, the bodyworker Keith noted his client seemed distant and overwhelmed. While normally talkative, she told the therapist things were really hard, the birth had been difficult, and the baby wasn't sleeping. Keith asked if she felt depressed, and she said "maybe, it's all a blur." He asked if she could speak to her husband about this, and she agreed.

When he called her husband, he reported his concern regarding her depression and strongly advised seeing her doctor as soon as possible. In Keith's follow-up phone call to her, she thanked him for saving her life, as she had been severely depressed. She was on medication and had new postpartum family support for the next few months. Keith reflected after the call that he was glad he had trusted his instincts; she had been in serious trouble with depression.

Complementary and alternative medicine (CAM) can have a role in adjunct treatment for perinatal depression. A review of supplements, exercise, massage, acupuncture, and light therapy finds antidepressive benefits in some studies, yet there is not enough current evidence for these CAM approaches as stand-alone therapy, and more research is needed (Deligiannidis and Freeman 2014). Pharmacological, medical, psychological, and social support may all be helpful for depression.

FOURTH TRIMESTER CONSIDERATIONS

Individuals receive "Congratulations!" with a birth. However, a popular cultural saying is that a person's body is supposed to "snap back" or "bounce back" after pregnancy. Ten months of pregnancy does not typically snap back to pre-pregnant appearance and function. Providers can bring increased awareness to the postpartum issues that affect birthing individuals to educate them as to potential concerns and areas for asking for help regarding pelvic health.

The immediate postpartum period is of significant importance. The first 12 weeks after birth is termed the "fourth trimester" as the individual's body is trying to achieve a sense of normalcy and homeostasis after birth. Everything from their pain levels to muscle strength, to function, to pelvic health, sexual health, and hormonal balance is changing at this time. Unfortunately, our society does not typically give too much time or thought to the postpartum period as now the focus has shifted from the pregnant person to the baby—but who cares for the birthing parent? Who has their best interest at heart? Who is there to ensure that proper healing is taking place, that they can get back to moving and doing, that they can perform normal daily activities, have a sex life, and be a parent and, most importantly, that their mental health and stability is prioritized?

Below are a few postpartum considerations that any birthing parents unfortunately will go months or sometimes years without knowing but are common and can impact them significantly.

1. *Incontinence:* Incontinence is the involuntary loss of urine or feces. While fecal incontinence is less common it typically occurs with severe levator ani injuries as well as OASIS injuries. Urinary incontinence is what most women will report and involves the loss of urine, which might occur with activity, the onset of an urge, at nighttime (bedwetting or enuresis), and even with the presence of a prolapse. There is a misconception that an individual who has a cesarean birth can somehow avoid pelvic floor dysfunction. While spontaneous vaginal delivery was associated with urinary incontinence and pelvic organ prolapse (Blomquist *et al.* 2018), cesarean births, although having lower risk, do not exclude an individual from dealing with these issues, especially if there was an attempt at a vaginal delivery prior to the cesarean.

2. *Pelvic organ prolapse (POP):* POP is the descent of the pelvic organs. This condition, like the former, is present more often in cases with levator ani injuries and OASIS injuries. Individuals typically present with any of the following: complaints of heaviness at the perineum or lower abdomen, symptoms that worsen at the end of the day, increased urgency, difficulty initiating a urine stream (and even a bowel movement) as well as incomplete emptying of bowel or bladder, painful intercourse, and the sensation of something falling out of the pelvis.

   There are four grades of prolapse: Grades 1 to 4. Symptoms may include a bulge sensation and possible problems with bladder, bowel, and sexual functioning with a grade 2, symptoms most likely at grade 3, and requiring medical intervention at grades 3 and 4. (See Chapter 8 for more details regarding POP.)

3. *Painful intercourse:* When resuming sex postpartum, some women have pain with the resumption of penetrative intercourse (dyspareunia). However, dyspareunia is an issue that should be addressed by a pelvic health professional. Many women experience symptoms related to perineal trauma or scar tissue, restrictions in tissue including skin and muscle, as well as decreased lubrication. If the birthing individual is breastfeeding it should be noted that estrogen levels decrease with breastfeeding, which can impact vaginal lubrication, leading to a feeling of dryness and discomfort. One simple solution is using a vaginal lubricant to address this issue, as well as the use of positioning, foreplay, and other factors (see Chapter 13).

   Another issue affecting sexual function may be scar tissue from perineal trauma, perineal tearing, episiotomies, prolonged birth, or the dreaded "husband stitch." This is an additional stitch or two that is added when suturing a perineum to ensure that the vaginal opening is "tighter" and yields more pleasure for the husbands/partners. Unfortunately, it has been associated with increased scar tissue in the area, perineal pain, and pain with intercourse, all non-conducive to the husband/partner receiving more sex.

   Besides painful intercourse there is also the reluctance that many birthing individuals feel, specifically cis-gendered females, for penile–vaginal intercourse after having a baby due to fear as well as the insecurities pertaining to the post-birth body. Many individuals decline or avoid intimacy because they feel less confident and positive about their postpartum bodies. Additionally, there is the concept of context and the fact that there is just not enough time for new parents to have sex due to the fatigue, lack of sleep, postpartum mental health, and increased business associated with a new family.

4. *Abdominal or pelvic pain:* This might be due to tissue restrictions or scar tissue as a result of physical trauma due to birth including a prolonged labor. One of the issues that might be responsible for pelvic pain is hemorrhoids as they are characterized by pain, bleeding, itching, and even burning. Hemorrhoids are actually inflamed blood vessels, but they are a true "pain in the butt" for those who have to deal with them. They are also compounded by constipation and straining which can add more pressure and increased irritation. Improved hydration and fiber in the diet as well as proper toileting hygiene including avoiding straining and elevating the feet through a stool can be helpful.

5. *Diastasis rectus abdominis (DRA):* This is a separation of the rectus abdominis (six-pack muscles) that occurs during pregnancy and persists postpartum. In the latter portion of the third trimester some individuals may note a separation of the abdomen, and some may notice "vaulting" at the upper abdomen when excessive stress is placed at these muscles or the region. After birth, DRA may persist. If the abdominal separation above and below the umbilicus (belly button) is greater than two finger widths, then the individual would be considered as having a DRA (see Chapter 6).

The above-mentioned issues tend to be the most commonly reported ones and many women go for quite some time without resolution. A team of providers can help support health in the postpartum journey, and direct care for perineal injuries, scar tissue, and pelvic floor dysfunction is the provision of optimum care.

EXERCISING WHILE PREGNANT AND POSTPARTUM

Exercise postpartum is a "hot topic" for many, but the focus should be the safe return to activity. Many persons feel great, without pain or symptoms, yet when they attempt exercise along comes the leaking, the prolapse, and the pain.

Of utmost importance is working with a fitness professional who understands the pregnant and postpartum body, is familiar with working with postpartum clients, and understands how to scale and appropriately address quality of movement (Table 5.2). Also of importance is knowledge of a client's history of exercise, injuries, and desired fitness goals (Boxes 5.13 and 5.14).

Table 5.2 Postpartum fitness considerations

Exercise item	Example	Example
Load	Body weight or weight lifted	Half squat with 10 lb dumbbell
Tempo	Speed of motion and holding time	Squat in 5 seconds, hold 5, up 5
Volume	Repetitions, sets	15 squats x 2 sets
Time	Time for reps and sets	15 squats x 2 sets in 3 minutes
Range	Motion excursion	Chair squat vs full squat
Stability/ mobility	Stability to mobility to compound exercise	Single leg squat to lunge to jump and hop

(Lo 2020)

Box 5.13 Patient case: Renee ♥

Renee was a mom seen at 9 months postpartum; she attempted running but noticed urinary leaking (incontinence) and was referred to pelvic floor physical therapy (PT). Her PT evaluation included movement assessment, external pelvic assessment, and internal myofascial assessment. She was found to have pelvic floor muscle weakness, coordination limitations, as well as general lower extremity weakness.

A program was outlined including increasing pelvic floor awareness and pelvic floor strengthening in a variety of positions including sitting, standing, and other functional positions (see Chapter 9 regarding awareness/strengthening for urinary incontinence (UI)). Additionally, she was trained in posterior chain (glutes, hamstrings, hip) strengthening along with gradual pre-run drills, a variation of speed and time with exercises before progressing to running. The program produced goal attainment of running without leakage. This mom ended up running her fastest mile time and was on track to run her first 5k, which she completed a month after concluding therapy and was able to do so under 30 minutes.

Postpartum fitness demonstration weightlifting (Figures 5.15–5.19):

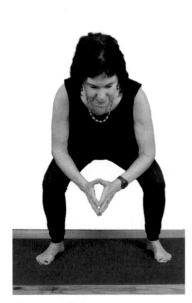

Figure 5.15 Squat.

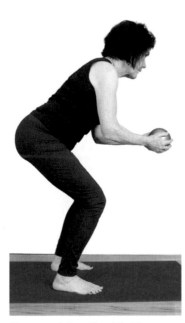

Figure 5.16 Standing hip hinge squat with rows.

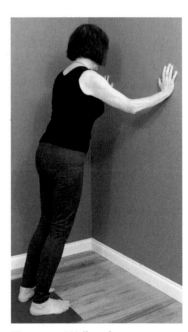

Figure 5.17 Wall push-up.

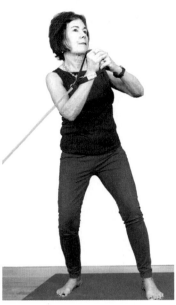
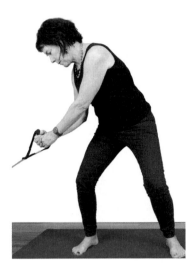

Figure 5.18 Resisted trunk rotations.

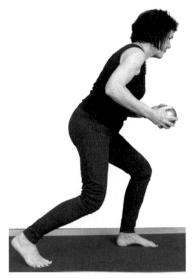

Figure 5.19 Lunges.

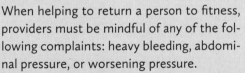

Box 5.14 Exercise contraindications

When helping to return a person to fitness, providers must be mindful of any of the following complaints: heavy bleeding, abdominal pressure, or worsening pressure.

Any complaint of pain with activity and any complaint of something "falling out" of the vagina, or any visible protrusions or leaking of urine or feces—these symptoms should be screened by a health care provider.

Pregnancy, the birth process, and the postpartum fourth trimester experience are unique to each individual. Care providers and health and fitness professionals can provide resources, training, and intervention as needed at each stage. Ideally, individuals have a healthy social and medical community for support along the journey.

Education regarding perinatal health conditions is lacking and many postpartum moms may be in part traumatized by unexpected bodily changes that persist after birth. Disparities exist regarding access to care, with preventable infant and maternal morbidity and mortality. Local and global needs can be met by care providers and governments working together to provide access to care and resources to support birth and postpartum health. Doulas and midwives can play a vital support role in each stage.

Consideration of resiliency, and coaching resiliency with support for the entire somato-emotional, physical, and spiritual aspects of pregnancy, can support pregnant, birthing, and postpartum moms throughout their journey. Movement therapy and bodywork can be wonderful conservative care and holistic options for health and wellness.

REFERENCES

23andme (2021) "Haplogroups Explained." Accessed 11/6/2021 at https://blog.23andme.com/ancestry-reports/haplogroups-explained.

Aasheim, V., Vika Nilsen, A. B., Reinar, L. M., and Lukasse, M. (2017) "Perineal techniques during the second stage of labour for reducing perineal trauma." *Cochrane Database System Review, 6* 6, CD006672.

Bahrami, M. H., Rayegani, S. M., Fereidouni, M., and Baghbani, M. (2005) "Prevalence and severity of carpal tunnel syndrome (CTS) during pregnancy." *Electromyography and Clinical Neurophysiology 45*, 2, 123-125.

Bergink, V., Kooistra, L., van den Berg, L., Wojnene, H., *et al.* (2011) "Validation of the Edinburgh depression scale during pregnancy." *Journal of Psychosomatic Research 70*, 385-389.

Bidwell, P., Thaker, R., Sevdalis, N., Silverton, L., *et al.* (2018) "A multi-centre quality improvement project to reduce the incidence of obstetric anal sphincter injury (OASI): Study protocol." *BMC Pregnancy and Childbirth 18*, 1, 331.

Blomquist, J. L., Munoz, A., Carroll, M., *et al.* (2018) "Association of delivery mode with pelvic floor disorders after childbirth." *JAMA Network 320*, 23, 2438-2447.

Buhrer, M. (2016) "The cycle of socioeconomic oppression of marginalized communities through poor access to reproductive health services." www.lonestar.edu.

Burch, J. (2003) "Visceral manipulation: A powerful new frontier in bodywork." *Massage Therapy Journal.*

Cantu, R. I. and Grodin, A. J. (2001) *Myofascial Manipulation.* Gaithersburg, MD: Aspen Publishers.

Caudwell-Hall, J., Atan, I. K., Martin, A., Rojas, R. G., *et al.* (2017) "Intrapartum predictors of maternal levator ani injury." *Acta Obstetricia Gynecologica Scandinavica 96*, 44, 426-443.

Deligiannidis, K. M. and Freeman, M. P. (2014) "Complementary and alternative therapies for perinatal depression." *Best Practice & Research Clinical Obstetrics & Gynaecology 28*, 1, 85-95.

Dikmen-Yildiz, P., Ayers, S., and Phillips, L. (2017a) "Depression, anxiety, PTSD, and comorbidity in perinatal women in Turkey: A longitudinal population-based study." *Midwifery 55*, 29-37.

Dikmen-Yildiz, P., Ayers, S., and Phillips, L. (2017b) "The prevalence of posttraumatic stress disorder in pregnancy and after birth: A systematic review and meta-analysis." *Journal of Affective Disorders 208*, 634-645.

Duley, L. (2009) "The global impact of pre-eclampsia and eclampsia." *Seminars in Perinatology 33*, 3, 130-137.

Ferraz, Z., Parra, J., Areia, A. L., Vasco, E., and Moura, P. (2017) "Acute onset neurological disorders during pregnancy: A literature review." *Revista Brasileira De Ginecologia E Obstetrícia 39*, 10, 560-568.

Gruber, K. J., Cupito, S. H., and Dobson, C. F. (2013) "Impact of doulas on healthy birth outcomes." *Journal of Perinatal Education 22*, 1, 49-58.

Harvey, M.-A., Pierce, M., Walter, J.-E., Chou, Q., *et al.* (2015) "Obstetrical anal sphincter injuries (OASIS) and

repair." *Journal of Obstetrics and Gynaecology Canada 37*, 12, 1131-1148.

Howell, E. A., Egorova, N. N., Balbierz, A., Zeitlin, J., and Hebert, P. L. (2016) "Site of delivery contribution to Black-white severe maternal morbidity disparity." *American Journal of Obstetric Gynecology 215*, 2, 143-152.

Jukic, A. M., Baird, D. D., Weinberg, C. R., McConnaughey, D. R., and Wilcox, A. J. (2013) "Length of human pregnancy and contributors to its natural variation." *Human Reproduction 28*, 10, 2848-2855.

Kozhimannil, K. B., Vogelsang, C. A., Hardeman, R. R., and Prasad, S. (2016) "Disrupting the pathways of social determinants of health: Doula support during pregnancy and childbirth." *Journal of American Board of Family Medicine 29*, 3, 308-317.

Lo, A. (2020) "The female athlete seminar." Accessed 6/7/2022 at https://physiodetective.com/courses/female-athlete-tfa.

Meister, R. L., Cahill, A. G., Conner, S. N., Woolfolk, C. L., and Lowder, J. L. (2016) "Predicting obstetric anal sphincter injuries in a modern obstetric population." *American Journal of Obstetrics and Gynecology 215*, 3, P310.E1-310.E7.

Mongelli, M., Wilcox, M., and Gardosi, J. (1996) "Estimating the date of confinement: Ultrasonographic biometry versus certain menstrual dates." *American Journal of Obstetrics and Gynecology 174*, 1, 278-281.

Mota, P., Pascoal, A. G., Vaz João, C. F., Veloso, A., and Bø, K. (2018) "Diastasis recti during pregnancy and postpartum." In S. Brandão, T. Da Roza, I. Ramos, and T. Mascarenhas (eds) *Women's Health and Biomechanics: Where Medicine and Engineering Meet.* Cham: Springer International Publishing.

Odent, M. (2019) "Physiological birth preparation." *Journal of Prenatal and Perinatal Psychological Health 33*, 3, 183.

Ondeck, M. (2019) "Healthy birth practice #2: Walk, move around, and change positions throughout labor." *Journal of Perinatal Education 28*, 2, 81-87.

Owens, D. C. and Fett, S. M. (2019) "Black maternal and infant health: Historical legacies of slavery." *American Journal of Public Health 109*, 10, 1342-1345.

Perales, M., Artal, R., and Lucia, A. (2017) "Exercise during pregnancy." *Journal of the American Medical Association 317*, 11, 1113-1114.

Poyatos-León, R., García-Hermoso, A., Sanabria-Martínez, G., Alvarez-Bueno, C., *et al.* (2015) "Effects of exercise during pregnancy on mode of delivery: A meta-analysis." *Acta Obstetricia et Gynecologica Scandinavica 94*, 10, 1039-1047.

Reitter, A., Halliday, A., and Walker, S. (2020) "Practical insight into upright breech birth from birth videos: A structured analysis." *Birth 47*, 2, 211-219.

Rizzardo, R., Magni, G., Andreoli, C., Merlin, G., *et al.* (1985) "Psychosocial aspects during pregnancy and obstetrical complications." *Journal of Psychosomatic Obstetrics & Gynecology 4*, 1, 11-22.

Sharma, V. and Sharma, P. (2012) "Postpartum depression: Diagnostic and treatment issues." *Journal of Obstetrics and Gynaecology Canada 34*, 5, 436–442.

Stuart-Parrigon, K. and Stuart, S. (2014) "Perinatal depression; an update and overview." *Current Psychiatry Reports 16*, 9, 468.

Vale de Castro Monteiro, M., Pereira, G. M. V., Aguiar, R. A. P., Azevedo, R. L., Correia-Junior, M. D., and Reis, Z. S. N. (2016) "Risk factors for severe obstetric perineal lacerations." *International Urogynecology Journal 27*, 1, 61–67.

Wetzler, G. (2010) "Visceral and obstetric physical therapy." Combined sections meeting, American Physical Therapy Association.

FURTHER RESOURCES

Centers for Disease Control and Prevention (2022) Healthy Pregnant or Postpartum Women. Accessed 6/17/2022 at www.cdc.gov/physicalactivity/basics/pregnancy/index.htm.

Edinburgh Postnatal Depression Scale (EPDS) (2022) Perinatal Services BC. Accessed 6/17/2022 at www.perinatalservicesbc.ca/health-professionals/professional-resources/health-promo/edinburgh-postnatal-depression-scale-(epds).

Hoyert, D. L. (2022) *Maternal Mortality Rates in the United States, 2020*. NCHS Health E-Stats. Accessed 6/17/2022 at www.cdc.gov/nchs/data/hestat/maternal-mortality/2020/maternal-mortality-rates-2020.htm.

Preeclampsia and Eclampsia (2022) National Institute of Child Health and Human Development. Accessed 6/17/2022 at www.nichd.nih.gov/health/topics/preeclampsia.

Spinning Babies: www.spinningbabies.com

CHAPTER 6

Diastasis Rectus Abdominis

Help, What Happened to My Abdominals?

This chapter presents diastasis rectus abdominis (DRA), the abdominal myofascial condition that is often ignored by health care providers in the perinatal time. Anatomical details, risk factors, potential co-morbidities, and expert evaluation and treatment techniques will be profiled.

Expert sequencing formats for DRA and associated core muscle groups, the transverse abdominis (TRA), pelvic floor muscles (PFM), and spinal multifidi, are presented. Integrated core concepts of motor control were introduced in earlier chapters, and therapeutic program guidelines follow through into subsequent chapters. Pelvic girdle pain, pelvic organ prolapse, urinary incontinence, fecal incontinence, and overall stability and mobility are intimately influenced by core control. The deep abdominal core myofascial structure of the transverse abdominis is the primary focus of this chapter.

DRA

DRA is a thinning and separation of the linea alba, the midline fascial structure that is the insertion site of all of the abdominal muscles. This may or may not cause a protrusion of the abdominal wall.

DRA at six months postpartum (Mota *et al.* 2015). While focused on the perinatal time, DRA may also occur in males, and non-birthing females. In males, it may be associated with increased risk for abdominal aortic aneurysm (De'Ath *et al.* 2010).

Incidence

DRA is a perplexing problem for many individuals, primarily pregnant and postpartum women, occurring in 33–100 percent of women (Axer, Keyserlingk, and Prescher 2001; Boisannault and Blaschak 1988; Mota *et al.* 2015; Spersted *et al.* 2016) (Box 6.1). There is a natural resolution of DRA in the postpartum time in some individuals, with a finding of only 39 percent displaying

> **Box 6.1 Nulliparas and primiparas**
>
> In a survey of 150 nulliparous (never pregnant) women, Beer *et al.* (2009) concluded that a normal finding was that a separation in the linea alba may be 22 mm wide at 3 cm above the umbilicus and 16 mm wide at 2 cm

below the umbilicus. Therefore, a small separation is considered as normal in nulliparas.

For women experiencing their first birth (primiparas), 100% exhibited DRA in the last trimester. At six months postpartum, only 39% displayed a DRA (Mota *et al.* 2015).

Anatomy

The abdominal wall muscles include the rectus abdominis, the internal and external oblique muscles, and the transverse abdominis (TRA). The TRA forms the deepest fascial connection into the linea alba. The TRA is formed from lateral bands of the latissimus dorsi and fascia that connect the sides of the trunk with the anterior myofascial structures.

The deepest abdominal myofascial structures, such as the TRA, are all linked to structures above (diaphragm), the sides (quadratus lumborum and latissimus), into the spine (thoracodorsal fascia, multifidus), and the pelvic floor below. The abdominal wall needs to work in symphony with the pelvis, spinal muscles, and the limbs for agility, power, and stability at rest.

The linea alba extends from the xiphoid process to the pubic symphysis and may be viewed as a central zipper. The thinning and separation during pregnancy most often occurs near the umbilicus yet may extend from the xiphoid to the pubic symphysis (Boissonault and Blaschak 1988). Small to large separations may occur in the linea alba, from less than 1 cm wide, up to several centimeters or more in width (Figure 6.1). Along with the DRA, the entire rib cage may be flared up and outwards, with an increased "infrasternal angle" from 90 degrees to over 100 degrees or even 120 degrees or more (Figure 6.2).

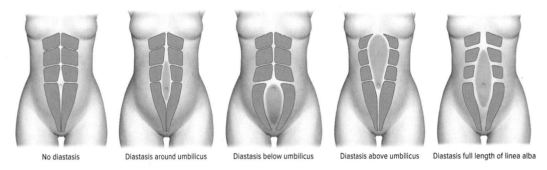

| No diastasis | Diastasis around umbilicus | Diastasis below umbilicus | Diastasis above umbilicus | Diastasis full length of linea alba |

Figure 6.1 DRA variations: Normal, 2 cm. Small lower gap, 3 cm infraumbilical. Medium upper gap, 4.5 cm xiphoid to umbilical. Large gap, 8 cm xiphoid to pubic symphysis.

Along with the DRA, the entire rib cage may be flared up and outwards, with an increased "infrasternal angle" from 90 degrees to over 100 degrees or even 120 degrees or more. This represents a lengthened external oblique muscle group (Spitznagle 2010) (Boxes 6.2–6.4). The infrasternal angle should narrow with exhalation and widen with inhalation, but not stay at a widened position with exertion or at rest.

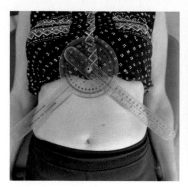
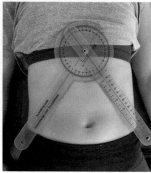

Figure 6.2 Infrasternal angle: Small flare in a multipara, 100 degrees (L);
Narrowed angle in a nullipara, 70 degrees (R).

Box 6.2 Recognize and respond to the emotional state

A woman may be experiencing a sense of loss in relation to perinatal fitness limitations, and abdominal contour changes that can occur with DRA. Providers may allay fear and worry by stating, "You have a separation in your abdominals that is common postpartum, and we will provide manual therapy, exercise, bracing or taping options, and habit training that can help the abdominals become stronger." This statement will identify the condition as common and provide information about treatment that is reassuring.

Box 6.3 Jessica's story: the belly bulge with DRA

Several months postpartum with her second baby at age 37, Jessica was having mid and low back pain as well as pelvic pain. She felt weak, and she was tested by a physical therapist (PT) and found to have a four-finger-width DRA (more information on this follows). The therapist found a large gap at her umbilicus, as well as a few inches above and below. Jessica reported she felt a sense of shock finding out that her abdominals had a separation! She felt vulnerable with the large gap in her rectus abdominis muscle.

She received minimal instruction from the therapist on what exercise to do, as the therapist admitted she did not know what protocols were best. Jessica researched this diagnosis and its protocols with minimal success. She strained her neck with a head lift exercise, and she still looked pregnant. She suffered embarrassment over her contour when changing at the gym. Her treatment that was successful follows.

Box 6.4 Co-morbidities

Co-morbidities that women's health specialists report as associated with DRA include low back pain, 80.7%, pelvic pain, 59.5%, and urinary incontinence at 59.4% (Keeler et al. 2012; Parker, Miller, and Dugan 2009). Spitznagle, Leong, and Van Dillen (2007) found DRA existing as a co-morbidity in 52% of older women presenting to a uro-gynecology clinic with signs of pelvic floor dysfunction including urinary incontinence, fecal incontinence, and pelvic organ prolapse (POP). Co-morbidities, other medical conditions that may occur with DRA, are the subject of research with Bø et al. (2015) finding that at six months postpartum younger women (average 28.7 years) had no associated pelvic organ prolapse, urinary incontinence, or differences in pelvic floor muscle (PFM) strength compared to those without DRA. Based on conflicting evidence from different studies, it is clear that more research is needed regarding potential co-morbidities and DRA (Sperstad *et al.* 2016).

Risk factors

The primary risk factor for DRA is pregnancy. Other risk factors include:

- older maternal age
- Asian or European ethnicity
- inconsistent exercise
- incorrect abdominal and/or weightlifting programs
- abdominal surgery
- multiparity
- obesity.

(Beer et al. 2009; Chiarello, Zellers, and Sage-King 2012; Liaw et al. 2011; Spitznagle, Leong, and Van Dillen 2007)

EVALUATION OF DRA, OVERVIEW

Listed below are the considerations that can help target treatment.

- Is there a DRA, and if so, how wide, and how deep? This is the "gap."
- Can they generate tension with the left and right sides of the gap with a head lift or curl up attempt?
- Does this DRA affect overall trunk control with limitations in movement and performance, and pain?
- Has an individual lost functional fitness power with activities of daily living and recreational functions?
- Are they in a state of postpartum trauma, feeling broken and without a guide for healing?
- How is the individual presenting with DRA breathing? Is the rib cage rigid, or mobile, are the ribs flared up and out from pregnancy?
- How is the entire lumbopelvic core performing?

Visual screening: A bulge or doming?

The first method to assess the abdominal wall is a simple visual screening technique for DRA with regards to the observed contour of the abdomen at rest and during a supine position head lift. With movement, a bulge may be observed near the umbilicus, or a doming or distension outward in a larger round or oval separation in the abdomen.

Digital palpation

A digital palpation test checks for the separation of the linea alba in supine to start.

The digital screening test with palpation starts in supine, with the "examiner" using two fingers to palpate for a separation of the linea alba (Figure 6.3). Gently pressing inwards one-half to one inch at the umbilicus, the head and trunk should be lifted with arms stretched towards knees, clearing the scapular spine (Figure 6.4). The examiner's palpating fingers will feel the lateral bands of the linea alba come together with midline or not. Fingertip palpation may suffice for screening (Keeler *et al.* 2012) (Box 6.5). More fingers may be added to grossly assess the width of the DRA of two, three, four, or more fingertips.

> Box 6.5 Measuring DRA
> Medical examiners may use palpation of the linea alba to assess the inter-recti distance (IRD) separation at the umbilicus, and 4.5 cm

above and 4.5 cm below the umbilicus. Further measures above and below may be taken if a significant gap over 2.5 cm is found. Measurements may also be taken with a tape measure or real time ultrasound (RUSI) (Bø *et al.* 2015; Lee, Lee, and McLaughlin 2008) (Box 6.6). However, these measurements do not indicate overall function or performance potential.

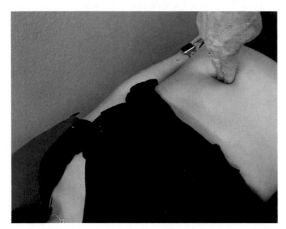

Figure 6.3 Palpation of linea alba at rest. Two fingers palpation at umbilicus.

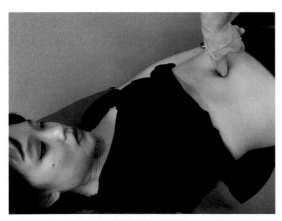

Figure 6.4 Palpation of linea alba with a curl up, lifting the head up and shoulder blades off the mat.

Box 6.6 RUSI: accurate   ᴼᴼ
RUSI screening is the most accurate clinical standard for measurement of the gap, and

its highest reliability is in assessment above the umbilicus (Benjamen, Van de Water, and Peiris 2016; Mota *et al.* 2015; Van de Water and Benjamen 2016) (Figure 6.5). RUSI is also used to monitor muscle appearance, mobility, and timing in movement. However, the expense of the equipment makes it prohibitive for many clinics, so the fingertip screening is often used to assess the gap. Specialty medical training seminars train health care professionals in the utilization of RUSI equipment.

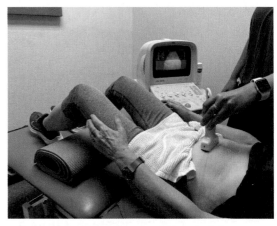

Figure 6.5 Real time ultrasound (RUSI) of the linea alba and the inter-recti distance (IRD) during a curl up. Lateral abdominal placements of the soundhead are also used to identify oblique and transverse abdominus function.

Research studies have focused on measuring changes in the gap, with closing the gap as the "holy grail" in a definition of treatment success. However, "closing the gap" is not needed for full function, and may not correlate with stability, nor fitness power. Functional testing should be done regarding multiplanar exertion. Assessment of how the entire spine, trunk, and abdomen work together for exertion is crucial in considering the client's key functional goals. (Lifting toddlers can be very demanding, for one thing, and they only become heavier over time.)

DRA INTERVENTIONS: EXERCISE, SUPPORT GARMENTS, AND TAPING

Therapeutic exercise

Therapeutic exercise is the optimum foundation for treatment. The underlying physiology in DRA treatments is to stimulate collagen synthesis and strengthen the entire core. Multiple exercise protocols can produce positive results with improved lumbar, pelvic, hip, and abdominal muscle control. There is not one sole exercise format to correct DRA, and while early research focused on measuring and closing the inter-recti distance (IRD), current research (Lee and Hodges 2016) and clinical expert consensus (Lee and Hodges 2019) considers the combined function of the abdominals and overall function in terms of generating tension in the myofascial trunk and abdominal structures.

Understanding core integrated motion control

TRANSVERSE ABDOMINIS: FUNCTIONAL CONTROL

Transverse abdominis (TRA) functions to generate tension in the bands of the rectus abdominis and provide a firm anchor for the abdominals to contract. The fibers of TRA pull laterally and firm the midline fascia. TRA works with the rectus abdominis, internal and external obliques, diaphragm, spinal multifidus, and the pelvic floor muscles to provide lumbopelvic stability. These interconnected myofascial groups provide stiffness for postural support in weight bearing, load transfers (lifting, pushing, pulling, and carrying), and movement control. These muscle groups also work together to display control in lengthening, elongating activities for human function.

Studies of TRA in relation to its synchrony with the multifidus and pelvic floor muscles (PFM), and during intra-abdominal pressure, clarify its role (Junginger *et al.* 2010). The TRA pre-sets and contracts before and during activity (Sapsford and Hodges 2001), and it works in synchrony with the PFM. The TRA can be viewed as critical to the support of the abdominal and trunk as a "closed canister" (Lee and Lee 2011). Expert functional analysis may also discern if the upper, middle, or lower abdominal muscle group is firing for force closure, or where deficiencies occur (Lee and Hodges 2019).

TRA should be trained clinically with the PFM and deep spinal muscles, the multifidus (Badillo *et al.* 2012; Hampton and Rader 2018). Exercise programs should screen for and train progressive tasks with abdominal, trunk, and other muscles (Hodges, Sapsford, and Pengel 2007; Lee and Lee 2011). Clients may seek a closure of the gap, and an overall toning with a focus on appearance (Box 6.7). However, addressing activities of daily living (ADL) and fitness limitations (such as pain and weakness in lifting a child) can provide a platform for overall fitness training that is task specific and progressive.

> ## Box 6.7 Varied core exercises help DRA
>
> A systematic review of exercise for DRA found exercises targeting the abdominals and core demonstrated a 35% reduction in incidence of DRA (Benjamen *et al.* 2014). Traditional strength training exercises such as planks and curl ups can produce beneficial changes in abdominal strength and improved disability scores in comparison to a supine program (Walton *et al.* 2016).

Binders, belts, and corsets

Binders and belts may help approximate the separated bundles of the recti and provide a sense of safety and stability to moms (Figure 6.6). The spinal muscles and sacroiliac (SI) joint rely on the stiffening effect of abdominal bracing for stability and motion, and a binder may help support the spine and SI by a relative stiffening effect. Women's health therapists' consensus favors the use of an adjustable binder (Keeler *et al.* 2012; Schulte *et al.* 2019) (Box 6.8).

The use of exercise, posture, and body mechanics, and an abdominal support garment in a woman with a large DRA, demonstrated closure from 11.5 cm to 2.0 cm at the umbilicus (Litos 2014, 2019).

Therapists must consider that binding the abdomen too tightly may cause a downward pressure on the pelvic organs and create or aggravate pelvic organ prolapse. To optimize intra-abdominal pressure with a binder, styles with upper and lower support bands may be used rather than full coverage binding.

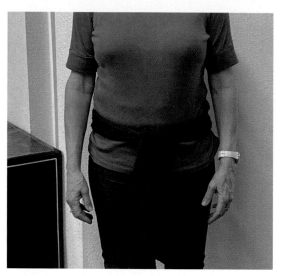

Figure 6.7 Scarf wrap binder.

Taping

Kinesio® Tape may be beneficial for some individuals in providing a sense of support and proprioception (Box 6.9). However, clinical techniques of application vary, and compliance may also vary, due to client preference, comfort, and skin irritation.

Tape may be applied in a letter X fashion above and below the umbilicus (Figure 6.8). A simpler tape application may utilize two transverse bands.

Box 6.8 A simple scarf may help support 🦋

A scarf wrapped around the abdomen with pressure where needed may feel great and increase core power (Figure 6.7). A long scarf may simply appear as a fashion statement, and it can easily be tightened or loosened for comfort throughout the day. This may be comforting and soothing in the perinatal time.

Here are examples of abdominal binders:

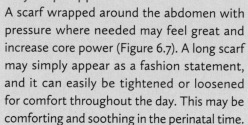

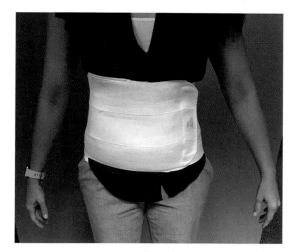

Figure 6.6 Basic abdominal binder.

Box 6.9 Tape and exercise 👓

A pilot study by Tuttle *et al.* (2018) used Kinesio® Tape and exercise in one of the protocols. Targeted TRA exercise and use of Kinesio® Tape were performed at six weeks up to three months postpartum. TRA was trained in the supine, side-lying, quadruped, and sitting position. Ten repetitions of a light TRA contraction were performed in each position, 3–4 x a week. (Subjects were trained to initially vocalize "haa" or "shh" while lightly drawing in navel towards spine, to hold neutral spine, and not hollow or overexert other muscles, or bulge-distend.)

A reduced inter-recti difference (IRD) was most significant in the taping group that also performed exercise (1.31 +– 0.20 mm change). This study represents a possible first step in DRA rehabilitation exercise, which would then be expanded into multiple other exercise formats.

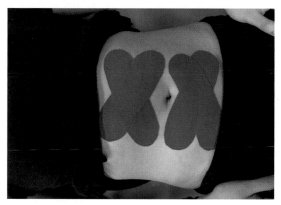

Figure 6.8 Kinesio® Tape TRA.

Hypopressive exercise

The abdominal-hypopressive technique (AHT), also known as "hypopressive exercise," is a format that is used primarily in Europe for DRA (Box 6.10). It is thought to activate primarily TRA, as well as utilize fascial connections from the pelvis and abdomen into the diaphragm. The technique involves respiratory control sequencing: a controlled inhale and a full exhale followed by a further drawing in of the abdominal wall. Pelvic floor muscles may be cued during hypopressive exercise (Stupp *et al.* 2011), and changes in the IRD have been observed (Gomez *et al.* 2018).

Hypopressive training sequences postures with respiratory techniques and muscle recruitment. It is a complex exercise format that requires a skilled instructor and progression into many postures (Nicole 2018). Instruction may include:

- assuming a posture that braces the spine and upper extremities, with an elongation through the spine

- next, an inhalation with TRA and external obliques engaged
- followed by a full exhalation, followed by an apnea (breath hold) technique drawing in the abdomen, requiring a closed glottis.

Box 6.10 AHT performance: progressive training

The AHT may be likened to the Ujaii breath in yoga, followed by a further full exhale and then a sucking up and in of the abdominals but with the glottis closed. One may sense the pelvic floor lift and an energetic "rush" as the abdominals and diaphragm lift up and in. However, clients often require several sessions to train the coordination of muscle groups with respiratory control.

Surgery for DRA

Surgery is rarely needed for DRA, yet it is an option, albeit with surgical risk factors (Box 6.11). A case report describes a successful surgery that was performed due to postpartum functional weakness, and lack of fitness performance benefit from a limited PT intervention of four months. (Surgical repair is typically delayed for at least a year postpartum.) In this study, despite a partial closure of the diastasis (6.52 cm to 3.58 cm), the individual had an inability to perform adequately for fitness testing (curl up and other testing) and full work function for her military career. She received an abdominoplasty with no reported complications, which allowed her to return to full function. Post recti repair she wore an abdominal binder for four weeks, returned to active duty at 21 days, and received ongoing PT for an additional six months (Gallus, Goldberg, and Field 2016).

Box 6.11 DRA surgery: cosmetic or medical?

In the United States, most insurance coverage denies surgery for DRA, considering the surgery cosmetic (Rosen *et al.* 2019). The authors report that the insurers do not understand "the necessity of abdominoplasty to relieve symptoms of patients with severe debilitation." Therapist and educator Diane Lee has devoted a book to the clinical decision making regarding the factors to consider and when it is likely indicated that surgery is required (Lee 2017).

SURGICAL COMPLICATIONS

Risk factors and complications from surgical intervention for DRA are high. A comprehensive review by Hickey, Finch, and Khanna (2011) indicated surgical complications from diastasis repair are as high as 40 percent including skin necrosis and wound dehiscence, infections, postoperative pain and nerve damage, and diastasis recurrence. The most common complication is the development of a seroma. The review concluded that surgical corrections are primarily cosmetic, and that diastasis does not carry a risk of progression to herniation. More research is needed to clarify the best surgical techniques.

Manual therapy for DRA

Manual therapy facilitation techniques are useful to help clients activate muscles and improve performance. Manual facilitation techniques may consist of touch or pressure on a muscle group, or tapping, or assisting pressure into a joint. For example, a hand over the abdomen while a client is in quadruped with a lax abdomen may be cued to "draw in or lift" to help engage the muscle group (Box 6.12).

Direct myofascial work to the trunk may also help to "remodel" the myofascial trunk, and apparently reduce a "gap" in one session as screened via RUSI. This technique was discussed in an expert webinar (Schulte *et al.* 2019) yet has not been researched.

Box 6.12 Remodeling the myofascial trunk

Consider the overall body pattern of an individual, what is displayed by their posture? Consider if they are "gripping" with their back, too rigid, and tend to favor spinal extension. Is there spasm and guarding in the multifidus and other muscles? Manual therapy providing a sweeping forward into ease for the abdominals may assist abdominal wall activation and lessen a "gap." Consider a shirt pulled too tight in the back, which may tug at the front.

Decisions in abdominal/core training

There are two seemingly opposite concepts in core training pertinent to DRA and core rehabilitation. One program emphasizes drawing in and firming the abdominals. The second concept emphasizes generating intra-abdominal pressure, which may cause distension outward in the abdomen.

Classic rehabilitation programs train a light abdominal muscle engagement, a drawing-in maneuver, and holding a firm, but not bulging or doming, abdominal wall. In optimal function, the navel lifts upwards and inwards slightly, in coordination with the diaphragm.

Programs may emphasize generating intra-abdominal pressure with the abdominal tensioning while a slight abdominal and trunk muscle distension occurs. Performing an eccentric abdominal wall activation with abdominal "bracing" and generating intra-abdominal pressure may be facilitated by first drawing in, and then second, firming, or a sense of swelling and fullness in the trunk. Generating pressure into the abdomen with a slight lengthening and firming of the muscles typically is a more complex maneuver, while not significantly distending or bulging outwards.

These concepts need to be considered for each client as to what allows optimum performance and function. Muscles need to contract, to shorten, which is a concentric contraction. Yet muscles also need to lengthen with control, which is eccentric muscle work. Concentric and eccentric muscle work is an interplay of the coordinated diaphragms in the body: the vocal, respiratory, and pelvic. Both techniques may be beneficial.

Training for DRA ideally addresses inner and outer core integration (Dufour *et al.* 2019). Inner unit core is listed in "initial" sequencing in Table 6.1 below. Outer units of the trunk and limbs are engaged in quadruped alternate extremity raises and functional activity training, lifting, pushing, pulling, and carrying exercises (Box 6.13). Individualized programs can promote a functional return of activities of daily living, fitness, and recreation.

DIFFICULTIES WITH CORE TRAINING

Overexertion patterns and incorrect effort during attempted abdominal/core recruitment may display any combination of the following:

- a tendency to spinal flexion, with either the head pulling down or tail tucking under or both occurring
- a hollowing of the obliques at the anterior superior abdomen
- an excessive outward bulging with distension of the lower and mid abdomen
- the umbilicus may lower and distend, along with an undesirable bulge or doming
- breath-holding during abdominal recruitment and generating pressure may cause a rise in intra-abdominal pressure which creates undesired symptoms such as pain, urinary incontinence, and/or prolapse aggravation.

> **Box 6.13 TRA attempt and** **pressure downwards**
> Bø, Sherburn, and Allen (2003) found 30% of subjects caused a descent of the pelvic floor region while attempting an abdominal drawing-in maneuver.

COORDINATION OF MUSCLE GROUPS: WHERE TO START?

What muscles are not firing during stability tests? There may be substitution patterns as listed above. Clients need to be assessed during static holds and mobility, as in the rehabilitation schools and developmental sequencing listed in Chapter 3, as well as in a client's functional performance goals.

The following are initial sequencing options in core training, with coordinated respiratory and intra-abdominal pressure regulation. This is not a cookbook, but rather considers how to begin with a client sensing, identifying, and activating a specific muscle group. Subsequently, the client learns co-contraction with other muscle groups and works with successive challenges for stability and mobility control.

MULTIFIDUS AND TRA EXERCISE

Holding "neutral spine" during exercise should be trained, and many clients tend towards spinal flexion or extension postures. The multifidus is recognized as the spinal core and it controls holding static postures and exertion, as well as multiplanar motion. Ideally the multifidus fires along with the TRA and PFM.

Starting a program with anterior–posterior pelvic tilting, and finding the midpoint or neutral between the two, is often the easiest format to train the multifidus. Clients that excessively tilt the pelvis anteriorly may benefit from initial cuing to engage a slight posterior tilt, in order to engage the abdominal muscles with mat exercises. Or those that tuck under excessively to "lift the tail" a little and "poke the booty out" a little.

SEQUENCING EXERCISE FORMATS

Clinical experience shows that once some clients recruit the PFM, they are then unable to engage the TRA. A current women's health review reinforces the critical interplay of the PFM and TRA (Werner and Dayan 2019) (Box 6.14).

Logical exercise sequencing may be initiated by first addressing the weakest link, such as the PFM, and then adding co-contractions and functional training as tolerated. Multiple positions may be tried to assess the weakest link, and activate that muscle group, and then add co-contractions (Table 6.1).

Box 6.14 Expert therapy: provider study

For bodyworkers, movement therapists and health care providers offering client care with these conditions, the provider learning curve may be long. Consistent study and compassionate client-centered care yields positive results! This exercise sequencing format may be "too much information" for some readers, as well as providers who do not test for pelvic symptoms during exercises. Yet the following chapters will expand upon pelvic health problems and increase provider awareness and skill. Women are "always postpartum," and can benefit from exercise progressions at any point in their life, even starting at menopause or later. These sequences apply to men as well!

Table 6.1 Options for postpartum stability sequencing sample
10 reps each, 3 sets, 3–4 x a week; see cuing verbal instructions below

Level of ex	DRA; TRA	PFM	Multifidus
Initial, gravity eliminated	Supine, side-lying, prone 1–5 sec	Supine, side-lying, prone 1–5 sec	Supine, side-lying, prone 1–5 sec
Initial	Seated, quadruped 1–5 sec	Seated, quadruped 1–5 sec	Seated, quadruped 1–5 sec
Intermediate	Supine, side-lying, prone, seated or quadruped 5–10 sec holds, +PFM	Supine, side-lying, prone, seated or quadruped 5–10 sec holds, +TRA	Supine, side-lying, prone, seated or quadruped 5–10 sec holds, +TRA +PFM
Intermediate	Quadruped alternate extremity raises Hip hinge squat, lunge, reach	Quadruped alternate extremity raises Hip hinge squat, lunge, reach	Quadruped alternate extremity raises Hip hinge squat, lunge, reach
Advanced	Lift, push, pull, weights, neutral spine	Lift, push, pull weights, neutral spine	Lift, push, pull weights, neutral spine
Advanced	Agility, trunk rotation, matrix lunge series	Agility, trunk rotation, matrix lunge series	Agility, trunk rotation, matrix lunge series

Cuing instructions:

1. TRA: Inhale, and as you exhale gently vocalize "shh" or "haa" and note a light drawing in and firming of the abdominals.

2. PFM: Inhale, and as you exhale lightly "wink" or draw in the pelvic muscles as if stopping pee or a fart. Imagine you are lifting a gemstone with the pelvic muscles.

3. Multifidus: Assume a position where your spine is elongated, tall. Imagine your back is expanding, swelling, and your tailbone is slightly lifted.

Advanced movement sequences such as those in Figures 6.9–6.13 can help work diagonal, rotational components with core control.

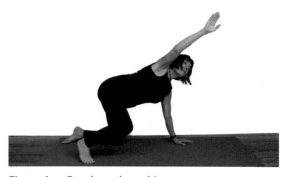

Figure 6.12 Quadruped reaching.

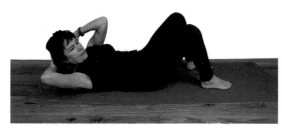

Figure 6.9 Diagonal curl ups.

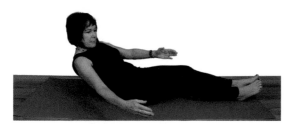

Figure 6.10 Roll back with rotation.

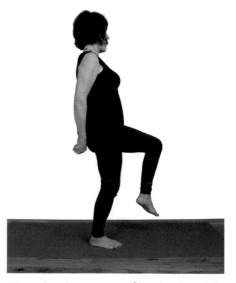

Figure 6.13 A movement flow, lumbopelvic hip stability in single limb stance, moving a weight behind the back with slight spine extension, eccentric abdominals, to moving the weight in front, concentric abdominals.

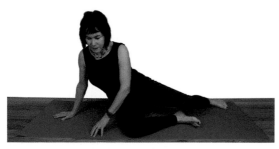

Figure 6.11 Side sitting to a partial side plank.

Putting it all together, clients may be cued to gently "zip the zipper." First, elongating the spine (multifidus), while gently winking pelvic sphincters (PFM), and then drawing up and in to the belly button (TRA).

Performance goals in athletes such as return to tennis or triathlon participation in 6–12 months will require sport specific training in addition to these rehab exercises. Trunk control with rotation and single limb stance, agility, or other functions requires neuromuscular re-education in a progression that develops concentric and eccentric control.

Utilization of the stabilization series sequence of exercises starting with heel slides, knee drop-outs, hip bridges, quadruped posturing, and other exercises (see Chapter 3, the exercise stabilization series levels 1–3) can help train TRA, PFM, and multifidus, and therefore restore critical foundations in rehab for trunk control (Boxes 6.15 and 6.16). These are based on developmental sequence kinesiology that need to be re-booted for optimizing performance. Individuals gifted with coordination and muscle recruitment may not require stabilization series training.

Box 6.15 Initial formats: ramp up to tolerance

Finding the best recruitment pattern for TRA for a starting program can guide an accurate home program at doses as listed in the TRA, PFM, and multifidus exercise chart. Overwork of too many repetitions in too rapid a succession over days may cause thoracic, lumbar, and other sites of pain.

Box 6.16 Patient case: Jessica ♥

Jessica was tested with the digital abdominal palpation technique by a PT three years after beginning her DRA protocol, and the therapist found there was no palpable separation. Her early program consisted of an abdominal drawing-in maneuver, and the technique of the head lift and approximation of the rectus bundles. She had advanced to heel slides, knee drop-outs, diagonal crunches, Pilates roll backs, planks, bridge to single leg bridge, and quadruped extremity raises. She had initially sagged her abdomen in the plank pose, and experienced low back pain during workouts in her first year of exercise. Jessica performed her exercises 4 x a week. A test for her IRD with RUSI 15 years postpartum found no visible gap with screening above, at, and below the umbilicus. Jessica's abdomen no longer had a bulge or pregnant appearance, yet her weight fluctuated in an 8 lb. range postpartum and weight gain produced a central or apple shaped distribution which was not common before pregnancy. She accepted the new shape as part of her life experience as a mom. She felt powerful in her core and able to do everything she wanted for physical function.

SUMMARY

In summary, DRA is a common occurrence. Multiple methods may be offered to enhance function, performance, and power. Cosmetic appearance is often improved. Consideration of client preferences for exercise and personal goals will allow providers to create individualized rehabilitation formats for optimizing function with DRA. Women's overall quality of life may be improved by targeting deep core training in the postpartum time frame (Thabet and Alshehri 2019).

Through the depths of suffering and the grit in healing, transformation may occur. The wounded become the teachers, healed and wise, guiding the way and easing paths for others towards victory.

(Maureen Mason)

REFERENCES

Axer, H., Keyserlingk, D., and Prescher, A. (2001) "Collagen fibers in linea alba and rectus abdominis sheaths. I. General scheme and morphological aspects." *Journal of Surgical Research 96*, 1, 127–134.

Badillo, S., Cathcart, D., Bobb, V., Litos, K., and Steffes, S. (2012) *SOWH APTA OB Fundamentals 2012 course and lab manual*, San Diego, CA, USA.

Beer, G., Schuster, A., Seifert, B., Manestar, M., Mihic-Probst, D., and Weber, S. (2009) "The normal width of the linea alba in nulliparous women." *Clinical Anatomy 22*, 6, 706–711.

Benjamen, D. R., Van de Water, A. T. M., and Peiris, C. L. (2014) "Effect of exercise on diastasis of the rectus abdominis in the antenatal and postnatal periods, as systematic review." *Physiotherapy 100*, 1, 1–8.

Bø, K., Berghmans, B., Morkved, S., and Van Kampen, M. (2015) *Evidence-Based Physical Therapy for the Pelvic Floor: Bridging Science into Clinical Practice*. London: Elsevier.

Bø, K., Sherburn, M., and Allen, T. (2003) "Transabdominal ultrasound measurement of pelvic floor muscle activity when activated directly or via a transverse abdominis muscle contraction." *Neurourology and Urodynamics 22*, 6, 582–588.

Boissonault, J. and Blaschak, M. (1988) "Incidence of diastasis rectus abdominis during the childbearing year." *Physical Therapy 68*, 7, 1082–1086.

Chiarello, C. M., Zellers, J. A., and Sage-King, F. M. (2012) "Predictors of Inter-recti distance in cadavers." *Journal of Women's Health Physical Therapy 36*, 3, 125–130

De'Ath, H. D., Lovegrove, R. E., Javid, M., Peter, N., *et al.* (2010) "An assessment of between-recti distance and divercation in patients with and without abdominal aortic aneurysm." *Royal College of Surgeons of England Annals 92*, 7, 591–594.

Dufour, S., Bernard, S., Murray-Davis, B., and Graham, N. (2019) "Establishing expert based recommendations for the conservative management of pregnancy-related diastasis rectus abdominis: A delphi concensus study." *JWHPT 43*, 2.

Gallus, K., Goldberg, K., and Field, R. (2016) "Functional improvement following diastasis repair in an active duty navy female." *Military Medicine 181*, e952–e954.

Gomez, F. R., Camargo, F. J. S., Cores, A. C., Nunez, S. P., and Costa, L. C. (2018) "Effect of hypopressive abdominal exercise program on intero rectus abdominis distance in postpartum." *British Journal of Sports Medicine 52*, 2.

Hampton, E. and Rader, H. (2018) "Pelvic floor function, dysfunction and treatment, Level 2B." Herman and Wallace Pelvic Rehabilitation Institute lab course January 19–21, 2018.

Hickey, F., Finch, J., and Khanna, A. (2011) "A systematic review on the outcomes of correction of the recti." *Hernia 15*, 6, 607–614.

Hodges, P., Sapsford, R., and Pengel, L. (2007) "Postural and respiratory functions of the pelvic floor muscles." *Neurourology and Urodynamics 26*, 3, 362–371.

Junginger, B., Baessler, K., Sapsford, R., and Hodges, P. W. (2010) "Effect of abdominal and pelvic floor tasks on muscle activity, abdominal pressure, and bladder neck." *International Urogynecology Journal 21*, 1, 69–77.

Keeler, J., Albrecht, M., Eberhardt, L., Horn, L., Donnely, C., and Lowe, D. (2012) "Diastasis rectus abdominis: A survey of women's health clinical practice specialists for current clinical practice postpartum women." *Journal of Women's Health Physical Therapy 36*, 3, 131–142.

Lee, D. (2017) *Diastasis Rectus Abdominis: A Clinical Guide for Those Who Are Split Down the Middle*. San Francisco: Blurb, Inc.

Lee, D. and Hodges, P. W. (2016) "Behavior of the linea alba during a curl up task in diastasis rectus abdominis: An observational study." *Journal of Orthopaedic and Sports Physical Therapy 46*, 7, 580–589.

Lee, D. and Lee, L.-J. (2011) *The Pelvic Girdle: An Integration of Clinical Expertise and Research*, 4th ed. Edinburgh: Churchill Livingstone.

Lee, D., Lee, L., and McLaughlin, L. (2008) "Stability, continence and breathing, the role of fascia following labor and delivery." *Journal of Bodywork and Movement Therapy 12*, 4, 333–338.

Liaw, L. J., Hsu, M. J., Liao, C. H., Liu, M. F., and Hsu, A. T. (2011) "The relationship between inter-recti distance measured by ultrasound imaging and abdominal muscle function in postpartum women: A 6-month follow up study." *Journal of Orthopaedic and Sports Physical Therapy 41*, 6, 435–443.

Litos, K. (2014) "Progressive therapeutic exercise program for successful treatment of a postpartum woman with a severe diastasis rectus abdominis." *Journal of Women's Health and Physical Therapy 38*, 2, 58–73.

Litos, K. (2019) Personal communication re. DRA and exercise protocols.

Mota, P., Pascoal, A., Carita, A., and Bø, K. (2015) "Prevalence and risk factors of diastasis recti abdominis from late pregnancy to 6 months postpartum, and relationship to lumbopelvic pain." *Manual Therapy 20*, 1, 200–205.

Nicole, S. (2018) Hypopressive Exercise and Yoga Workshop hosted at Del Mar Yoga, San Diego.

Parker, M., Millar, A., and Dugan, S. (2009) "Diastasis rectus abdominis and lumbopelvic pain and dysfunction; are they related?" *Journal of Women's Health Physical Therapy 33*, 15–22.

Rosen, C. M., Ngaage, L.M., Rada, E. M., Slezak, S., *et al.* (2019) "Surgical management of diastasis recti: A systematic review of insurance coverage in the United States." *Annals of Plastic Surgery 83*, 4, 475–480.

Sapsford, R. and Hodges, P. (2001) "Contraction of the pelvic floor muscles during abdominal maneuvers." *Archives of Physical Medicine and Rehabilitation 82*, 1081–1088.

Schulte, L., Lee, D., Weibe, J., Dufour, S., *et al.* (2019) *The Diastasis Recti Re Cap*. Institute for Birth Healing, Instituteforbirthhealing.com (Expert opinion webinar).

Sperstad, J., Tennifjord, M., Hilde, G., Engh, M., and Bø, K. (2016) "Diastasis recti abdominis during pregnancy and 12 months after childbirth: Prevalence, risk factors and report of lumbopelvic pain." *British Journal of Sports Medicine 50*, 1092–1096.

Spitznagle, T. (2010) "Diagnosis and treatment of movement impairments associated with musculoskeletal pelvic pain syndromes." Three-day seminar, Herman and Wallace Pelvic Rehabilitation Institute, San Diego, CA, USA.

Spitznagle, T., Leong, F., and Van Dillen, L. (2007) "Prevalence of diastasis recti abdominis in a urogynecologic population." *International Urogynecology 18*, 321–328.

Stupp, L., Resende, A., Petricelli, C., Nakamura, M., Alexandre, S., and Zanetti, M. (2011) "Pelvic floor muscle and transversus abdominis activation in abdominal hypopressive technique through electromyography." *Neurourology and Urodynamics 30*, 8, 1518–1521.

Thabet, A. A. and Alshehri, M. A. (2019) "Efficacy of deep core stability exercise program in postpartum women with diastasis recti abdominis; a randomized controlled trial." *Journal of Musculoskeletal Neuronal Interact 19*, 1, 62–68.

Tuttle, L. J., Fasching, J., Keller, A., Milan, P., *et al.* (2018) "Noninvasive treatment of postpartum diastasis recti abdominis: A pilot study." *Journal of Women's Health Physical Therapy 42*, 2, 65–75.

Van de Water, A. and Benjamen, D. (2016) "Measurement methods to assess diastasis of the rectus abdominis muscle (DRAM): A systematic review of their measurement properties and meta-analytic reliability generalization." *Manual Therapy 21*, 41–53.

Walton, L. M., Costa, A., LaVanture, D., McIlrath, S., and Stebbins, B. (2016) "The effects of a six week dynamic core stability plank exercise program compared to a traditional supine strengthening program on diastasis recti abdominis closure, pain, Oswestry disability index (ODI) and pelvic floor disability index scores (PFDI)." *Physical Therapy and Rehabilitation 3*, 3.

Werner, L. and Dayan, M. (2019) "Diastasis recti abdominis diagnosis, risk factors, effect on musculoskeletal function, framework for treatment and implications for the pelvic floor." *Current Women's Health Reviews 15*, 2, 86–101.

CHAPTER 7

Pelvic Girdle Pain

This chapter considers biomechanics, current research, expert opinion, and physiological/biological rationale for bodywork and movement therapies for pelvic girdle pain (PGP). Therapeutic exercise protocols and other considerations are presented for improving function and reducing pain.

DEFINITION

Often starting in pregnancy, pelvic girdle pain (PGP) is pain that is located from the posterior iliac crest and gluteal folds posteriorly into the anterior pelvic region in the range of the bony pelvis. (With an apology for what may be an abbreviation soup in this chapter, pregnancy related PGP is often termed PPGP in the scientific literature, or even PRPGP.) It is important to recognize PGP as a separate diagnosis and delineate it from low back pain (LBP). PGP often occurs with LBP in the perinatal time frame and may resolve or linger.

Symphysis pubis pain and sacroiliac (SI) pain are both components of what may fall under the heading of PGP. Symphysis site pain is also termed symphysis pubis dysfunction (SPD) (Leadbetter, Mawer, and Lindow 2004). In the last few decades research has emerged on PGP consensus standards for screening, descriptive anatomical delineation, and testing for SI, symphysis, and pubis regions (Albert, Godskesen, and Westergaard 2001, 2002; Cook et al. 2007). PGP may involve the right, or left, or both SI joints, and/or the symphysis pubis. Women reporting more joints involved versus only one are likely to have a poorer prognosis on the recovery spectrum (Albert et al. 2001) (Box 7.1).

> **Box 7.1 PGP: specialty care needed**
> Like many pelvic health conditions, PGP is not an area that is readily recognized by medical and/or holistic wellness providers. Individuals suffering with this condition may have a difficult journey finding appropriate care and may suffer with limitations in rest and play activities.

PGP: PELVIC BIOMECHANICS

How is the pelvic ring stable, what holds the bones together? Structurally, form and force closure are two key components in a locking motion of the SI joint and symphysis pubis, required for stability. In standing, biomechanical studies identify a locking motion of sacral flexion or nutation, and iliac extension or counternutation. The "form" of interlocking articular surfaces and taut ligaments, as well as "force" of compression and shearing from muscle, fascia, and gravitational forces, creates stability (Vleming *et al.* 2012). Overstretched or strained ligaments as well as weakened muscle support systems can contribute to instability and pain, especially in the "unloaded" position of tasks such as turning over in bed or lifting legs off the ground. PGP may be directly related to instability in form and force closure, and/or other factors (Figures 7.1 and 7.2) (Box 7.2).

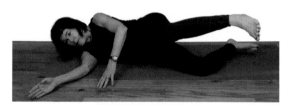

Figure 7.1 Rolling twist: painful?

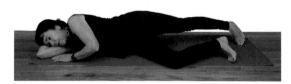

Figure 7.2 Toe tap Pilates: painful?

Box 7.2 Patient case: Naomi, her PGP, and instability

A few months postpartum with baby number two at age 32, Naomi was having difficulty with walking and exertion, with varied pains around the pubic area, groin, low back, and tailbone area. Naomi had felt pains in these areas while pregnant, but they were of a low level, but then were flared postpartum. She felt depressed and as if she had lost herself, as she had been an avid fitness enthusiast prior to her pregnancies.

Seeking help, she saw two physical therapists (PTs) and a personal trainer, and the pains were aggravated from these treatments, which she felt were too high level for her. She was asked to perform a hip bridge, and then a single leg bridge exercise; she experienced a flash of pain across her back and her pelvis tilted to the side. Hamstring spasms and cramping stopped her from bridging after a few repetitions as well. She described twinges and aches around the pelvic ring, from the symphysis pubis as well as the tailbone region and radiating pain down the back of the left leg to the calf and top of the foot. Pain became a daily reminder for her that things were different, as she had sensations of a sense of something "shifting" and sometimes a sharp stabbing ache in the symphysis pubis or SI joint. Lying in bed on her side or turning in bed was often the worst pain. Her muscles did not relax to allow her to lie on her back unless she placed a rolled towel across the low back. The bed was no longer a sanctuary of refreshment and recharge, and she suffered sleep deprivation and fatigue.

She had a loss of power with activities. Stair climbing, hill walking, and lunges were painful and caused her iliotibial band and pelvic muscles to spasm. Of particular concern, her muscles became rigid or "locked up" after exertion. Pushing the stroller up a slight hill with two babies, her back and pelvic area began to spasm, and she barely made it home. How could she take care of her babies? She felt afraid to take excursions unless it was on a flat area. Flat surface stroller walks were the only safe options to prevent pain. Further details of her treatment are provided in this chapter.

Factors contributing to PGP

Pregnancy and birth dynamics may cause the symphysis pubis, and/or SI joint, to become mobile to the point of instability, and this is usually associated with muscle weakness as well. Pain and limited load transfer and exertion tolerance occur (Lee and Lee 2011). Asymmetrical motion of the SI joints has also been indicated as a pain generator. Mechanical, hormonal, as well as environmental and genetic factors impact the stability of the pelvic girdle.

Sensitization of tissue in the pelvic ring may also occur from thoracic, lumbar, and sacral nerve stretch and/or compression, as well as central sensitization. Associated local and distal myofascial slings can produce pain around the pelvic area. Mood and affective challenges from role changes, lack of sleep, and other co-morbidities such as bladder or bowel problems may further exacerbate pain.

Risk factors for PGP

PGP has been studied more in pregnancy than in the postnatal time frame. Recent research (Clinton *et al.* 2017) finds risk factors for antenatal PGP to include:

- the presence of orthopedic dysfunction
- a history of trauma or falls
- an increased BMI
- smoking
- prior pregnancy history
- a belief system that they have a negative prognosis for improvement in their PGP condition.

Belief systems are part of the framework of the biopsychosocial model and can have a positive or negative effect on treatment outcomes. Client evaluation and treatment for a condition such as PGP ideally considers biological, cognitive, affective, social, health history, and work history dynamics (Gatchel *et al.* 2007) (Box 7.3).

> **Box 7.3 Facilitating hope, recovery** 🦋
> Is there hope, is there a sense that recovery is possible? Is a cloud of depression and a sense of hopelessness present? Is the individual with PGP feeling stuck on an island? Or do they know someone who has been helped with treatment? Provider storytelling of prior cases that have benefitted from treatment can help create hope and participation.

Incidence rates

Specific areas of the SI, symphysis pubis, and pelvis have been reported to impact 20–54 percent of women (Albert, Godskesen, and Westergaard 2002; Gutke, Ostagaard, and Oberg 2006; Wu *et al.* 2004).

Pain classification

ANTENATAL PGP

Pain can be classified into four groups:

- double-sided SI pain at 6.3 percent
- pelvic girdle syndrome with pain in both SI joints and the symphysis, 6.0 percent
- one-sided SI pain at 5.5 percent
- symphysiolysis (symphysis pain) at 2.3 percent.

(Cook et al. 2007; Godskesen and Westergaard 2002)

The use of this classification schema is the most specific descriptive diagnostic system (Boxes 7.4 and 7.5).

Box 7.4 PGP: find the causes

Knowing what is hurting, and why, is the key to helping and healing for individuals with PGP. Bodywork and movement therapy can exacerbate or help ameliorate PGP, but there is no cookbook approach! Targeting the drivers for the symptoms is key, and this entails screening and re-testing over time.

Box 7.5 Clinical practice guidelines (CPG)

CPG are the best standards for evaluation and treatment, based on extensive review of the best evidence-based studies. CPG for PGP in the antenatal period give a grade of B (moderate evidence) to consideration of postural influences on pain, a grade of C (weak evidence) is assigned to manual therapy intervention for PGP antenatally, and grade D (conflicting evidence) for the use of support belts and exercise. More research is needed to clarify best practices in the antenatal time frame (Clinton *et al.* 2017).

Prevention of PGP in pregnancy

A study providing preventative programs in early pregnancy up to 20 weeks (Eggen *et al.* 2012) found "only minor influence on the prevalence and severity of LBP and PGP in pregnancy." However, research further along in pregnancy, in antenatal weeks 20 to 36, found significantly less lumbopelvic pain than a control group (25 percent versus 37 percent), as well as significantly improved functional status scores (Morkved *et al.* 2010). Other research found a 10-week program of stability ball exercises, progressive core exercises, and/or yoga produced significant improvement in pain and functional status (Belogolovsky *et al.* 2015). Further research with posture, body mechanics, and movement education instruction as an intervention, or combined with an exercise program, produced reductions in pain (Guan *et al.* 2021).

Postpartum PGP: PP-PGP

What percent of women have continued PP-PGP? Research findings vary, from 8.5 percent (Albert *et al.* 2001) to 10–20 percent (Bergstrom, Persson, and Mogren 2014; Clinton *et al.* 2017). Unfortunately, some women will have a persistent low level of disability and/or pain related to the pelvic girdle up to 1–2 years postpartum (Simonds *et al.* 2022).

Symphysis pubis dysfunction

Symphysis pubis dysfunction (SPD) may occur during pregnancy or postpartum (Leadbetter, Mawer, and Lindow 2006). A 1 cm separation of the left and right symphysis pubis is common during pregnancy and may not cause pain or dysfunction. How much of a separation may need help, even surgery? Remarkably, small or large separations may cause pain and dysfunction, but case studies listed here point out that pain is not simply based on measured anatomical variance! SPD pain may occur in the absence of pubic separation, or may be associated with a separation. An X-ray or CT scan may be used postnatally to measure a separation.

POSTNATAL SPD: CASES

Postnatal SPD may be 2 percent in the perinatal time up to six months postpartum based on a questionnaire of women with pain reported at their medical visits (Owens, Pearson, and Mason 2002) (Boxes 7.6–7.10).

- A separation of 9.5 cm anteriorly and 3–5 mm separation of the SI joint has been described in a case report where improvement was noted with treatment utilizing a binder, a walker, and physical therapy, with the authors stating, "Conservative management including analgesia, rest, and a pelvic binder is a reasonable method of management" (Jain and Sternberg 2005).
- An ultrasound study of SPD found that

at more than three years postpartum a subject with a relatively small gap (10 mm) had SPD whereas an individual with a larger gap (35 mm) was pain free (Scriven, Jones, and McKnight 1995).

Box 7.6 Client evaluation for PGP

Medical screening in PGP reviews health history, surgeries, trauma to the pelvic area, birth dynamics, pain profiles, limitations or impairments, symptoms, and goals. An examination of gait, and functional tasks, can identify movement impairments in PGP. Tests of strength, flexibility, and endurance identify limitations. Provocative mechanical testing of the lumbar spine and hips, as well as the specific pelvic girdle joints, should be provided within the limits of client tolerance. There may be associated pudendal, sciatic, and/or femoral neuropathies, with an accompanying "drop foot" gait and/or the presence of a limp. The presence of diastasis rectus abdominis, pelvic organ prolapse, levator ani or coccyx pain, postpartum depression, and other co-morbidities may limit testing to be provided over the course of two or more sessions to not aggravate symptoms.

Box 7.7 PGP validated tests

Recent research (Simonds, Abraham, and Spitznagle 2022) identifies that the most important tests to identify PGP are the active straight leg raise (ASLR) and the posterior pelvic pain provocation test (P4), described below (Figures 7.3–7.8). The ASLR and P4 tests should be used in context of all other evaluation and examination components.

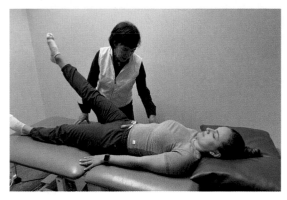

Figure 7.3 ASLR.

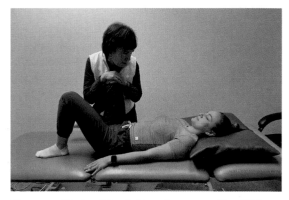

Figure 7.4 Post pelvic girdle pain provocation (P4).

Other tests that may be useful include:

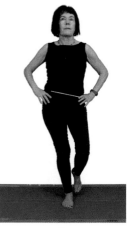

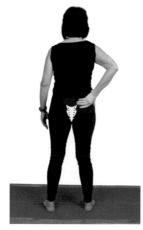

Figure 7.5 Single limb stance and hip drop: positive Trendelenburg.

Figure 7.6 Palpation long dorsal ligament.

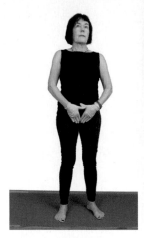

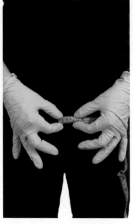

Figure 7.7 Palpation symphysis pubis.

Figure 7.8 Tape measure over symphysis pubis.

FUNCTIONAL TESTING: HOW ARE THEY MOVING?

Functional testing of the client with PGP includes screening the following (Box 7.11):

- Sit to stand: Is upper extremity assistance required?
- Gait: Is there heel strike and push off and trunk rotation? Is there stability of the pelvis? Is there a stable swing phase, or is there increased "double support" time?
- Single limb stance test. A positive test for weakness of the gluteus medius and other muscles is a hip drop on the unsupported side, termed positive Trendelenburg.
- Standing kinetic tests: Active motions of the thoracic and lumbar spine, the

sacrum, ilium, trochanters, femoral condyles, and ankle/foot complex create a picture of kinetic chain function and pain drivers.

- Rolling over and turning in bed: This may be one of the most difficult motions due to the "open chain" nature of this activity.
- Floor to half kneel to standing function: Some individuals cannot transfer their weight and generate sufficient support to move upright without upper extremity assistance. Individuals may keep their legs together to move from kneeling to standing as a pain limiting maneuver.

Box 7.11 PGP and stair climbing 🦋
Individuals in two-story homes may need to live downstairs while in initial pain, or even years following childbirth. Per pain and instability, clients may need a railing, or need to sidestep, to reduce forces through the pelvic ring.

POSTURE SCREENING

Moms often carry babies on one hip and are prone to lateral shifts of the rib cage over the pelvis as well as other pelvic girdle asymmetries. Obliquities and asymmetries of the spine, rib cage, and pelvis may be found on postural and palpation screens. These include right and left side differences with elevated iliac crests, anterior or posterior iliac rotations, and sacral and coccyx asymmetries. These asymmetries may be corrected with manual therapy, exercise, and client follow up with postural and ergonomic self-care (Box 7.12).

Box 7.12 Patient case: Naomi's ❤
PGP: intake details
Naomi's intake screening identified that she had experienced a few hard falls on her pelvis and spine with athletic functions. She had experienced pre-pregnancy LBP and left leg sciatica as well, related to a bending and twisting lifting incident. Mechanical testing was positive for SI and symphysis pubis pain, as well as movement impairments of instability in single leg stance, demonstrating lumbar extension and rotation. She had pain in her lumbar, SI regions, and symphysis pubis with stair climbing and rolling on the mat. Her core muscles, TRA, multifidus, and PFM were weak and unable to hold sustained contractions. She also wanted to be able to have pain-free sex (her symphysis pubis and SI hurt during sexual activity).

EXPECTATIONS FOR RECOVERY

Vollestad and Stuge (2009) studied prognostic indicators for recovery from PGP postpartum and found that the subject's belief in their possibility for recovery, as well as the ASLR test, had the highest correlation with their disability and pain symptoms. Disability ratings (Salen, Spangfortþke, and Nordemar 1994) have been found to correlate with ratings on the active straight leg raise test (ASLR) as well as the posterior pelvic provocation test (P4) (Robinson *et al.* 2010). Recent research (Simonds, Abraham, and Hill 2018) in a small postpartum sample found a significant correlation with Oswestry Disability Index (ODI) scores and PGP assessed at intervals up to three months postpartum.

Deering *et al.* (2018) identified fatigue in the lumbopelvic stabilizing muscles that lasted 26 weeks postpartum compared to nullipara muscle function (Box 7.13). This study pioneered an ASLR Fatigue Test, and independent of pain production, postpartum females had poorer endurance than controls.

Box 7.13 Education, expectations, and programming

In light of prolonged postural weakness post-partum, clients may need care for well over six months, and care providers need not tell clients they will have continued chronic pain or permanent loss of function! Client education as to a potential six-months to one-year program will lower initial expectations and can help promote adherence towards long-term achievement of goals. Home program therapeutic exercise prescriptions with monthly advanced challenges and adherence tracking systems may provide the most cost-effective long-term specialty care.

INTERVENTION FOR PGP

Therapeutic programs for PGP can include:

- education for postural habits and ergonomics
- exercises for functional stability, mobility, strength, and endurance
- manual therapy for myofascial pain, and correcting alignment of the pelvis, rib cage, and spine towards symmetry
- training in specialty pelvic support belts.

EXERCISE FOR PGP

A recent systematic review found specific stabilizing exercises and a non-elastic SI support belt to be effective for interventions for SI dysfunctions in pregnant and nonpregnant adults (Sharma *et al.* 2014). Other research found significant improvement utilizing exercise intervention for unilateral SI pain in a study of 25 women, though the participants were not a specific postpartum population (Brizzolara *et al.* 2018).

Endurance

Therapeutic exercise programs for PGP must build strength and endurance for functional activities and address local stabilizers as well as global muscle systems (Sahrmann, Azevedo, and van Dillen 2017). From lifting the legs in supine, to rolling over in bed, getting out of bed and walking, reaching, squatting, and lifting for infant care and ADL, stability and mobility are required from the trunk and spine into the extremities, and must be considered in goal and program planning.

Rapid fatigue and then compensatory spasm often occur in the first several weeks of treatment. Customized exercise programs with less extensive workouts 2 x a day, 6 x a week can help re-set foundations. Stabilization exercise series of 3–5 repetitions (stop before cramping) can be built up to sets of 30 repetitions x 2–3 to build endurance.

Posture and symmetry

Education for postural habits, ergonomics, promoting symmetry, and support can be trained. Sitting in a symmetrical position with a neutral spine, versus in a slumped position with legs crossed, will help reduce pain. For play activities on the floor, sitting on a footstool with the knees lower than the hips is preferable to floor sitting. Performing the "log roll" maneuver to get in and out of bed, with a deliberate activation of the deep stabilizers (PFM, TRA, and multifidus), may be pain reducing (Figures 7.9–7.11).

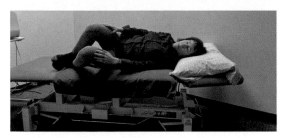

Figure 7.9 Log roll to side.

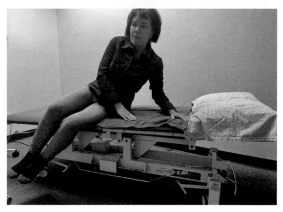

Figure 7.11 Push up with arms to sit.

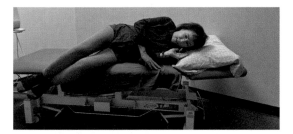

Figure 7.10 Side-lying to drop knees LE off bed together.

PGP TREATMENT WITH BELTS: EXTERNAL SUPPORT

Some find comfort and relief in reduced PGP with stabilization belts, although recent research (Brizzolara *et al.* 2018) suggests there is not enough evidence for stabilization belts to be a part of clinical practice guidelines (Box 7.14). Other research has demonstrated reduced SI mobility (Damen *et al.* 2002) and improved ASLR ability (Mens *et al.* 1999) with belt use.

region, reinforcing gluteal, piriformis, long dorsal ligament, and other structures.

If a belt is too tight it may create a compression of myofascial and nerve structures in the pelvic area, such as meralgia paresthetica (Patijn *et al.* 2011). Clients may exercise with belts on if they desire. Application of an SI belt while supine, prior to getting out of bed, may help with this ADL task which is often painful in this population (Box 7.15).

> **Box 7.14 SI stability enhancement**
> Snijders, Vleeming, and Stoeckart (1993) demonstrated that in biomechanical analysis in cadaver studies, the SI joint is a relatively flat surface and therefore is vulnerable to shearing forces. Pelvis stability relies on muscular, joint, and fascial integrity, which are compromised in pregnancy and birth. The authors conclude that symptom reduction of pain postpartum with an SI belt is due to enhanced stability to the joint across the SI

> **Box 7.15 SI belt**
> SI belts may be relatively lifesaving for a few months, or longer as needed, and detective work with the client as to when they are most in need of their belt as well as gradual weaning from the belt with guidance is appreciated.

SURGICAL FIXATION FOR PGP

Some individuals such as those with multi-level laxity or connective tissue disorders may require surgical fixation (Box 7.16). Postpartum continuation of disabling pelvic pain, and frequently LBP as well, may not respond to conservative care (van Zwienen *et al.* 2004). Fixation surgery with plates, screws, and other devices applied to stabilize the pelvis can produce improved function and reduce pain. Surgical fixation of the pelvic ring may be provided at the symphysis pubis, SI joints, or both. Complication rates from pelvic fixation surgeries are relatively high at 18–29 percent and therefore conservative care with a pelvic specialty team should first be offered.

Box 7.16 Surgery for PGP: help, yet possible complications

A small study (Kibsgard, Roise, and Stuge 2014) included eight patients with high disability rating and pelvic girdle pain requiring surgery. Symphysis stabilization was performed, and unilateral anterior approach for SI stabilization. Outcome measures were documented pre-operatively, and postoperative outcomes at three, six, and twelve months. Significant changes were seen in Oswestry disability scores, and visual analog pain scores. The SF-36 was utilized for social functioning assessment, and this demonstrated improvement. However, surgical complications occurred including nerve damage as well as infection and the authors concluded more research is needed.

A larger study (Smith *et al.* 2013) of 263 patients undergoing either minimally invasive or open fixation of the SI joint found better results from the less invasive technique. Post-surgical complications occurred in 18–21% of patients, including neuropathy, infections, pain at the joint, buttock, or leg, trochanteric bursitis, falls, and other adverse events. This study finds a strong trend towards minimally invasive surgery and recommends more long-term follow up and outcome measures.

DISCUSSION

Individualized programming

Program instruction for clients with multiple problems can be complex. Finding pain-free exercise routines is critical to reduce anxiety and fear-avoidance behavior, as well as to build endurance. Encouraging psychological, social, and health care team support is also important to address the broader biopsychosocial needs.

Consider Table 6.1 with options for strength formats and recognize that multifidus, TRA, and PFM are all recognized as deep stabilizers for the pelvic ring, along with the ligamentous system. Starting with these three muscle groups and working into the lumbopelvic neutral with multifidus, PFM activation via the stabilization series (Chapter 3) may be effective in terms of client tolerance and ease of execution, as well as pain reduction. Advancing to a lunge matrix, multiplanar mobility, agility, and sport training are long-term considerations and goals with extensive programming needs.

Therapeutic exercise: Clinical opinion

Closed chain exercise is the best tolerated, with sample exercises listed below. Long-term clients with financial/insurance/travel constraints can be seen once a month to update, expand, correct, and reinforce home exercise, posture, ergonomics, and strategies for outings and return to fitness activities.

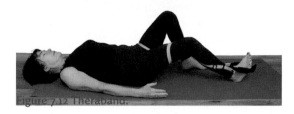

Heel slides: A critical eye is needed to screen for pelvic rotation, lumbar stability, and knee inclination into a typically valgus pattern. Direct pressure of the heel into the mat during leg extension will activate concentric gluteal contraction while the psoas muscle is eccentrically controlling the descent of the femur. Cuing co-contraction of the latissimus dorsi with upper extremities exerting a light isometric press to the mat, in addition to multifidus activation for a neutral lordosis, will help link upper and lower myofascial slings during heel slides (Figure 7.12).

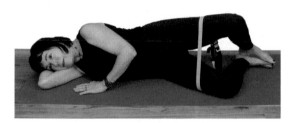

Figure 7.13 Clam foot into wall, t-band.

Clams: Hip external rotator exercise can be performed with foot pressure into a wall. In side-lying, the client lightly presses both feet into a wall, and activates the hip external rotator and abductor group by lifting the top knee a few, to several, inches (Figure 7.13).

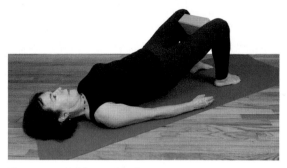

Figure 7.14 Bridge and ball.

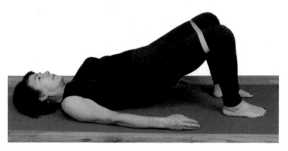

Figure 7.15 Bridge and Pilates ring.

A gentle ball squeeze and/or engaging the hip abductor/external rotators Pilates ring hold between the distal thighs during bridging may help activate PFM and abdominal control and promote pain reduction (Figures 7.14 and 7.15).

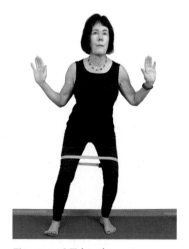

Figure 7.16 T-band squat.

A functional fitness program can include a sit to stand pattern, and then return to a seated posture with eccentric control. Sit to stand and the return to sit is basically a squat exercise. Squats are needed for ADL and fitness and may be trained in a small mini squat or yoga "chair pose," to train a hip hinge lift with reaching (Figure 7.16).

Piriformis, hip flexor, adductor, and lumbar stretches can prevent rebound spasm and pain. In the case of instability syndromes, modification of stretches towards smaller excursions can promote a pain-free experience and increase program compliance.

FLUID MOTION

Flowing movements such as yoga asana sequences, or dancing, contain movements of the lumbopelvic hip area which are often challenges for the client with PGP. The use of imagery and visualization can be helpful in training fluidity of motion and ease (Franklin *et al.* 2003). Yoga can be utilized to establish joint stabilization via posture locks, and concentric and eccentric control with pacing asana and pranayama in a scaffolding format as an individual builds stamina and skill (Garner 2016).

SUMMARY

Kanakaris, Roberts, and Giannoudis (2011), in their review of PGP, state, "The scientific and clinical implications of PPGP require the multidisciplinary interaction of a wide number of health-related specialties, including obstetrics and gynaecology, general medicine, orthopaedic surgery, physiotherapy, rheumatology and clinical psychiatry," and this writer would add: any informed and compassionate movement therapist and bodyworker.

The review by Verstraete, Vanderstraeten, and Parewijck (2013) states, "It is obvious that PPGP is a complex disorder." And further on states that the "aim of this multidimensional and multidisciplinary approach is to increase the women's self-knowledge and self-efficacy, so pain and disability can be minimized. To inform the gynecologist/obstetrician about the severity, etiology, and treatment options of PPGP is an important step in recognition" (Box 7.17).

> **Box 7.17 Patient case: Naomi's treatment**
>
> Naomi struggled with PGP of a significant nature for over three years. She began a lumbopelvic stabilization protocol and recalls it took over 12 months for her to feel stable and pain free. She blended stabilization exercises with Pilates reformer workouts and modified yoga asanas. In her late 40s, she rarely notes "twinges" in her symphysis pubis unless she rapidly abducts her leg or lunges; however, with a warmup, light to moderate agility activity is tolerated pain free. Foundation exercises she performs 4–5 times per week include planks, press ups, quadruped alternate extremity raises, Pilates' "the swimmer" and prone knee bends, quadruped to down dog preparation, cat camel, child's pose, bridges, single limb bridges, side planks, double knee to chest, roll backs seated to supine, and clams. She also dances a few times a week for ten minutes to move "all the parts" in a flowing pattern.

PGP may improve rapidly or require longer term care. The clients' key functional goals should be considered foremost in all aspects of care. Providers can speak of hope, resiliency, and restoration of comfort and power as benefits from rehabilitation and celebrate joy with clients with whom they help to restore function.

REFERENCES

Albert, H., Godskesen, M., and Westergaard, J. (2001) "Prognosis in four syndromes of pregnancy-related pelvic pain." *Acta Obstetricia et Gynecologica Scandinavica 2001*, 80, 505–510.

Albert, H. B., Godskesen, M., and Westergaard, J. G. (2002) "Incidence of four syndromes of pregnancy-related pelvic joint pain." *Spine 27*, 24, 2831–2834.

Belogolovsky, I., Katzman, I., Christopherson, N., Rivera, M., *et al.* (2015) "The effectiveness of exercise in treatment of pregnancy-related lumbar and pelvic girdle pain: A meta-analysis and evidence-based review." *Journal of Women's Health Physical Therapy 39*, 2, 53–64.

Bergstrom, C., Persson, M., and Mogren, I. (2014) "Pregnancy-related low back pain and pelvic girdle pain approximately 14 months after pregnancy-pain status, self-rated health family situation." *BMC Pregnancy and Childbirth 14*, 8.

Brizzolara, K., Wang-Prince, S., Roddey, T., and Medley, A. (2018) "Effectiveness of adding a compression belt to lumbopelvic stabilization exercises for women with sacroiliac joint pain, a feasibility randomized clinical trial." *Journal of Women's Health Physical Therapy 42*, 2, 313–314.

Clinton, S., Newell, A., Downey, P. A., and Ferriera, K. (2017) "Pelvic girdle pain in the antepartum population: Physical therapy clinical practice guidelines linked to the international classification of functioning, disability, and health from the section on women's health and the orthopedic section of the American Physical Therapy Association." *Journal of Women's Health Physical Therapy 41*, 2, 102–125.

Cook, C., Massa, L., Harm-Ernandes, I., Segneri, R., *et al.* (2007) "Interrater reliability and diagnostic accuracy of pelvic girdle pain classification." *Journal of Manipulative and Physiological Therapeutics 30*, 4, 252–258.

Damen, L., Spoor, C. W., Snijders, C. J., and Stam, H. J. (2002) "Does a pelvic belt influence sacroiliac laxity?" *Clinical Biomechanics 17*, 495–498.

Deering, R., Senefeld, J., Pashiben, T., Neumann, D., Cruz, M., and Hunter, S. (2018) "Fatigability of the lumbopelvic stability muscles in women 8- and 26-weeks postpartum." *Journal of Women's Health Physical Therapy 423*, 128–138.

Dufour, S. and Daniel, S. (2018) "Understanding clinical decision making in pregnancy-related pelvic girdle pain." *Journal of Women's Health Physical Therapy 42*, 3, 120–127.

Eggen, M., Stuge, B., Mowinckel, P., Jensen, K., and Hagen, K. (2012) "Can supervised exercises including ergonomic advice reduce the prevalence and severity of low back pain and pelvic girdle pain in pregnancy? A randomized controlled trial." *Physical Therapy 92*, 6, 781–790.

Franklin, E. (2003) *Pelvic Power: Mind/Body Exercises for Strength, Flexibility, Posture, and Balance for Men and Women*. Hightstown, NJ: Princeton Book Company.

Garner, G. (2016) *Medical Therapeutic Yoga: Biopsychosocial Rehabilitation and Wellness Care*. Edinburgh: Handspring.

Gatchel, R. J., Peng, Y. B., Peters, M. L., Fuchs, P. N., *et al.* (2007) "The biopsychosocial approach to chronic pain: Scientific advances and future directions." *Psychological Bulletin 133*, 4, 581–624.

Guan, J., Hamnett, C., Jakucionis, S., Hameed, F., *et al.* (2021) "Can an outpatient exercise program for pregnancy related pelvic pain improve pain and function versus education? A feasibility study." *Journal of Women's Health Physical Therapy 45*, 2, 68–75.

Gutke, A., Ostagaard, H., and Oberg, B. (2006) "Pelvic girdle pain and lumbar pain in pregnancy: A cohort study of the consequences in terms of health and functioning." *Spine 31*, 5, 149–155.

Jain, N. and Sternberg, B. (2005) "Symphyseal separation." *Obstetrics and Gynecology 105*, 5, 1229–1232.

Kanakaris, N., Roberts, C., and Giannoudis, P. (2011) "Pregnancy related pelvic girdle pain: An update." *BMC Medicine 9*, 15.

Kibsgard, T. J., Roise, O., and Stuge, B. (2014) "Pelvic joint fusion in patients with severe pelvic girdle pain—a single subject research design study." *BMC Musculoskeletal Disorders 15*, 85.

Leadbetter, R. E., Mawer, D., and Lindow, S. W. (2004) "Symphysis pubis dysfunction: A review of the literature." *Journal of Maternal-Fetal and Neonatal Medicine 16*, 6, 349–354.

Leadbetter, R. E., Mawer, D., and Lindow, S. W. (2006) "The development of a scoring system for symphysis pubis dysfunction." *Journal of Obstetric Gynecology 26*, 1, 20–23.

Lee, D. and Lee, L.-J. (2011) *The Pelvic Girdle: An Integration of Clinical Expertise and Research*, 4th ed. Edinburgh: Churchill Livingstone.

Mens, J., Vleming, A., Snijders, C., Stam, H., and Ginai, A. (1999) "The active straight leg raise test and mobility of the pelvic joints." *European Spine Journal 8*, 468–473.

Morkved, S., Salvesen, K. A., Schei, B., Lydersen, S., *et al.* (2010) "Does group training during pregnancy prevent lumbopelvic pain? A randomized clinical trial." *Acta Obstetricia et Gynecologica Scandanavia 86*, 3.

Owens, K., Pearson, A., and Mason, G. (2002) "Symphysis pubis dysfunction—a cause of significant obstetric morbidity." *European Journal of Obstetrics and Gynecology 105*, 2, 143-146.

Patijn, J., Mekhall, N., Hayek, S., Lataster, A., vann Kleef, M., and Van Zundert, J. (2011) "Meralgia paresthetica, evidence based medicine." *Pain Practice 11*, 3, 302-308.

Robinson, H. S., Mengshoel, A. M., Bjelland, E. K., and Vollestad, N. K. (2010) "Pelvic girdle pain, clinical tests and disability in late pregnancy." *Manual Therapy 15*, 280-285.

Sahrmann, S., Azevedo, D. C., and van Dillen, L. (2017) "Diagnosis and treatment of movement impairment syndromes." *Brazilian Journal of Physical Therapy 21*, 6, 391-399.

Salen, B. A., Spangfortþke, L., and Nordemar, R. (1994) "The disability rating index: An instrument for the assessment of disability in clinical settings." *Journal of Clinical Epidemiology 47*, 12, 1423-1435.

Scriven, M., Jones, D., and McKnight, L. (1995) "The importance of pubic pain following childbirth: A clinical and ultrasonographic study of diastasis of the pubic symphysis." *Journal of the Royal Society of Medicine 88*, 28-30.

Sharma, A., Sharma, S., Steiner, L., and Brudvig, T. (2014) "Identification and effectiveness of physical therapy interventions for sacroiliac dysfunction in pregnant and nonpregnant adults: A systematic review." *Journal of Women's Health Physical Therapy 38*, 3, 110-117.

Simonds, A., Abraham, K., and Hill, C. (2018) "Disability, pelvic girdle pain, and depressive symptoms in the first three months postpartum." *Journal of Women's Health Physical Therapy 42*, 3, 139-147.

Simonds, A., Abraham, K., and Spitznagle, T. (2022) "Executive summary of the clinical practice guidelines for pelvic girdle pain in the postpartum population." *Journal of Women's Health Physical Therapy 46*, 1.

Smith, G., Capobianco, R., Cher, D., Rudolf, L., *et al.* (2013) "Open versus minimally invasive sacroiliac joint fusion; a multicenter comparison of perioperative measures and clinical outcomes." *Annals of Surgical Innovation and Research 7*, 14.

Snijders, C. J., Vleeming, A., and Stoeckart, R. (1993) "Transfer of lumbosacral load to iliac bones and legs. Part 1: Biomechanics of self-bracing of the sacroiliac joints and its significance for treatment and exercise." *Clinical Biomechanic 8*, 285-294.

van Zwienen, C. M., van den Bosch, E. W., Snijders, C. J., and van Vugt, A. B. (2004) "Triple pelvic ring fixation with severe pregnancy related low back and pelvic pain." *Spine 29*, 478-484.

Verstraete, E., Vanderstraeten, G., and Parewijck, W. (2013) "Pelvic girdle pain during or after pregnancy: A review of recent evidence and a clinical care path proposal." *Facts, Views and Vision. Issues in Obstetrics, Gynecology and Reproductive Health 5*, 1, 33-43.

Vleming, A., Schuenke, M., Masi, A., Carreiro, J., Danneels, L., and Willard, F. (2012) "The sacroiliac joint: An overview of its anatomy, function, and potential clinical implications." *Journal of Anatomy 221*, 6, 537-567.

Vollestad, N. and Stuge, B. (2009) "Prognostic factors for recovery from postpartum pelvic girdle pain." *European Spine Journal 18*, 718-726.

Wu, W. H., Meijer, O. G., Ugeki, K., Mens, A. M. A., *et al.* (2004) "Pregnancy-related pelvic girdle pain (PPP): I, Terminology, clinical presentation, and prevalence." *European Spine Journal 13*, 7, 575-589.

CHAPTER 8

Pelvic Organ Prolapse

This chapter will help to enlighten readers on the topic of pelvic organ prolapse (POP). Risk factors associated with pelvic floor dysfunction (PFD) and current paradigms in conservative care will be presented.

INTRODUCTION TO PELVIC ORGAN PROLAPSE

Pelvic organ prolapse (POP) is a pelvic health condition that is little known by the general public, and it can be surprising and even shocking to those who experience the condition (Box 8.1). It is primarily a postpartum condition characterized by the descent of the pelvic organs towards the vaginal and/or rectal opening. It can also occur in the non-birthing population. Most often, the bladder is lowered, also the rectum may be lowered and, less likely, is uterine descent (Hunskaar *et al.* 2005). Multiple therapeutic methods with movement, bodywork, and lifestyle habits can assist in healing this condition, yet in the most complex cases surgical support may be needed.

A view of therapeutic interventions may include:

- therapeutic exercise to strengthen weak lumbopelvic core muscles
- training synergy with the respiratory and pelvic diaphragms, and the lumbopelvic core
- ribcage, diaphragm, spine, hip, and abdominal wall mobilizations to reduce compression

- biotensegrity-focused soft tissue manual and visceral work
- decompression and gravity assist posturing and exercise programs
- functional fitness, ergonomics, and posture training
- training in pelvic floor equipment electrical stimulation, dilators, or wands.

Necessary medical intervention treatment may include:

- pharmaceuticals, typically hormone replacement therapy
- support devices; pessaries
- surgery to optimize organ positioning and functioning.

> **Box 8.1 Mind–body–spirit care with POP clients**
> Individuals presenting for POP treatment may be somewhat disembodied or numb from acknowledging sensations around the pelvic area, as a coping mechanism. They

may have catastrophic thinking when a "diagnosis" is initially made. They may have no knowledge about the prevalence of POP, and the potential benefits of conservative care. Education as to POP drivers and success stories can facilitate client engagement in a program.

Conservative care can be of tremendous help, yet it is typically not a "quick fix." Treatment requires a 3 D view of an individual and all their myofascial support systems.

POP terminology

Terms identifying the organ involved in POP include bladder: cystocele; uterus: uterine prolapse; and the rectum: rectocele. Additionally, there may be vaginal vault prolapse, and another type of POP with multiple tissue regions involved, termed enterocele (Figure 8.1). POP is most often recognized by the sufferer as a bulge sensation, or pelvic heaviness or pressure.

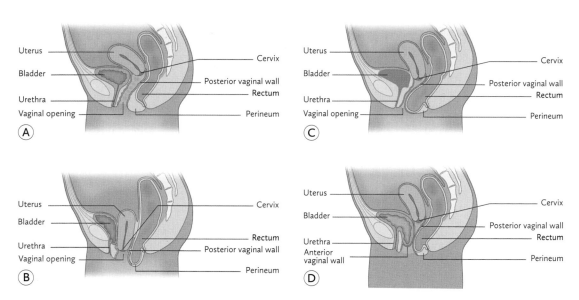

Figure 8.1 Prolapse types: A. Normal pelvic organ positioning; B. Entire prolapse of organs; C. Rectocele; D. Cystocele and rectocele.

Staging POP

POP may be medically graded in relation to organ descent towards or beyond the hymen. Stages I and II may not cause symptoms, but in stages III and IV there is a descent beyond the vaginal or rectal opening, with structures extending beyond the hymen. Stages III and IV create the presence of a visible bulge that causes multiple symptoms and may need surgery (Figure 8.2 and Boxes 8.2–8.4).

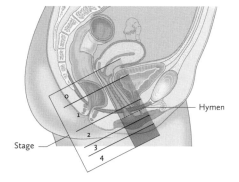

Figure 8.2 Prolapse staging.

Box 8.2 POP Q: specialty examination

More exacting testing by medical specialists uses the POP Q test. Exact ratings of POP are obtained via analysis of multiple measurements taken in relation to the descent of internal pelvic structures towards the hymen with the POP Q test (Bump *et al.* 1996; Madhu *et al.* 2018; Pham *et al.* 2011).

Box 8.3 A postpartum patient case: POP story

Monica had experienced a childbirth at age 36 with a 9 lb. baby, and then again at age 40 with a baby weighing 8 lb. 8 oz. Monica felt on odd pressure in her pelvic area postpartum baby no. 1, and it was infrequent but then more noticeable after baby no. 2. Her self-described "weird" symptoms at three months postpartum included pressure in the perineum in the vulvar and vaginal areas, with a sense of heaviness and bulging. This pressure sometimes turned into sharp pain in the perineum later in the day. She had to get off her feet and recline to reduce the discomfort. Sometimes her bladder leaked, sometimes it was hard to empty. Bowel function was strange for her as she noted sensations of incomplete emptying, pressure, and a bulge sensation with defecation, leading to severe straining. Sex was painful as she attempted to restore intimacy, and sometimes there was a new pressure sensation or obstruction that made things uncomfortable, even causing a sudden cessation of sexual activity at times. Her pelvic pressure feeling literally made her feel like her bottom was dropping out at times. She had to leave a postpartum workout due to pelvic pressure during squats and lunges. She recalls a sense of sadness and fatigue at this time, as well as shame, feeling she alone had these problems. In spite of all this, she remembers she was in the "love bubble" of new motherhood and felt such joy holding her babies, nursing over their first years of life, tending to all their needs, and being off work to embrace family life.

Box 8.4 Biopsychosocial (BPS) aspects of POP

From a BPS view, Monica was suffering with biological, social, and environmental factors, as well as psychological factors, all contributing to her pain and function loss. Biological changes included childbirth related pelvic floor myofascial trauma, and likely had hormone changes and vaginal atrophy postpartum, associated with nursing. Social factors included isolation due to inability to perform group exercise. Environmental factors included a lack of maternal health care education regarding POP and PFD, and a lack of postpartum doctor screening and intervention. Psychological elements included shame, depression, and lowered self-esteem. Monica was suffering from biological, environmental, psychological, and social factors in her postpartum "fourth trimester."

POP and PFD

POP symptoms may be very mild and cease over time as postpartum estrogen levels rise and the bladder, uterus, and bowel return to a higher position in the pelvic bowl, yet often there is asymptomatic prolapse. POP is considered as one type of PFD, yet there may be associated problems with pain, bladder, bowel, and sexual dysfunction. POP may cause other types of PFD, with tissue descent or bulge causing obstructed urination, defecation, and sexual activity. Individuals presenting for medical care for urinary incontinence, fecal incontinence, and pelvic pain should be screened for POP. Those with POP may also have low back pain (LBP), diastasis rectus abdominis, and pelvic girdle pain.

RISK FACTORS AND INCIDENCE RATES

POP is most often found in postpartum females, yet it may occur post gynecologic surgery such as hysterectomy (Palm 2017) and/or in the menopause transition. The risk for POP increases across the decades, with the incidence of 0.9 percent at ages 30–39, 2.8 percent at ages 40–49, 4.7 percent at ages 50–59, 7.5 percent at ages 60–69, and 11.1 percent at ages 70–79 (Olson *et al.* 1997).

Lifestyle/health history risk factors for POP include:

- a high impact activity profile
- heavy lifting demands (Woodman *et al.* 2006)
- multiparity, older age, large birth weight infant
- history of multiple abdominal surgeries.

Associated POP co-morbidities include:

- hypermobility syndromes (Al-Rawi and Al-Rawi 1982)
- constipation
- respiratory disease history (allergies, asthma, bronchitis, chronic cough)
- high BMI
- vaginal atrophy.

Perinatal factors

During pregnancy, mechanical and hormone factors combine to create a downward force on the pelvic organs, associated with a softening and lengthening of muscles and ligaments. There may be hidden pelvic nerve stretch or compression damage in the perinatal time frame (Bellews, Nitz, and Schoettelkotte 2015; Smith, Hosker, and Warrel 1989), in addition to muscle weakening and lengthening (Braekken *et al.* 2010; Smith *et al.* 1989; Vakali *et al.* 2005). Perinatal pelvic floor muscle and nerve injuries can cause pain, weakness, and loss of function.

Birth events which increase POP risk include large birth weight babies, long second stage labor, birth interventions such as vacuum extraction and/or forceps assistance, vaginal tearing or episiotomy, and multiparity. POP may occur post cesarean birth, but it is less likely. The demands for lifting and carrying of infants with a weakened, over-stretched pelvic floor can aggravate POP. Childcare challenges include frequent bending, squatting, and lifting.

Studies of intra-abdominal pressure have found that the greatest pressure is generated in lifting with a squat from the floor level, versus receiving weight transferred into the arms when upright (Gerten *et al.* 2008). Limiting full squats or training the lumbopelvic core for this function should be part of postpartum training.

Vaginal atrophy

Nursing is advocated as the optimum method for infant nutrition care as well as maternal–child bonding, yet temporary reductions in circulating hormones, notably estrogen, are associated with vaginal atrophy (VA) and POP. Similar hormone reductions occur at menopause and are associated with increased incidence of POP in that time frame. VA is identified with perineal tissue inspection, and it involves a loss of tissue strength, elasticity, and hydration, recognized anatomically as a thinning of the epithelial layer of the urogenital triangle, and associated tissue reddening and heightened pain receptors firing with touch, pressure, and stretch. VA is associated with pelvic pain and may appear as a burning, sharp, stinging sensation with attempted sexual relations (Goetsch 1999). VA can be treated, at a doctor's discretion, with estrogen. With the cessation of nursing and a return of menses, VA can lessen as estrogen levels stabilize (Box 8.5).

> **Box 8.5 Natural healing, for some**
> POP can resolve somewhat from status at birth and early postpartum into the cessation of nursing.

Women often struggle with weight retention postpartum. Higher weight is associated with POP in some studies (Hunskaar *et al.* 2005), yet central adiposity may impact the risk more than BMI score alone (Gerten *et al.* 2008).

Genetics are associated with POP. A twin study (Buschbaum *et al.* 2006) of parous and nulliparous older twins found similar levels of POP in the post-menopausal time frame.

Hypermobility syndromes and the associated ligamentous laxity create an increased risk for POP. A study of those with the connective tissue disorder Ehlers-Danlos syndrome identified an incidence rate of POP surgery in those with a mean age of 46 at a 38 percent prevalence compared with POP surgery in the general population at 16 percent (Smith *et al.* 1989) (Box 8.6).

> **Box 8.6 Anatomic changes**
> **in the levator ani**
> The levator ani (LA) muscle group is a supporting sling from the pubic bone, sweeping posterior to the ischium, ilium bones, and sacrum. The LA supports the bladder, uterus, and bowel. The intersection of the left and right sides of the LA forms a V-shaped myofascial landmark, the hiatus. The levator hiatus demonstrates a lengthening, widening, and lowering postpartum (Braekken *et al.* 2010; Friedman *et al.* 2015; Vakili *et al.* 2005). The levator hiatus is the focal point for research on structural changes in PFM that are associated with POP.

POP SIGNS AND SYMPTOMS

Many women have asymptomatic POP. One study found symptoms of POP were reported at 3–6 percent, whereas on examination POP was diagnosed at 41–50 percent (Barber and Maher 2013). Symptoms may be subtle with an occasional sensation of pressure or bulge, or a sense of heaviness. As POP advances, there may be a more profound presentation with discomfort sitting and walking, due to the "bulge." Women may "feel or visually observe a bulge as something coming out of the vagina, have difficulty inserting a tampon, and have sensations of heaviness, pressure, fullness or aching, most often during physical activity" (Womenshealth.gov 2019). A sense of "bother" has been identified as the concern that leads women to seek treatment (Hunskaar *et al.* 2005).

EVALUATION

POP screening: nosy questions
Individuals with PFD symptoms should be questioned as to specific symptoms (partial list).

- Is a pressure or bulge felt or noticed?
- Is there a sensation of heaviness?
- Is there a need to strain and/or perform

digital splinting or pressure to assist urination or defecation?

- Is there any feeling of incomplete bladder or bowel emptying?
- Do they need a special maneuver to allow for emptying?

Women may feel shame and have difficulties relating to others and divulging POP symptoms to health care providers (Dunivan *et al.* 2014) (Box 8.7).

> **Box 8.7 Medical screening details**
>
> The above items and other symptoms are screened in the pelvic floor distress inventory (PFDI) which covers urinary distress, pelvic organ distress, and colorectal distress (Barber *et al.* 2011). The PFDI is a valid and reliable tool for identifying symptoms and tracking change over time.

After history and symptom screening such as the PFDI, a provider may proceed with an examination of posture, respiration patterns and rib/thoracic mobility, spinal and hip flexibility and strength, and then perineal and pelvic floor muscle (PFM) assessment.

Pelvic examination

Pelvic examination includes visual inspection of the perineum, assessment of sensation, the presence of spasm, tenderness, or pain, and/or referred pain, and a PFM test strength. A general assessment for the level of prolapse may be performed, with the examiner noting the presence of a bulge in the anterior wall, typically the bladder, a bulge in the center of the vaginal column, typically the uterus, and/or a bulge in the posterior wall, the rectal area. Symptoms may be tested with a cough, and a bearing down or Valsalva as if straining to eliminate, and observe for a bulge. Real time ultrasound is also used in assessment and may indicate correct effort or dyssynergia during attempted PFM contraction. (POP staging and/or the POP Q test is performed by specialists as in the prior descriptions.)

Client goals

The client's functional limitations such as activity restrictions may all be used to create short and long-term goals with a plan of care with the client's input on their key issues or concerns, and their key functional goals. Women may feel shame and have difficulties relating to others and divulging POP symptoms to providers (Dunivan *et al.* 2014) (Box 8.8).

POP TREATMENT

Education and resources for POP

Following an evaluation, a treatment plan is developed which may include:

- education and habit training on reducing downward pressure into the abdomen, with great attention to respiratory and PFM synergy
- strengthening the lumbar, pelvic, hip, and abdominal myofascial systems in a progressive format
- training in optimal body mechanics and posture
- addressing strategies for community and recreation participation
- teamwork with the doctor regarding pharmaceutical, pessary, and/or surgical options

- education and support in the use of an Impressa® bladder support device, soft cup, or pessary
- discussion regarding surgical options and benefits/risks/preparation considerations
- addressing psychosocial factors as needed/referrals.

Box 8.8 Self-care strategy

Those struggling with POP may tell others they have a "hernia" to avoid having to share private matters, as well as to avoid requests for heavy lifting and other exertional tasks. (POP is not technically a hernia, and the term hernia is not used by specialty providers for describing POP.)

Therapeutic exercise for POP

Accurate PFM training is a foundation of POP treatment. Neuromuscular re-education in multiple positions is necessary to optimize the synergy between the PFM and the respiratory diaphragm.

Borello-France *et al.* (2007) found that there is a correlation of less severe prolapse with higher pelvic muscle testing scores, and higher levels of prolapse with weaker individuals. A study (Braekken *et al.* 2010) demonstrated a lift of the levator hiatus following six months of specific pelvic floor muscle training therapy, including 18 PT sessions. The bladder was elevated 3 mm and the rectum 4–5 mm. This study points towards a resilience model for improving the position of the levator hiatus, utilizing RUSI, and conservative care with extensive exercise training support (Box 8.9).

Box 8.9 Research supports exercise for POP

In the text *Evidence-Based Physical Therapy for the Pelvic Floor* (2015), Bø et al. found exercise and conservative care studies demonstrated improved POP staging as assessed via POP Q, reduced bother, reduced sensation of bulge, increased PFM strength, and improved quality of life.

HYPOPRESSIVE EXERCISE

The hypopressive exercise technique may be useful to assist PFM training, and in theory help reduce POP. The abdominal hypopressive technique (AHT) is described as used more in European countries currently (Stupp *et al.* 2011) (Box 8.10). (See Chapter 6.)

Box 8.10 Hypopressive and pelvic exercise benefits

Bernardes *et al.* (2012) studied POP, and standard PFM exercise versus hypopressive exercise. Results included an increased cross-sectional anatomy of the levator ani after 12 weeks of exercise in a PFM strengthening group, as well as a hypopressive exercise group, as measured by ultrasound, compared to a control population (Bernardes *et al.* 2012). There may be similar benefits in anatomical changes that improve structural support from a standard PFM strengthening as well as a hypopressive program.

The following photos illustrate exercises that may benefit postural alignment, strength, neuromuscular control, and reduce intra-abdominal pressure through optimum core control, for the client with POP (Figures 8.3–8.15). Additionally, decompression during rest and/or exercise can help reduce POP symptoms in some individuals (sample):

YOGA AND EXERCISE FOR POP

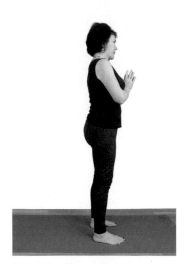

Figure 8.3 Mountain.

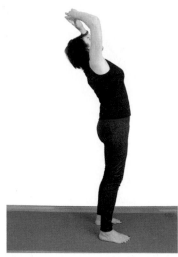

Figure 8.4 Back bow.

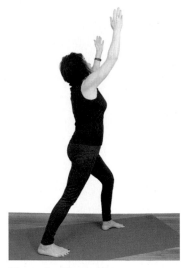

Figure 8.5 Warrior I.

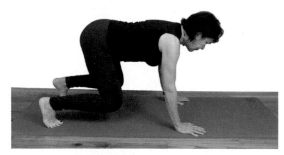

Figure 8.6 Down dog preparation.

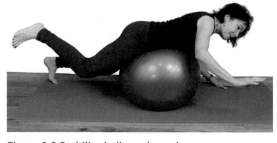

Figure 8.8 Stability ball quadruped.

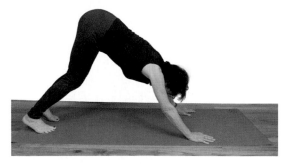

Figure 8.7 Down dog.

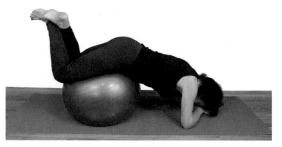

Figure 8.9 Child's pose, supported hips on ball.

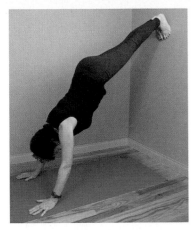

Figure 8.10 Handstand.

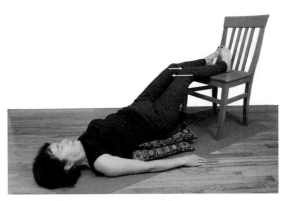

Figure 8.13 Decompression and exercise, rolling legs in.

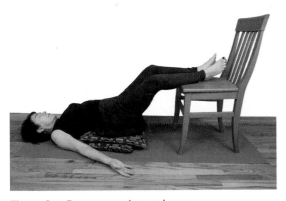

Figure 8.11 Decompression and rest.

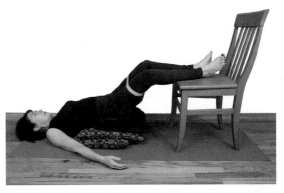

Figure 8.14 Decompression and resistive exercise.

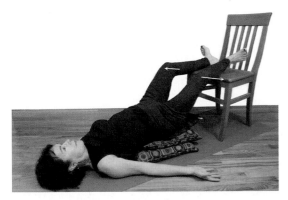

Figure 8.12 Decompression and exercise, rolling legs out.

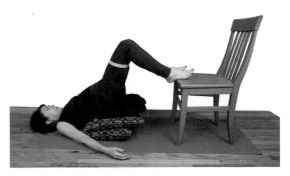

Figure 8.15 Decompression, hip bridge, and resistance exercise.

PILATES

Pilates has great application for treatment of POP as it is a low impact workout that can be energizing and also centering. Routines on the mat or reformer can create a sense of flow, and advancement to standing closed chain hip abduction and adduction can engage adductors and PFM, TRA, and multifidus in holding and eccentric/concentric work.

BIOFEEDBACK AND ELECTRICAL STIMULATION

Modalities such as biofeedback and/or electrical stimulation can help train, strengthen, and guide a correct PFM exercise practice protocol. Biofeedback can monitor external and/or internal PFM contraction and train quick flick and endurance contractions. Electrical stimulation can help weak muscles engage and up train for endurance contractions, typically sets of 10–30 second holds to build endurance. These modalities are validated as assisting prolapse rehabilitation yet are not stand-alone POP treatments (Ahadi *et al.* 2017; Yang *et al.* 2017). Models are available for home rental use or purchase (currentmedicaltechnology.com, perifit.co), as well as progressive vaginal weights for strengthening (intimaterose.com).

DECOMPRESSION AND POP

Historically, women have used inversion positioning to reduce POP. Clinically, some women report that during their exercises in positions with the hips elevated (such as down dog) they note a sense of a shift internally that may last for hours following the practice (Box 8.11). In this regard, exercise and decompression have the potential to reduce the main symptom of POP, which is a sensation of a bulge (Figure 8.16).

> ### Box 8.11 Bottoms up for POP self-care
> A sense of a "shift" internally may last for hours following recumbent/inversion

exercise. POP symptoms may be cumulative over a few days' time, and recumbent and inversion postures may also help to provide rest and to recharge energy levels.

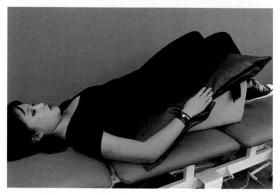

Figure 8.16 Decompression with a wedge and pillows.

Individualized decompression instruction may utilize gravity assist to help reduce pressure and perhaps even shift organs superiorly, for 5 to 15 minutes, once to a few times per week. However, women working full time with careers and/or household management and childcare may not have time for decompression/inversion protocols and may need pessary use and/or surgery to allow a high impact lifestyle.

Pessaries and other support devices

Pessaries are devices that are worn internally in the vaginal canal to provide support (Figure 8.17 and Box 8.12). Pessaries are the preferred method of non-surgical treatment of POP, yet not all women are candidates for pessaries due to anatomical variances in ability to retain the pessary comfortably, and some cannot independently insert and remove the pessary. Pessaries are similar to an orthotic in a shoe to assist foot alignment, and they have been used since recorded medical history (Shah, Sultan, and Thakar 2006). They represent a relatively low cost, low risk treatment for POP as well as stress urinary incontinence.

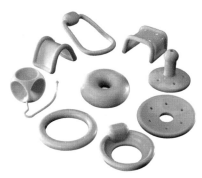

Figure 8.17 Pessary devices.
Image provided courtesy of CooperSurgical, Inc.

Box 8.12 Pessary use for POP

Pessary utilization may assist the individual with POP via mechanical support to limit distension, drop, or bulge. A pessary is usually made of silicone that is inserted vaginally by a specialty provider. Varied shapes are offered and tried for comfort and retention. Shapes include rings, cubes, and other options. Some women may self-insert the pessary for pelvic health self-care. Women unable to insert or remove a pessary visit their doctor for monthly or less frequent pessary removal, pelvic re-evaluation, pessary cleaning, and re-insertion.

Vaginal estrogen may be prescribed to assist tissue health with pessary use, and it may lead to greater satisfaction and longer term pessary use (Dessie *et al.* 2016; Harvey-Springer 2019).

PESSARY CHALLENGES

A recent review (de Albuquerque Coelho, de Castro, and Juliato 2016) found that "the pessary can produce a positive effect on women's quality of life and can significantly improve sexual function and body perception." However, researchers found a median rate of pessary discontinuation at 49.1 percent. Problems included discomfort, inability to apply and remove the pessary, inability

to retain the pessary, and a desire for surgery. Yang *et al.* (2018) identified lack of success with pessaries correlating with higher symptom rating on the colorectal section of the PFDI.

Other devices that may provide support in the case of mild prolapse include the tampon-like Impressa® bladder support device and/or the soft cup. Health care provider instruction in POP support devices is advised to optimize comfort and present complications such as tissue erosion or toxic shock syndrome which can be associated with pessary use.

Splinting and perineal support to assist function

Women with POP may be able to use perineal pressure, and even internal vaginal support or "splinting," to assist in bladder, bowel, or pessary control (Haylen *et al.* 2016; Palm 2017). Specific techniques may be instructed by a pelvic health care provider and found in the text *Pelvic Organ Prolapse: The Silent Epidemic* (Palm 2017).

MANUAL THERAPY

Manual therapy can facilitate muscle awareness, neuromuscular re-education, and reduce restrictions in tissue from scars and myofascial changes associated with childbirth (Chaitow and Lovegrove Jones 2012) (Box 8.13). Visceral mobilization for organ specific mobility can assist in balancing myofascial planes across three dimensions, and this can be beneficial in some cases of POP (see Chapter 4, Box 4.24). Visceral mobilization for POP is clinically helpful, and is based on the embryologic origins of structures, as explained by Ramona Horton (2015).

> ### Box 8.13 Facilitating the PFM
> Sometimes women cannot fully contract their PFM and obtain a "lift" during attempted exercise; this can be observed to change to an improved status with even one session of manual myofascial and visceral therapy work.

BIOTENSEGRITY MANUAL WORK

Recent evidence portrays a remarkable case series where over 80 percent of patients with POP benefitted from manual therapy with a biotensegrity focused approach (Crowle and Harley 2021). Staging of POP was improved in these cases, with 36 percent attaining a "complete recovery of organ position and shape." Biotensegrity considers a multidimensional web of compression and tensile elements that is dynamic and adaptable. The researchers utilized biotensegrity principles to treat areas of stiffness, such as episiotomy scars, with myofascial release. This is the first research on this method to appear in a case series on POP.

Surgery for POP

Women may require surgery for POP (Box 8.14). Surgical results may be positive and allow improved function and quality of life. The American Urogynecology Society (AUGS) advocates for advanced female pelvic reconstruction training of surgeons, as well as teamwork collaboration with other health care providers for patient support. Optimal preparation for surgery would include pelvic floor muscle strengthening, vaginal estrogen if indicated, cessation of high impact activity,

addressing constipation and bowel health, and a pessary trial. However, the current need for repeat surgery for POP stands at 29.2 percent (Olson *et al.* 1997).

> ### Box 8.14 Vital surgery for some individuals
> Surgical methods require the use of mesh, as pelvic muscles and ligaments cannot be suspended by sutures alone. Yet mesh types vary and there may be complications. The patient support group Association for Pelvic Organ Prolapse (APOPS) recognizes the necessity of certain types of mesh that are necessary in specialty surgery in the case of lax "native" connective tissue, and advocates for continued use (AUGS Practice Bulletin 2017).

Ideally, comprehensive conservative care practices are offered and implemented prior to treatment. Factors such as high impact sport, frequent Valsalva with exertion, constipation, weak PFM, scar tissue, estrogen deficiencies and associated muscle weakness, and frequent prolonged flexed postures can all create pressure into the pelvic organs and are aggravating factors for POP (Boxes 8.15 and 8.16).

> ### Box 8.15 Patient case: Monica
> Monica received specialty pelvic therapy when her second child was one year old; she was shocked to find out her pelvic muscle strength was 1/5! She was trained in PFM, TRA, and multifidus strengthening, as well as body mechanics and decompression options. She reports 90% reduced POP related bulge symptoms. She also was prescribed vaginal estrogen 2 x a week. She uses pressure reduction with a recumbent exercise, as well

as the use of inversion postures with yoga. She was prescribed a pessary and needed to try three types until she found a comfortable style. She self-manages the insertion and removal of the pessary based on her activity level. However, if she sits bent over her computer for hours, and walks a few hours several days in a row, as well as developing constipation, and not using her pessary, the bulge sensation can return. She felt the "total program" for her success included the combined PFM/core training, lifting mechanics, postural attention, nutritional and behavioral changes to reduce constipation, and minimal dose hormone replacement.

Box 8.16 Critical self-care

Moms have to be heroes for self-care, for making it to treatment in the midst of their own family life chaos and schedule demands, as well as enduring pain and functional activity loss.

FOURTH TRIMESTER CHALLENGES

The barriers are high to receiving postpartum care via the health care system (Matambanadzo 2014; Tully, Stuebe, and Verbiest 2017) due to lack of education and limited to no programming standards for perinatal conditions. A mom's self-care is typically low priority in the blur of the fourth trimester, and onward into toddler and childcare needs. Postpartum clients with PFD such as POP may present at any stage, from new motherhood, perimenopause, or later.

SUMMARY

POP treatment may be complex; however, expert conservative care may reduce symptoms (Braekken 2010; Hagen and Stark 2011; Wiegersma *et al.* 2017) and even optimize organ positioning, mobility, and function (Crowle and Harley 2021). Women may develop self-care and fitness routines for POP that enhance their general health and wellness throughout their life. Care providers are encouraged to consider a resilience model with POP and utilize team members to optimize care. Pelvic health providers can experience great satisfaction in offering education and paths for healing for each individual woman presenting for treatment.

REFERENCES

Ahadi, T., Taghvasdoost, N., Aminimoghaddam, S., Forogh, B., *et al.* (2017) "Efficacy of biofeedback on quality of life in stages I and II pelvic organ prolapse: A pilot study." *European Journal of Gynecology and Reproductive Biology* 215, 242–246.

Al-Rawi, Z. and Al-Rawi, T. (1982) "Joint hypermobility in women with genital prolapse." *The Lancet 319*, 8287, 1439–1441.

AUGS (2017) "Pelvic organ prolapse, female pelvic medicine and reconstructive surgery." *Practice Bulletin 23*, 4.

Barber, M. D. and Maher, C. (2013) "Epidemiology and outcome assessment of pelvic organ prolapse." *International Urogynecology Journal 24*, 1783–1790.

Barber, M. D., Chen, Z., Lukacz, E., Markland, A., *et al.* (2011) "Further validation of the short version of the pelvic floor distress inventory (PFDI) and pelvic floor impact questionnaire (PFIQ)." *Neurourology and Urodynamics 30*, 4, 541–546.

Bellews, J., Nitz, A., and Schoettelkotte, B. (2015) "Postpartum femoral nerve palsy: A case study and the role of electrophysiologic testing and neuromuscular electrical stimulation." *Journal of Women's Health Physical Therapy 39*, 3, 109–114.

Bernardes, B., Resende, A., Stupp, L., Oliveira, E., *et al.* (2012) "Efficacy of pelvic floor muscle training and hypopressive exercises for treating pelvic organ prolapse in women; a randomized controlled trial." *Sao Paulo Medical Journal 130*, 1, 5–9.

Bø, K., Berghmans, B., Morkved, S., and Van Kampen, M. (2015) *Evidence-Based Physical Therapy for the Pelvic Floor, Bridging Science into Clinical Practice.* London: Elsevier.

Borello-France, D., Handa, V., Brown, M., Goode, P., *et al.* (2007) "Pelvic floor muscle function in women with pelvic organ prolapse." *Physical Therapy and Rehabilitation Journal 87*, 4, 399–407.

Braekken, I., Majida, M., Engh, M., and Bo, K. (2010) "Can pelvic floor muscle training reverse pelvic organ prolapse and reduce prolapse symptoms? An assessor blinded, randomized controlled trial." *American Journal of Obstetrics and Gynecology 203*, 2, 170–177.

Bump, R. C., Mattiasson, A., Bø, K., Brubaker, L. P., *et al.* (1996) "The standardization of terminology of female pelvic organ prolapse and pelvic floor dysfunction." *American Journal of Obstetrics and Gynecology 175*, 10–17.

Buschbaum, G. M., Duecy, E., Kerr, L., Huang, L., Perevich, M., and Guzick, D. (2006) "Incontinence and pelvic organ prolapse in parous/nulliparous pairs of identical twins." *Obstetrics and Gynecology 108*, 6, 1388–1393.

Chaitow, L. and Lovegrove Jones, R. (2012) *Chronic Pelvic Pain and Dysfunction, Practical Physical Medicine.* Edinburgh: Churchill Livingstone.

Crowle, A. and Harley, C. (2021) "Biotensegrity focused therapy for pelvic organ prolapse: A nonrandomized prospective clinical case series." *Journal of Women's Health Physical Therapy 45*, 3, 135–142.

de Albuquerque Coelho, S. C., de Castro, E. B., and Juliato, C. R. T. (2016) "Female pelvic organ prolapse using pessaries: A systematic review." *International Urogynecology Journal 27*, 1797–1803.

Dessie, S. G., Armstrong, K., Modest, A. M., Hacker, M. R., and Hota, L. S. (2016) "Effect of vaginal estrogen on pessary use." *International Urogynecology Journal 27*, 9, 1423–1429.

Dunivan, G., Anger, J., Alas, A., Weislander, C., *et al.* (2014) "Pelvic organ prolapse: A disease of silence and shame." *Female Pelvic Medicine and Reconstructive Surgery 20*, 6, 322–327.

Friedman, B., Slothers, L., Lazare, D., and MacNab, A. (2015) "Positional pelvic organ prolapse evaluation using open, weight-bearing magnetic resource imaging." *Canadian Urological Association Journal 9*, 5–6, 197–201.

Gerten, K., Richter, H., Wheeler, T., Pair, L., *et al.* (2008) "Intra-abdominal pressure changes associated with lifting: Implications for postoperative activity restrictions." *American Journal of Obstetrics and Gynecology 198*, 3, P306.E1–306.E5.

Goetsch, M. (1999) "Postpartum dyspareunia: An unexplored problem." *Journal of Reproductive Medicine 44*, 11, 963–968.

Hagen, S. and Stark, D. (2011) "Conservative prevention and management of pelvic organ prolapse in women." *Cochrane Database of Systematic Reviews 12*, CD003882.

Harvey-Springer, R. (2019) "Pessary—Tips and Tricks." Urogynecology for the Advanced Provider, AUGS, The LINE Hotel, Austin, April 11–13, 2019.

Haylen, B., Maher, C., Barber, M. C., Camargo, S., *et al.* (2016) "An International Urogynecological Association (IUGA)/International Continence Society (ICS) joint report on the terminology for female pelvic organ prolapse (POP)." *International Urogynecology Journal 27*, 165–194.

Horton, R. C. (2015) "Clinical review: The anatomy, biological plausibility, and efficacy of visceral mobilization in the treatment of pelvic floor dysfunction." *Journal of Pelvic, Obstetric and Gynecological Physiotherapy 117*, 5–18.

Hunskaar, S., Burgio, K., Clark, A., Lapitan, M., *et al.* (2005) "Epidemiology of Urinary Incontinence (UI) and Faecal Incontinence (FI) and Pelvic Organ Prolapse (POP)." 3rd International Consultation on Incontinence and International Continence Society, Montréal, QC, Canada.

Madhu, C., Swift, S., Maloney-Geany, S., and Drake, M. J. (2018) "How to use the pelvic organ prolapse quantification (POP-Q) system?" *Neurology and Urodynamics Sounding Board 37*, S6.

Matambanadzo, S. (2014) "The Fourth Trimester." *University of Michigan Journal on Law Reform 48*, 1, 117. http://repository.law.umich.edu/mjlr/vol48/iss1/3

Olson, A., Smith, V., Bergstrom, J., Colling, J., and Clark, A. (1997) "Epidemiology of surgically managed pelvic organ prolapse and urinary incontinence." *Obstetrics and Gynecology 89*, 4, 501–506.

Palm, S. (2017) *Pelvic Organ Prolapse: The Silent Epidemic*, 3rd ed. Atlanta: POP Publishing and Distribution.

Pham, T., Burgart, A., Keller, K., Mueller, E. R., *et al.* (2011) "Current use of pelvic organ prolapse quantification by AUGS and ICS members." *Female Pelvic Medicine Reconstructive Surgery 17*, 67–69.

Shah, S. M., Sultan, A. H., and Thakar, R. (2006) "The history and evolution of pessaries for pelvic organ prolapse." *International Urogynecology Journal Pelvic Floor Dysfunction 17*, 2, M170–175.

Smith, A., Hosker, G., and Warrel, D. (1989) "The role of partial denervation of the pelvic floor in the aetiology of genitourinary prolapse and stress incontinence of urine. A neurophysiological study." *British Journal of Obstetrics and Gynecology 96*, 24.

Stupp, L., Resende, A., Petricelli, C., Nakamura, M., Alexandre, S., and Zanetti, M. (2011) "Pelvic floor muscle and transversus abdominis activation in abdominal hypopressive technique through electromyography." *Neurourology and Urodynamics 30*, 8, 1518–1521.

Tully, K., Stuebe, A., and Verbiest, S. (2017) "The fourth trimester: A critical transition period with unmet maternal needs." *American Journal of Obstetrics and Gynecology 217*, 1, 37–44.

Vakili, B., Zeheng, Y. T., Loesch, H., Echols, K. T., *et al.* (2005) "Levator contraction strength and genital hiatus as risk factors for recurrent pelvic organ prolapse." *American Journal of Obstetrics and Gynecology 192*, 1592–1598.

Wiegersma, M., Panman, C. M., Berger, M. Y., De Vet, H. C. W., *et al.* (2017) "Minimally important change in the pelvic floor distress inventory—20 among women opting for conservative prolapse treatment." *American Journal of Obstetrics and Gynecology 216*, 4, 397.E1–397.E7.

Womenshealth.gov (2019) "A fact sheet from the Office of Women's Health: Pelvic organ prolapse." Available at https://owh-wh-d9-dev.s3.amazonaws.com/s3fs-public/documents/fact-sheet-pelvic-organ-prolapse.pdf.

Woodman, P. J., Swift, S. E., O'Boyle, A. L., Valley, M. T., *et al.* (2006) "Prevalence of severe pelvic organ prolapse in relation to job description and socioeconomic status: A multicenter cross-sectional study." *International Urogynecology Journal 17*, 340–345.

Yang, J., Han, J., Zhu, F., and Wang, Y. (2018) "Ring and Gellhorn pessaries used in patients with pelvic organ prolapse: A retrospective study of 8 years." *Archives of Gynecology and Obstetrics 298*, 3, 623–629.

Yang, S., Sang, W., Feng, J., Zhao, H., Li, X., *et al.* (2017) "The effect of rehabilitation exercises combined with direct vagina low voltage low frequency electric stimulation on pelvic nerve electrophysiology and tissue function in primiparous women: A randomized controlled trial." *Journal of Clinical Nursing 26*, 23–24.

FURTHER RESOURCES

CMT (2022) Accessed 5/1/2022 at https://www.cmtmedical.com.

Kegel Exercises: A Complete Guide (2022) Accessed 5/1/2022 at https://www.intimaterose.com/pages/how-to-do-kegel-exercises.

Pelvic Organ Prolapse Quantification (POP-Q) System (2022) Accessed 5/1/2022 at https://www.physio-pedia.com/Pelvic_Organ_Prolapse_Quantification_(POP-Q)_System.

Perifit (2022) Accessed 5/1/2022 at https://perifit.co.

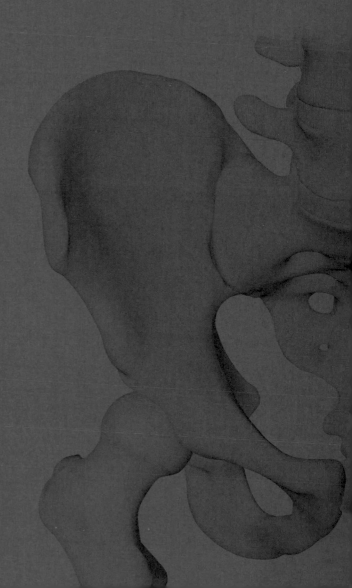

PELVIC CHALLENGES AND HEALTH ACROSS THE AGES

CHAPTER 9

Urinary Incontinence

This chapter presents the varied types of urinary incontinence: UI. Paradigms for UI screening, evaluation, and treatment options are portrayed. Key lifestyle habits and pelvic floor muscle training will be presented for readers to gain self-care and client care options.

UI is a common, yet troubling, condition entailing the involuntary loss of urine. It is a myth that it is just a problem for old folks. However, it is a major factor in family decisions to place elders in nursing homes. UI affects women more than men, due to anatomic and endocrine influences, as well as the myofascial stresses of pregnancy and childbearing. UI occurs in 26 percent of female athletes, and up to 75 percent for those in high impact sports (Pires *et al.* 2020). Males are more likely to experience UI at older ages, due to a combination of factors.

Incontinence occurs in women with increasing frequency over the lifespan, affecting 17 percent of women over age 20, 37.5 percent at ages 30–50, and in elderly women in nursing homes, up to 77 percent (Lukacz *et al.* 2017). Sadly, most UI is untreated, with 75 percent not seeking care, and of those seeking medical care (25%), less than half are provided with screening and intervention (Lukacz *et al.* 2017) (Box 9.1).

> **Box 9.1 Private shame, lack of care**
>
> It is common for women to not seek care, possibly due to their ease and convenience with continence pad use (prior experience with menses), but also due to factors such as shame and a lack of confidence, as well as medical providers' lack of training and skill.

CO-MORBIDITIES AND UI

Obesity, depression, constipation, sleep apnea, alcohol, and tobacco use are all risks for UI. Conditions such as multiple sclerosis, Parkinson's disease, cancer, and diabetes are also associated with increased risk for UI. Autoimmune conditions such as interstitial cystitis and fibromyalgia have greater incidence of UI. Males and females may have sphincter injuries, spinal cord injuries, stroke, dementia, and other factors that can cause UI. Non-neurologic conditions include benign prostatic hypertrophy, bladder dysfunction (over or under active), urinary tract infection (UTI), and combined side effects of medications (polypharmacy) (Hester, Kretschmer, and Badlani 2017).

Associated complications of UI can include:
- skin irritation, bacterial overgrowth, and infections from continence pad use

- reduced activities for fear of leaks; reduced ADL, work, social, community, and recreational participation

- surgical intervention and postoperative aggravation of symptoms.

UI AND INFECTIONS

Bladder infections may aggravate the bladder walls and urethra and cause pain and leakage. Infections can spread to the kidneys and overall sepsis may occur, requiring hospitalization and multiple drug interventions. Balance problems may be associated with bladder infections and immune system challenges that are systemic. Medical intervention is critical to target infectious organisms and support recovery.

DEFINITIONS: TYPES OF UI

1. *Stress UI (SUI):* The involuntary urine loss with exertion. Rises in intra-abdominal pressure during laughing, coughing, sneezing, or exercise override the closure (shut off mechanism) of the bladder and urethra, creating leaks (Figure 9.1)
2. *Urge UI (UUI):* The sudden onset of a need to urinate, followed by an involuntary loss of urine (Figure 9.2)
3. *Mixed UI:* A combination of SUI and UUI symptoms
4. *Overflow UI:* Urine loss due to incomplete bladder emptying. Causes include poor bladder muscle (detrusor) contractility, and/or outlet obstruction leading to overflow
5. *Functional UI:* UI due to lack of sufficient mobility to make it to the toilet, and/or physical barriers to making it to a toilet.

(Khandelwal and Kistler 2013)

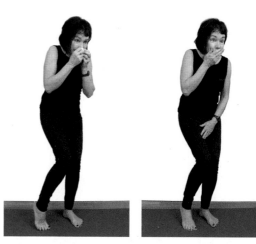

Figure 9.1 Sneeze SUI.   Figure 9.2 Urge UI.

OVERVIEW: URINARY INCONTINENCE SCREENING

Screening questions as to the nature of the leaks, the amount, and continence pad use help create a profile of the incontinence (Box 9.2). Activity of daily living (ADL), work, community, and recreation/sports limitations are screened. Sleep disturbance from nocturia (needing to urinate at night) is assessed. Childbirth history, surgeries, medication use, bowel profile (Bristol stool scale), and other health items are screened. Health history may reveal the onset and cause of the incontinence, and/or aggravating factors. The urination method can be questioned: Does the individual sit and relax the pelvic floor muscles (PFM) during urination, or do they hover over the toilet (females in a partial squat) or force urine out (females and/or males) with a bear down/ Valsalva?

- Is the individual able to breathe during PFM engagement?
- Is synergy present with the PFM and the diaphragm, such as an inhale and PFM relaxation, and an exhale and PFM contraction?
- Is dyssynergia present, a bearing down during attempted contraction?
- Is a global clenching of muscles present?
- Is pain present?

> **Box 9.2 Urinary distress**
> Outcome measures such as the urinary distress inventory (UDI) may be used to clarify symptoms and distress (Oregon Health & Science University 2019; Utomo *et al.* 2015).

Can they stop the flow?

A simple question may be asked: Are you able to stop and start your urine flow? Individuals receiving bladder treatment are often asked to provide a urine sample for their doctor, and they typically know if they can perform this "stop" function. (The stop/start of urine flow should not be used for bladder training as it disrupts the synergy between the bladder and PFM.) Those that can stop the flow have some awareness and control of their PFM.

How do they move and breathe?

Overall mobility, such as sit to stand performance, gait, posture, strength, respiratory function (rib/ diaphragm excursion), and range of motion are viewed for limitations.

Specialty testing with equipment

Testing with biofeedback and/or real time ultrasound (RUSI) can elucidate (Box 9.3):

- Is the individual able to contract the PFM, to hold the contraction, and to relax fully?

> **Box 9.3 Ultrasound imaging**
> **and biofeedback**
> With RUSI we view the bladder from the area above the pubic bone, and clients may stay dressed. A trans-perineal view may be used, requiring disrobing. With biofeedback, sensors are placed on the surface of the PFM externally, or internally in the vagina or rectum. Electrical signals from nerve firing during muscle contractions are picked up by sensors (electrodes), which via software programming are turned into a visual display. Feedback from muscle contraction versus relaxation may be viewed as a line graph, bar graph, smiling or sad face, a flower opening or closing, and other symbols. Both these modalities help empower awareness and control and are often fun for clients to use. Home biofeedback units are available as well. However, home biofeedback devices may be more challenging than performing an exercise protocol following expert instruction (Dufour *et al.* 2019). A recent review found PFM supervised exercise as superior to the use of biofeedback and other modalities (Abrams *et al.* 2017).

Incorrect effort and leakage

Research with the PFM and bladder control identifies incontinent women as having weaker PFM, less endurance, and even an incorrect effort. An incorrect effort visible on RUSI is bladder neck depression from downward pressure during attempted contraction. Correct contractions create a lift of the bladder and elongation of the bladder neck in a superior direction. The researchers state, "The observation that many women were performing PFM exercises incorrectly reinforces the need for individual PFM assessment with a skilled practitioner" (Thompson *et al.* 2006).

Direct testing of PFM

The PFM may be directly tested by specialist (Box 9.4), and this helps to decipher:

- Weakness: Are the PFM too weak, too loose, and unable to contract?
- Shortened, hypomobile: Are the PFM too tight, with no myofascial mobility, and unable to contract, lift, relax, or distend? This may be a "short pelvic floor."
- Is there tenderness, pain, or spasm present?

Box 9.4 Manual testing of PFM 👓

A manual muscle test may be provided with digital palpation directly to the internal PFM, with grading of 0–5 on the Oxford scale (Thompson *et al.* 2006). An alternative format is to use the International Continence Society rating with phrases that identify the muscles as "non-contracting" or "non-relaxing" PFM. With a non-relaxing PFM, an individual may contract and then lock up, not being able to relax. Non-contracting = 0 on the Oxford scale (ics.org). A strong PFM group can contract and lift up and in and hold for 5–10 seconds or more: Grade 5 on the Oxford scale.

Indication for necessary visceral work?

External and internal myofascial structures and organs can be assessed for their stiffness, glide, and balance with surrounding local, as well as distant, structures. Organ mobility testing and treatment can be performed with external and/or internal work, including bi-manual palpation and treatment. During visceral work, myofascial locations can be mapped and these enhance client awareness and appreciation of sensations, such as tenderness/stiffness in the obturator foramen and associated bladder sensations. Interested readers are referred to courses and textbooks, such as *Urogenital Manipulation* (Barral 2006).

TREATMENT OVERVIEW

Conservative care practices should be the first line of treatment, and strategies are presented here emphasizing education, lifestyle, habit training, pelvic floor muscle (PFM) exercise, nutrition, and manual therapy.

Treatment planning: up train or down train?

Screening and testing clarify what types of treatment are needed for the PFM.

UP TRAINING

In the case of a weak and/or lax-loose PFM group, facilitation and "up training" may be needed (Mazur-Bialy *et al.* 2020). Exploration of the best postures and cues to obtain a contraction, co-contraction strategies, and RUSI or biofeedback may be used. Sensory awareness such as the pelvic clock (Chapter 2), the use of wands or dilators (Chapter 4), electrical stimulation, as well as progressive vaginal weights may be used. Weights are used in a recumbent position to start, and if a transition to standing is attempted, weights are not retained if the PFM are weak and/or the vaginal ring muscle bulbospongiosis is lax. Light weights may be used in standing and progress to heavier weights to build strength and endurance; however, the PFM are not meant to constantly pull up heavy weights. Programming is individualized (Box 9.5).

Box 9.5 PFM function: detective work

Avoid "cookbook" approaches with Kegel exercises for UI. Routine verbal instructions to "do pelvic exercises" should not be provided without assessment of effort. An unrecognized "short pelvic floor" will fail at Kegel training for UI, as it cannot contract from a shortened state. For weak individuals that need strengthening, there is not one best way for individuals to perform PFM exercises (Mateus-Vasconcelos *et al.* 2017). Isolated PFM contractions with diaphragm breathing, PFM with abdominal co-contractions, hypopressive exercise, and functional training all can be useful in continence training. PFM training for bladder storage and emptying is a gold standard in UI treatment and may be easy, or complex, depending upon individual ability to control this hidden body area.

DOWN TRAINING

A taut, tight, relatively immobile PFM group may be electrically silent on biofeedback, and display no movement with RUSI, or with digital palpation. With a "short pelvic floor" (Chapter 4), "down training" can be provided with myofascial mobilization, respiratory exercises, and relaxation. Wands, dilators, and even partner training can assist in regaining mobility in a short PFM. Mobile PFMs can rebound, stretch, and lengthen eccentrically, which appears to help many with continence as well as pain reduction.

Associated tender and trigger points may be present with bladder pain syndromes of urgency, frequency, and UI. Lumbar, pelvic, and hip myofascial treatment can reduce these tender/ trigger points and the associated urinary distress symptoms (Fitzgerald *et al.* 2012; Wolf *et al.* 2020).

Intervention: hello PFM!

Teaching clients to "wink" their PFM can make them laugh. When we laugh, cough, or sneeze, a quick pre-set and contraction (wink) occurs in the PFM. Normally continence is maintained by automatic support at the bladder neck, urethra, and outlet at the urogenital diaphragm and external urogenital muscles. The PFM are optimally pre-set in relation to anticipated intra-abdominal pressure (IAP).

Training tips: PFM

Most individuals can sense if they can "wink" or contract the anus (external anal sphincter) because it is a stronger muscle group than the urogenital triangle. "Winking" the anus can help to connect with the PFM. Next, they can be cued to attempt to contract the muscles that stop urine, for males a cue to "pull up" the testicles, or for women to "stop the flow, lift up and in." A cue to "zip the zipper" from the back to the front, up to the belly button, can help some individuals engage. PFM exercises may be prescribed to build strength, power, and endurance. Individualized programs of PFM training may include:

- quick flicks, rapid 1 second PFM contractions, repeat 3 x, 3 reps (9 total)
- contract, hold for 5 seconds, relax for 5 seconds, repeat 3 x, 10 reps (30 total per day)
- contract and hold for 10 seconds, relax for 10 seconds, repeat 10 x.

Intervention: hello bladder!

The overall goal of any treatment is to reduce or stop leaks, and this involves saying "hello" to the bladder and all its "signals." Bladder filling, storage, and emptying are explained and attention to "bladder signals" is discussed. Ideally, individuals can sense bladder signals and urinate or "void" when it is one-half to three-quarters full. Those waiting too long are more likely to experience SUI or UUI due to maximum filling (Figures 9.3 and 9.4). Individuals can be asked to place a hand above the pubic bone and say "hello bladder," and start their day with an intention to appreciate and listen to the bladder and respond to signals.

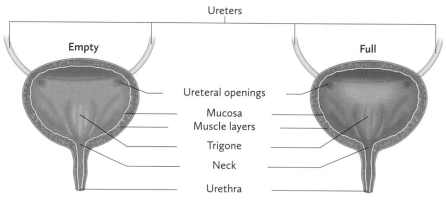

Figure 9.3 Bladder anatomy.

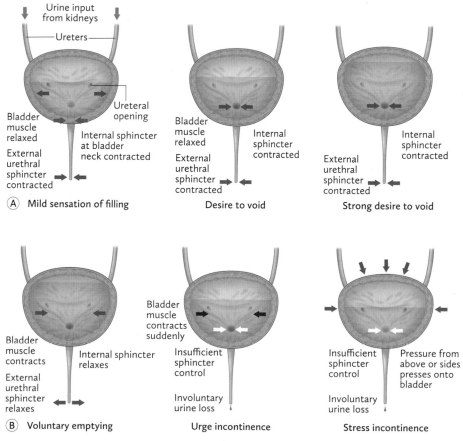

Figure 9.4 Bladder signals.

Lifestyle factors: habit training

Education and utilization of "bladder health" habits can markedly improve function. These habits include:

- noticing bladder signals during filling: minimal, moderate, maximum filling
- optimally urinating every 2–4 hours daily
- consuming optimum fluid, fiber
- eliminating bladder triggers including constipation, food and beverage irritants, such as spices, onions, citrus, coffee, alcohol, and other items
- using a proper urination technique, with PFM relaxation
- using "quick flicks" or deep PFM relaxation techniques to defer urges if voiding is too frequent
- recognizing medication side effects such as diuretics (Boxes 9.7–9.9).

Fluid

Hydration should be adequate to promote urine output an average of 5–7 times over a 24-hour period (Box 9.6). Drinking eight glasses of water a day may be sufficient. Hydration at 50 percent of body weight in ounces of water per day (e.g. a 160 lb. individual should drink 80 oz. per day) is optimal for some individuals. Hydration needs vary with age, ambient temperature, humidity, and fitness activity (Figure 9.5).

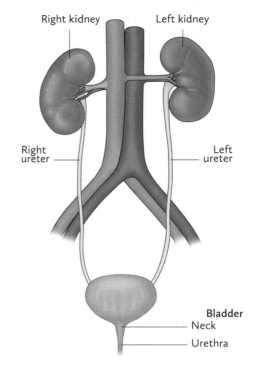

Figure 9.5 Kidneys and bladder.

Box 9.6 Dehydration, hydration

Signs of dehydration include low to no urine output, headaches, muscle cramps, fatigue, constipation, dry skin, mouth, and tongue, low blood pressure, and possible fainting. In older adults, swallowing difficulties (dysphagia), poor cognition, delirium, falls and subsequent fractures, and kidney failure can ensue (Beck *et al.* 2021). Optimum hydration will promote several voids over a 24-hour period. Overhydration and electrolyte imbalances (hyponatremia, low sodium) may occur in athletes drinking excess water. Hyponatremia in elders is typically associated with medications and certain diseases. Hyponatremia can be fatal (Henry 2015).

Box 9.7 Patient case: Earl ♥

Earl received pelvic physical therapy (PT) for UI after his prostatectomy, initially requiring four large continence pads a day. After four sessions, he only required a light continence pad daily, for a few small leaks per week, and he had good hydration and PFM control. He did not leak unless he waited too long to void or had GI distress of constipation or diarrhea. At his fifth PT session, he was angry, as his UI had returned, requiring two large pads per day. He was asked about his preceding activities before the leaks recurred; he had tended his grapefruit trees in his desert home and consumed 4–5 grapefruit per day for the last few days. He was provided with education reinforcing citrus as a "trigger" to the bladder, and a follow up session found he had returned to a few small leaks per week. However, he was upset to have to give up his beloved grapefruit.

Fiber

Twenty to 30 grams per day is a standard recommendation and may be gradually increased in those deficient.

Relaxed urination

Optimum urination involves the bladder wall muscle, the detrusor, contracting while the PFM relax. Males may "push" a little at the end, but ongoing pushing should not be necessary unless there is an obstruction to emptying. Pelvic organ prolapse, prostate swelling, or other conditions can create a need to strain and needs medical screening.

Timed voiding

Voiding on a schedule can help establish good routines, such as instructions to urinate every 2–3 hours in the daytime for those that tend to wait too long. Individuals who void too often, as in bladder urgency and frequency, can be guided in strategies to decrease voids.

Visualizing a serene emoticon of the bladder can be helpful in sensory-motor training. A content, calm bladder image accompanied by total body relaxation can help those with urgency frequency to wait 5–30 minutes for bladder re-training.

Bladder diaries

Bladder diaries require monitoring food, beverages, activities, and bladder urges, measured urine output, and stool output. Volumes in ounces or milliliters are recorded by catching urine in a measuring container. An alternate method is to count the number of seconds for a void. The recordings serve as an educational process for adults and can provide detective work as to reasons for leakage. Basic math can analyze maximum, minimum, and average void volumes.

Box 9.8 Patient case: Annette ♥

Annette presented for treatment with mixed UI symptoms, as well as pelvic and low back pain. She wore 2–3 large continence pads per day, over the last few years, and felt symptoms were worsening. At age 48 she had perimenopause symptoms of missed menses a few months at a time. She had pain with sex (dyspareunia) and constipation with output of 2–3 stools per week, Bristol #1–3 type. She drank 1–2 glasses of water per day. She had minimal awareness of her PFM, had a "short pelvic floor" on testing, and was unable to sense her bladder signals. She worked as a teacher and was a busy "soccer mom" with carpooling her three children to afterschool activities. Her bladder diary revealed she only urinated two times per day, and leaks followed 4–7 hours of no toilet use. Her treatment follows.

Pressure systems

An integrated view considers the pressure systems in the trunk, abdomen, and the influence of downward force into the pelvic area. A stiff, rigid thorax, rib cage, abdominal wall, and weak or stiff PFM group is a common finding in UI. Often, pressure systems above the bladder from myofascial taut tissue and/or breath holding and bearing down can override the compliance and reaction force of the system below, the fascial network including the PFM. The bladder and urethral supports may not meet the demands and hence a leak, small, medium, or large.

> Box 9.9 Patient case:
> Annette's treatment
> Annette, the teacher with mixed UI, received education in lifestyle habits and PT treatment, such as:
>
> - bladder signal sensation-scanning, ideally voiding every 2–3 hours
> - short PFM myofascial treatment, down training
> - constipation treatment including use of a colon massage, fluid, and fiber training
> - education on the role of estrogen changes in perimenopause, to discuss with her doctor if needed.
>
> Instead of daily leaks she reduced her leaks

> to once a week or less, a smaller volume leak, when she "got off track and did not poop for days and waited too long to pee."

Medical care for UI

Those with UI despite conservative care may be candidates for the use of medical care such as:

- medications
- intermittent catheterization
- support tampons or pessaries
- injections and/or
- surgeries.

(Lucas et al. 2012)

Pessaries can support the internal positioning of the bladder and the bladder neck.

Urethral support injections can stiffen the proximal urethra at the bladder neck. Bladder slings can help with continence. Those without ability to relax and store and/or empty may need intermittent catheterization, a bladder revision or cystectomy, requiring a diversion and an external collection device. Surgeries can be of great benefit and are appropriate for those with minimal to no benefit from conservative care, and ongoing moderate to severe UI. However, risks of infections, pain, and need for repeat surgical intervention exist and doctors will optimally follow the most current evidence-based guidelines for choice of procedures (Lukacz *et al.* 2017).

SUMMARY

In summary, UI is a troubling and often emotionally challenging health problem. Multiple conservative care practices require education and reinforcement for behavior change. Attention to bladder signals, reducing constipation and downward pressure into the bladder and urethra, therapeutic exercise, and manual therapy can promote synergy of the diaphragms (pelvic, respiratory, and vocal) and improve bladder control (Mazur-Bialy *et al.* 2020). Education and empowerment of individuals towards improved continence control can be reached with a multimodal approach by a team of care providers.

REFERENCES

Abrams, P., Cardozo, L., Wagg, A., and Wein, A. (eds) (2017) *Incontinence*. 6th ed. Bristol: International Continence Society.

Barral, J. P. (2006) *Urogenital Manipulation*. Seattle: Eastland Press.

Beck, A. M., Seemer, J., Knudsen, A. W., and Munk, T. (2021) "Narrative review of low-intake dehydration in older adults." *Nutrients 13*, 9, 3142.

Dufour, S., Fedorkow, D., Kun, J., Deng, S. X., and Fang, Q. (2019) "Exploring the impact of a mobile health solution for postpartum pelvic floor muscle training: A pilot randomized controlled feasibility study." *JMIR mHealth and uHealth 7*, 7, e12587.

Fitzgerald, M. P., Payne, C. K., Lukacz, E. S., Yang, C. C., *et al.* (2012) "Randomized multicenter clinical trial of myofascial physical therapy in women with interstitial cystitis/painful bladder syndrome and pelvic floor tenderness." *Journal of Urology 187*, 6, 2113–2118.

Henry, D. A. (2015) "In the clinic: Hyponatremia." *Annals of Internal Medicine 163*, 3.

Hester, A., Kretschmer, A., and Badlani, G. (2017) "Male incontinence: The etiology or basis of treatment." *European Urological Focus 3*, 4–5.

Khandelwal, C. and Kistler, C. (2013) "Diagnosis of urinary incontinence." *American Family Physician 87*, 8, 543–550.

Lucas, M. G., Bosch, R. J. L., Burkhard, F. C., Cruz, F., *et al.* (2012) "EAU guidelines on surgical treatment of urinary incontinence." *European Urology 62*, 6, 1118–1129.

Lukacz, E., Santigo-Lastra, Y., Albo, M., and Brubacker, L. (2017) "Urinary incontinence in women: A review." *JAMA 318*, 16, 1592–1604.

Mateus-Vasconcelos, E. C. L., Riberio, A. M., Antonio, F. I., Brito, L. G. O., and Ferreira, C. H. J. (2017) "Physiotherapy methods to facilitate pelvic floor muscle contraction: A systematic review." *Physiotherapy Theory and Practice 34*, 6, 420–432.

Mazur-Bialy, A. I., Kolomanska-Bogucka, D., Nowakowski, C., and Tim, S. (2020) "Urinary incontinence in women: Modern methods of physiotherapy as a support for surgical treatment or independent therapy, review." *Journal of Clinical Medicine 9*, 1211.

Oregon Health & Science University "Urinary Distress Inventory, Short Form (UDI-6)." Accessed 9/23/22 at https://www.ohsu.edu/sites/default/files/2019-06/Female-Urology-Questionnaire-6.pdf.

Pires, T., Pires, P., Moreira, H., and Viana, R. (2020) "Prevalence of urinary incontinence in high impact sport athletes: A systematic review and meta-analysis." *Journal of Human Kinetics 73*, 279–288.

Thompson, J. A., O'Sullivan, P. B., Briffa, N. K., and Neuman, P. (2006) "Assessment of voluntary pelvic floor muscle contraction in continent and incontinent women using transperineal ultrasound, manual muscle testing and vaginal squeeze pressure measurements." *International Urogynecology Journal Pelvic Floor Dysfunction 17*, 6, 624–630.

Utomo, E., Korfage, I. J., Wildhagen, M. F., Steensma, A. B., *et al.* (2015) "Validation of the urogenital distress inventory (UDI-6) and incontinence impact questionnaire (IIQ-7) in a Dutch population." *Neurourology and Urodynamics 34*, 1, 24–31.

Wolf, B. J., Joyce, C. J., McAlarnen, L. A., Brincat, C. A., *et al.* (2020) "Consideration of pelvic floor myofascial release for overactive bladder." *Journal of Bodywork and Movement Therapy 24*, 2, 144–150.

FURTHER RESOURCES

Haylen, B. (2022) ICS Glossary. Accessed 6/10/2022 at https://www.ics.org/glossary.

Urinary Distress Inventory, Short Form (UDI-6). (1995) Oregon Health and Science University. Accessed 3/7/2022 at https://www.ohsu.edu/sites/default/files/2019-06/Female-Urology-Questionnaire-6.pdf.

CHAPTER 10

Gastrointestinal Health, Pelvic Health, and Dysfunction

This chapter delves into the critical topic of digestive, colorectal, and pelvic health in relation to conservative care practices. Preparation for this chapter includes prior chapter information with topics such as:

- foundation knowledge in pelvic anatomy/physiology
- pelvic floor muscle (PFM) synergy with the diaphragms
- bladder and bowel function/dysfunction
- mechanisms in simple and complex pelvic pain.

Movement therapists, bodyworkers, and other care providers can help optimize health in these areas. Digestive processes, assimilation, and output are influenced by many factors and these topics thread through this book, with more detail in Chapter 14. Constipation, fecal incontinence, and/or pain may all occur in relation to gastrointestinal (GI) function. Therapies to enhance digestive processes and associated myofascial system functions will be a mainstay of this chapter.

THE GASTROINTESTINAL SYSTEM

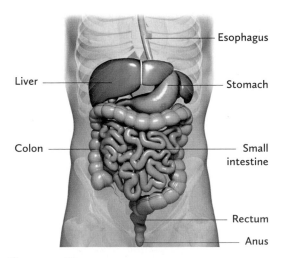

Figure 10.1 GI system.

The GI system is a vast interconnected thoroughfare, from the mouth to the exit in the pelvis at the anal sphincter (Figure 10.1). The GI system is our energy factory, breaking down, moving, and assimilating nutrients and creating metabolic products that support life. Our ability to eat, drink, digest, and create well-formed stool at the exit is regulated by many systems, but overall, this is an autonomic driven system that works under the radar of our awareness.

The second brain
The GI transit path relies on a "second brain" of sorts, with neural connections and processes that work independently of conscious control.

Smelling food, salivation, chewing, swallowing, and movement of food from the mouth to the esophagus, stomach, duodenum and small intestine, large intestine, rectum, and internal/external anal sphincters rely on a "second brain" of neural vascular and myofascial networks.

These functions work well when we are calm, relaxed, and feel safe. When we are stressed and the overall sympathetic nervous system tone is higher (fight, flight, freeze mode), digestive processes shut down to preserve vital organs.

SPHINCTER SITES

Upper GI tracts

Sphincter mechanisms exist all along the GI tract. The mouth is a sphincter which opens to receive food or clenches and turns away if there is dislike or disinterest in food. With food intake, salivation and chewing begin to break down food. Swallowing mechanics include the tongue rising and moving up against the palate, with a wave backwards towards the throat. The throat must relax and open to allow food a sufficient downward movement. Food then moves into the upper and lower esophagus, then the gastro-esophageal junction (lower esophageal sphincter), and into the stomach. Food is churned and broken down by stomach acid and enzymes. Next, "chyme," partially digested food, moves out of the stomach to the pylorus, which is a sphincter junction into the duodenum. The duodenum receives digestive enzymes from the gallbladder, liver, and pancreas to further help break down the food.

Lower GI tract

The tubular duodenum descends from the stomach and links to the jejunum at the duodenal–jejunal sphincter, where it transfers the further digested contents into the small intestine. Absorption of nutrients occurs in the small intestine, and next, the ileocecal valve transfers waste product to the large intestine, the colon. The colon hydrates or dehydrates waste as needed, with a water supply from the cecum, and ideally delivers an optimum consistency stool to the rectum to "sample." When all systems are "go," the bulk of stool moves along the ascending, transverse, and descending colon downward towards the sigmoid colon and the rectum.

Final sphincter control

The internal (smooth muscle) and external (volitional) anal sphincters are the final junction points below the rectum that prevent stool from exiting. The sense of a "need to go" is facilitated by peristalsis in the colon, with a small amount of stool moving towards the exit via internal sphincter relaxation, and an external anal sphincter contraction holding back stool. If toilet access is available and an individual is ready, stool emptying occurs with further peristalsis, and a relaxation of the internal and external anal sphincter. Otherwise, the rectum stores stool and an individual waits until a convenient time to eliminate (Mayo Foundation for Medical Education and Research 2020; National Institute of Diabetes and Digestive and Kidney Diseases 2017).

Abdominal wall firming and intra-abdominal pressure assists in elimination, with a bearing down mechanism, and PFM relaxation. A closed glottis (upper diaphragm), firm respiratory diaphragm (middle diaphragm), and relaxed and lengthened PFM muscle group (pelvic diaphragm) all coordinate to assist defecation. The bearing down mechanism is termed Valsalva (Teach Me Physiology 2022).

The "second brain" maintains homeostasis via pathways from digestive organs to the brain, spinal cord, and autonomic fibers of the sympathetic and parasympathetic systems to operate in balance. The autonomic system to the GI region, the "gut," is the enteric nervous system. The enteric nervous system is the regulator to the small and large intestines, and it is a network with relays between organs as well (Browning and Travagli 2014; Furness 2012).

GI PROBLEMS: OVERVIEW

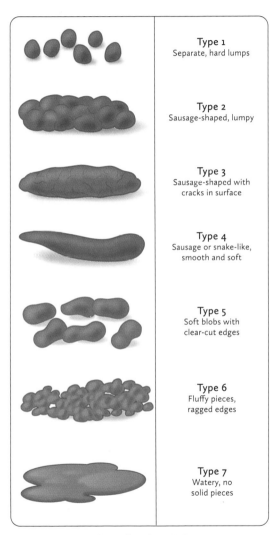

Figure 10.2 Bristol stool scale (BSS).

Constipation, irritable bowel syndrome, diarrhea, and fecal incontinence are problems that can be episodic or chronic and affect function and participation in all aspects of life (Figure 10.2).

GI problems typically affect more women than men, and this is due in part to obstetrical injuries suffered by women, and hormonal influences (Chey, Kurlander, and Eswaren 2015; Laine *et al.* 2011). Some GI conditions are of unknown etiology. If the underlying mechanisms and triggers are identified, these root problems may be treated.

Constipation

Constipation is a common condition that may include fewer than three stool outputs per week, hard or lumpy stools, straining or pain with defecation, a sense of obstruction/blockage to emptying, or sensations of incomplete evacuation (Rome Foundation 2016) (Box 10.1). Constipation occurs in approximately 30 percent of individuals with increasing incidence in elders (50%) and up to 70 percent in those institutionalized for nursing care (De Giorgio *et al.* 2015).

> **Box 10.1 Constipation types**
>
> Constipation types vary by normal transit, slow transit, or outlet obstruction. In normal transit, digestion moves along readily, yet insufficient fluid, fiber, and/or lifestyle habits lead to constipation. In slow transit there is increased time for digestive processes to occur and a delay in the ability to produce stool. A transit study can be performed with a pill which shows up on an X-ray over 24–48 hours, displaying the progress of contents through the colon (Song *et al.* 2012). Slow transit involves deficiencies in the motility of the colon, with limited peristalsis. Even with eating well, hydrating well, and exercising, transmit may be slow. In outlet obstruction

there is a lack of synergy between the abdominal wall and the pelvic floor muscles (PFM); the PFM contract during attempted defecation, blocking the outlet. This effort of PFM contraction versus relaxation is termed dyssynergic defecation and it is medically verified by a digital rectal exam, failed rectal balloon expulsion test, and also biofeedback and MRI testing (Bharucha and Wald 2019; Binford 2015; Mayo Foundation for Medical Education and Research 2020).

Factors associated with constipation may include (limited list):

- sedentary behavior; lack of exercise (Tantawy *et al.* 2017)
- insufficient fluid and/or fiber intake
- poor nutrition, such as excess meat, rice, bread, and other items
- pain with defecation, and learned withholding/avoidance
- pelvic floor muscle (PFM) and diaphragm dyssynergia
- sensory-motor dysfunction of the rectum
- immobility: wheelchair or bed-bound status, including post-surgical time frames
- medical: hypothyroidism, endocrine, exocrine, diabetes, autoimmune, orthopedic, and neurodegenerative diseases
- psychological/behavioral disorders: somatization, anxiety, depression, hostility, obsessive-compulsive, and psychosis
- medications including opioid pain relievers, antibiotics, antihistamines, bladder incontinence medications, and medications for mood disorders
- hemorrhoids, fissures, anal stenosis, rectocele, as well as reproductive, genital, colon/rectal cancers
- travel/schedule disruptions.

Irritable bowel syndrome

Irritable bowel syndrome (IBS) is a medically defined condition based on examination and identification of varied states of constipation and/or diarrhea, typically associated with bloating, gas, and pain (Borgnini *et al.* 2017). IBS is a chronic GI disease with varied presentations over time, with remissions, improvements, and relapses between the sub types listed below (Posserud, Ersyd, and Simren 2006).

Classifications of IBS include:

- IBS-C: constipation dominant
- IBS-D: diarrhea dominant
- IBS-Mixed: constipation and diarrhea.

(Chey et al. 2015)

Conditions associated with IBS can include (limited list):

- gut dysbiosis: alterations in the intestinal mucosa, gut microbiome, with autoimmune and systemic sequelae
- post infections, post medication/antibiotic regimes, post-surgical, or combinations of these elements
- fibromyalgia, chronic fatigue syndrome, and/or chronic pelvic pain
- upper GI symptoms of dysphagia, gastroesophageal reflux, and dyspepsia (Riedl *et al.* 2008)
- nutrition related conditions as in FODMAP and SIBO (see below)
- Adverse childhood experiences (ACE) scores and associated altered psychological states.

(Ju et al. 2020)

PHYSIOLOGICAL CHANGES IN IBS

IBS is related to alterations in visceral sensation, brain, and GI/gut dynamics, altered motility, psychological variables, and other contributing factors. Intestinal permeability, gut microbiome changes (both small and large intestines), and alterations in gut immune functioning are found in those with IBS (Sultan *et al.* 2021). Visceral-somatic reflexes and centralization of pain occur in IBS, with pain sensed during internal pressure, visceral stretching, and muscle activity related to digestion. Studies measuring GI visceral pressure, stretch, or muscle activity show brain activity is altered in those with pain towards hypersensitivity and pain signaling (Dickhaus *et al.* 2003; Mayer *et al.* 2001).

FLATAL AND FECAL INCONTINENCE

In IBS-D, there is typical bloating, cramping, pain, gut dysbiosis, and flatulence (gas) and fecal incontinence (FI) (loss of stool) can occur. It is difficult for the bowel to sense loose stool, as well as hold it back, therefore potential release of gas may actually include FI. Developing good habits for fluid and fiber intake are typically insufficient in IBS-D. Insoluble fiber contained in high residue food typically aggravates symptoms, yet soluble fiber is better tolerated and can shift BSS to #4–5 in some individuals. IBS-D type symptoms may be an indicator of inflammatory bowel disease, such as Crohn's disease and ulcerative colitis. These diseases are associated with BSS #6–7 and weight loss and require medical intervention (Anandam 2014; Chey *et al.* 2015). Food sensitivities may trigger symptoms, particularly in IBS-D. Clients often look for a quick fix to reduce symptoms in the form of medications. The standard American diet (SAD) with additives and emulsifiers can contribute to IBS.

Never trust a fart.

(Edward in *The Bucket List* (Reiner 2007))

Fermentation, FODMAP, SIBO

In digestion, food undergoes fermentation as sugars break down. However, some individuals have sensitivities to foods with fructose and similar compounds, recognized as FODMAP (De Roest *et al.* 2013) (Boxes 10.2 and 10.3). Those with FODMAP sensitivities may also have small intestine bacterial overgrowth (SIBO) (Borghini *et al.* 2017; Gandhi *et al.* 2021).

> **Box 10.2 Fermentation troubles**
> Apples, milk, multigrain whole wheat bread, honey, ripe bananas, peaches, and plums are FODMAP-containing foods. Reduced FODMAP intake can greatly improve digestive health. This is profoundly helpful for those with IBS!

Dietary intolerances can cause or exacerbate pelvic floor dysfunction (PFD). Bloating, gas, cramping, and difficulties in producing optimum stool will cause or exacerbate pelvic pain, bladder or bowel continence issues, constipation, pelvic organ prolapse, and also affect sexual functioning.

> **Box 10.3 Medical screening**
> Screening for GI disorders should include health history, an analysis of the BSS, and screening for PFD symptoms. Health history factors which may impact abdominal and pelvic health are numerous and may include genetics, abnormalities at birth, GI infections, surgeries, childbirth, use of certain medications, a history of trauma in youth (ACE score), malnutrition and/or inadequate nutrition, and food allergies or sensitivities. A medical screening referral is indicated with the presence of any *red flags* as presented in Chapter 4. With significant pain, bleeding, dehydration, prolonged constipation, or

other distress symptoms, lab tests may be necessary to check electrolyte levels, kidney, liver, and other metabolic functions, and radiology to rule out masses or obstructions.

PFM control

PFM screening questions and examinations (visual observation, palpation, mapping, muscle testing) may be provided. Tests for synergy, dyssynergia, PFM weakness/laxity, and/or tightness/spasm can identify impairments associated with PFD symptoms and provide a basis for an appropriate treatment plan. Up training and/or down training, associated lumbopelvic hip concerns, and general nervous system imbalances can also be integrated into goal planning.

TREATMENTS

Treatment for constipation

Initial treatment of simple constipation includes factors as listed (Box 10.4):

- optimal fluid intake to allow urination every 3–4 hours
- optimal fiber, soluble and insoluble: 20–30 grams per day
- reduction of binding foods such as rice, bread, and bananas
- physical activity with increased lifestyle and/or fitness programs
- recognition of bowel signals and transport to the toilet
- PFM synergy training with the abdominals and diaphragm in the "mechanics" for elimination.

Box 10.4 Improved compliance: tracking output

Symptom tracking as in BSS number, pain reductions, and improved health literacy with shopping and meal preparation can be encouraged and celebrated to enhance compliance.

More detailed constipation treatment may include specialist intervention:

- nutrition training optimizing a variety of healthy choices and exploring food sensitivities and allergies
- guidance in the use of over-the-counter laxatives, stimulants, and stool softeners
- specific exercise prescription, qigong, yoga, walking, or other aerobic exercise 140 minutes a week or more (Gao et al. 2019)
- a colon massage and other manual therapy (see below)
- biofeedback with ultrasound and external or internal sensors (Binford 2015)
- electrical stimulation protocols: TENS units and/or external anal/internal anal electrodes (Clarke et al. 2009; Ismail et al. 2009; Mahony et al. 2004).

Medical management can include, under specialty care:

- digestive aids such as bromelin, peppermint, and milk thistle (Post-White, Lada, and Kelly 2007) (Box 10.5)
- digestive enzymes such as amylase, lipase, protease, lactase, and sucrase (Denhard 2022)
- pharmaceutical interventions
- life-saving surgeries such as resections, ostomy creation (Byrne et al. 2014).

> **Box 10.5 Spices for constipation**
> Spices such as ginger, cinnamon, fennel, and turmeric may help increase digestive fire and are basic constituents of items such as chai (Mashhadi *et al.* 2013). Fennel and turmeric in capsule form has been shown to significantly reduce IBS symptoms over a two-month period (Di Ciaula *et al.* 2018).

Some individuals need a bowel program which is medically prescribed, such as the use of a stimulant and a stool softener two or three times a week to help with a clean-out. Others rely on enema schedules, and those with severely resistant constipation may use a weekly colonic as a maintenance system. Pharmaceuticals may help, and form the sole treatment of many medical providers, but also have side effects such as pain and diarrhea (Chey *et al.* 2015).

Nutrition for IBS-D, considering FODMAP and SIBO

IBS-D type profiles may have difficulty digesting and absorbing many types of food (Gandhi *et al.* 2021), and may need periods of a liquid diet. Research studies are now validating the significance of nutrition in IBS, with recognition that "the low FODMAP diet leads to clinical response in 50–80 percent of patients with IBS, in particular with improvements in bloating, flatulence, diarrhea, and global symptoms" (Staudacher and Whelan 2017).

Nutrition training can optimize healthy choices, exploring food sensitivities, and allergies. FODMAP outlines and recipes with foods to limit or eliminate, as well as likely tolerated foods, are listed in online resources (IBSdiets.org 2022). Clients may have catastrophic thinking when first learning about FODMAP and viewing a newly restrictive diet; however, over time they can adjust and often consume FODMAP items but in smaller quantities, as well as learn about an abundance of healthy options and new foods (Box 10.6).

> **Box 10.6 Holistic GI care: patience, time, healing**
> A "whole food" diet of unprocessed food often eliminates symptoms, along with digestive aids and a very slow uptake of probiotics under the supervision of specialists. This can be gradually implemented for most people willing and eager to improve health.
>
> It may take over a year to shift nutrition and lifestyle habits, change the gut microbiome, and improve intestinal and immune system functioning.

BODYWORK/MANUAL THERAPY AND EXERCISE FOR GI AND PFD

Manual therapy

Manual therapy (Box 10.7) can help GI and associated PFM regions with:

- a client focusing on recognition of sensations in the GI and pelvic areas, as in interoception; the client attains awareness of the internal sense of their body
- release of scar tissue and/or myofascial tension in associated structures from the spine/trunk, the extremities, and around viscera
- improved visceral mobility in relation to other organs and supportive myofascial structures, and improved organ motility (Barral 2007)
- generalized body relaxation towards parasympathetic balance.

Box 10.7 Manual therapy results

Manual therapy combined with visceral work can sometimes help the organs themselves to function, perhaps by assisting mind–body integration. This may be experienced by "bowel sounds," a gurgling sound, and a client's sensations of things "releasing" during myofascial and visceral manual therapy for GI problems. An outcome may be a "good poop" immediately following therapy in a constipated client.

Resiliency

Myofascial, neurovascular, and GI systems are capable of resiliency. Mapping the GI system with manual therapy can help clients connect with somatic integration, recognizing a great variety of symptoms in specific sites. The process of "saying hello" to sites along the GI tracts with manual "mapping" can engage clients in awareness and appreciation of their physical body and its vital functions. Mindfulness and relaxation training can be instructed during manual therapy work, enhancing parasympathetic "rest and digest" functions.

Somato-sensory awareness can help improve health in areas such as:

- noticing how cold beverages and ice may cause throat and stomach discomfort
- noticing digestive sensations in the small and large intestines in relation to nutrition, such as gas, bloating, and cramping after consuming food triggers
- noticing clarity of mind, reduced nasal stuffiness, and mucus production in relation to improved eating (Chaudhary 2016)
- noticing how negative mood and stress can cause or aggravate GI symptoms, and a reduced stress environment can make for a happy belly, calm belly, easy belly. (These phrases can be taught during down training/relaxation!)

Colon massage

A colon massage can be helpful in somato-sensory awareness, and once instructed, clients can perform this technique on themselves, or have a partner or family member assist (Figure 10.3). A general technique is to softly trace the colon from its right lower quadrant origin, up and across, and then downwards into the left lower quadrant, ten strokes to start. This may be followed by small circles moving to a greater depth, but in the comfort range. Visceral trained therapists can combine anterior and posterior holds, and even combined internal and external manual work. Multiple studies point to colon massage efficacy (McClurg and Lowe-Strong 2011; Sinclair 2011).

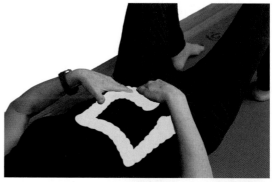
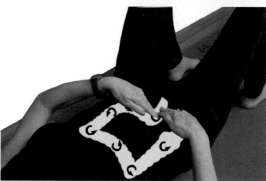

Figure 10.3 Colon massage.

Therapeutic exercise

Many types of exercise can reduce constipation as well as help improve IBS conditions. Walking and yoga are two key programs that can be readily accessible and have research to support their health benefits (Binford 2015; Ganesh *et al.* 2021; Kuttner *et al.* 2006; Taneja *et al.* 2004; Tantway *et al.* 2017).

Exercise intervention ideally will consider entire body function and dysfunction in formatting prescriptions. GI and pelvic functioning require control of the diaphragms (upper throat/ vocal, respiratory, and pelvic), adequate trunk, spine, and PFM strength and control. PFM also need the ability to relax, stretch, and open for elimination functions. Clients may need stretch and relaxation in one body area (such as the ribcage, spine, and abdominal wall) yet also require strength and endurance exercises in another area (such as weak PFM after childbirth or pelvic surgery). Mat exercise formats as displayed in Chapters 2, 3, and 4 (yoga/Pilates) are typical elements of prescribed programs.

MIND–BODY THERAPY AND NUTRITION

Combination approaches for GI and PFD can address cognitive behavioral therapy, relaxation/ stress management, and nutrition approaches. Research has shown a positive impact on improved quality of life scores and IBS symptom reduction with high compliance with the element of self-choice in programming (Zia *et al.* 2016). The case example listed in Chapter 14 demonstrates a multimodal approach to healing GI and PFD and includes manual therapy and exercise (Allison).

Complex cases and surgery

There are individuals who may require multiple medications and surgeries to function in regards to GI health. Medical intervention can be lifesaving in cases of inflammatory bowel diseases, bowel obstructions, cancer conditions, and autoimmune diseases. Medical cases may still benefit from follow up manual therapy, exercise, and nutrition training with individualized programming, including pain reductions, improved GI and PFM functioning, and overall mobility.

CONCLUSION

PFD and GI system dysfunction can be improved with detective work, problem solving, and a wide array of holistic interventions. Reduced bloating, cramping, pain, and gas, and improved BSS output, can be signs that the GI system is functioning better in its entirety.

Emerging evidence shows that mind–body approaches, improved nutrition, gut microbiome support, and the use of manual therapy and exercise can improve GI function and reduce PFD. A team of providers can offer treatments addressed in this chapter, with clients benefitting from improved overall health and vitality. Expressions of gratitude from clients who have "transformed" is the reward to care providers for a job well done.

REFERENCES

Anandam, J. L. (2014) "Surgical management for fecal incontinence." *Clinics in Colon Rectal Surgery 27*, 3, 106–109.

Barral, J. P. (2007) *Visceral Manipulation II*. Seattle: Eastland Press.

Bharucha, A. E. and Wald, A. (2019) "Chronic constipation." *Mayo Clinic Proceedings 94*, 11, 2340–2357.

Binford, J. (2015) "Physical therapy management of outlet dysfunction constipation and chronic pelvic pain." *Journal of Women's Health Physical Therapy 37*, 2.

Borghini, R., Donato, G., Alvaro, D., and Picarelli, A. (2017) "New insights into IBS-like disorders: Pandoras box has been opened: A review." *Gastroenterology Hepatology Bed to Bench 10*, 2, 79–89.

Browning, K. N. and Travagli, R. A. (2014) "Central nervous system control of gastrointestinal motility and secretion and modulation of gastrointestinal functions." *Comprehensive Physiology 4*, 4.

Byrne, J., Ambrosini, S. F., Jackson, Q. F., and Okrainer, A. (2014) "Laparoscopic versus open surgical management of adhesive small bowel obstruction: A comparison of outcomes." *Surgical Endoscopy 29*, 9, 2525–2532.

Chaudhary, K. (2016) *The Prime: Prepare and Repair Your Body for Spontaneous Weight Loss*. London: Penguin.

Chey, W. D., Kurlander, J., and Eswaren, S. (2015) "Irritable bowel syndrome: A clinical review." *Journal of the American Medical Association 313*, 9, 949–958.

Clarke, M. C. C., Chase, J. W., Gibb, S., Robertson, V. J., *et al.* (2009) "Improvement of quality of life in children with slow transit constipation after treatment with transcutaneous electrical stimulation." *Journal of Pediatric Surgery 44*, 6, 1268–1273.

De Giorgio, R., Ruggeri, E., Stanghellini, V., Eusebi, L. H., Bazzoli, F., and Chiarioni, G. (2015) "Chronic constipation in the elderly: A primer for the gastroenterologist." *BMC Gastroenterology 15*, 130.

De Roest, R. H., Dobbs, B. R., Chapman, B. A., Batman, B., *et al.* (2013) "The low FODMAP diet improves gastrointestinal symptoms in patients with irritable bowel syndrome: A prospective study." *International Journal of Clinical Practice 67*, 9, 895–903.

Denhard, M. (2022) "Digestive enzymes and digestive enzyme supplements." Johns Hopkins Medicine, Health. Accessed 9/23/22 at https://www.hopkinsmedicine.org/health/wellness-and-prevention/digestive-enzymes-and-digestive-enzyme-supplements.

Di Ciaula, A., Portincasa, P., Maes, N., and Albert, A. (2018) "Efficacy of bio-optimized extracts of turmeric and essential fennel oil on the quality of life in patients with irritable bowel syndrome." *Annals of Gastroenterology 31*, 6, 685–691.

Dickhaus, B., Mayer, E. A., Firooz, N., Stains, J., *et al.* (2003) "Irritable bowel syndrome patients show enhanced modulation of visceral perception by auditory stress." *American Journal of Gastroenterology 98*, 135–143.

Furness J. B. (2012) "The enteric nervous system and neurogastroenterology." *Nature Reviews Gastroenterology and Hepatology 9*, 286–294.

Gandhi, A., Shah, A., Jones, M. P., Koloski, N., and Taiiey, N. J. (2021) "Methane positive small intestinal bacterial overgrowth in inflammatory bowel disease and irritable bowel syndrome: A systematic review and meta-analysis." *Gut Microbes 13*, 1, e1933313-2–e1933313-16.

Ganesh, H. R. S., Subramanya, P., Raghavendra, R. M., and Udupa, V. (2021) "Role of yoga therapy in improving digestive health and quality of sleep in the elderly population: A randomized controlled trial." *Journal of Bodywork and Movement Therapy 27*, 692–697.

Gao, R., Tao, Y., Zhou, C., Li, J., *et al.* (2019) "Exercise therapy in patients with constipation: A systematic review and meta-analysis of randomized controlled trials." *Scandinavian Journal of Gastroenterology 54*, 2, 169–177.

IBSdiets.org (2022) "Low FODMAP diet information and other IBS diets." Accessed 9/23/22 at https://www.ibsdiets.org.

Ismail, K. A., Chase, J., Gibb, S., Clarke, M., *et al.* (2009) "Daily transabdominal electrical stimulation at home increased defecation in children with slow-transit constipation: A pilot study." *Journal of Pediatric Surgery 44*, 12, 2388–2392.

Ju, T., Naliboff, B. D., Shih, W., Presson, A. P., Liu, C., *et al.* (2020) "Risk and protective factors related to early adverse life events in irritable bowel syndrome." *Journal of Clinical Gastroenterology 54*, 1, 63–69.

Kuttner, L., Chambers, C. T., Hardial, J., Israel, D. M., *et al.* (2006) "A randomized trial of yoga for adolescents with irritable bowel syndrome." *Pain Research Management 11*, 4, S372–S373.

Laine, K., Skeldestad, F. E., Sanda, B., Horne, H., Spydslaug, A., and Staff, A. C. (2011) "Prevalence and risk factors for anal incontinence after obstetric anal sphincter rupture." *Acta Obstetricia et Gynecologica Scandinavica 90*, 4, 319–324.

Mahony, R. T., Malone P. A., Nalty, J., Behan, M., O'Connell, P. R., and O'Herlihy, C. (2004) "Randomized clinical trial of intra-anal electromyographic biofeedback physiotherapy with intra-anal electromyographic biofeedback augmented with electrical stimulation of the anal sphincter in the early treatment of postpartum fecal incontinence." *American Journal of Obstetrics and Gynecology 191*, 3, 885–890.

Mashhadi, N. S., Ghiasvand, R., Askari, G., Hariri, M., *et al.* (2013) "Anti-oxidative and anti-inflammatory effects of ginger in health and physical activity: Review of current evidence." *International Journal of Preventative Medicine 4*, 1, S36–S42.

Mayer, E. A., Craske, M., and Naliboff, B. D. (2001) "Depression, anxiety, and the gastrointestinal system." *Journal of Clinical Psychiatry 62*, 28–36.

Mayo Foundation for Medical Education and Research (2020) "Slide show: See how your digestive system works." Accessed 9/23/22 at https://www.mayoclinic.org/digestive-system/sls-20076373.

McClurg, D. and Lowe-Strong, A. (2011) "Does abdominal massage relieve constipation? Review." *Nursing Times 107*, 12, 20–22.

National Institute of Diabetes and Digestive and Kidney Diseases (NIDDK) (2017) "Your digestive system and how it works." Accessed 9/23/22 at https://www.niddk.nih.gov/health-information/digestive-diseases/digestive-system-how-it-works.

Posserud, I., Ersyd, A., and Simren, M. (2006) "Functional findings in irritable bowel syndrome." *World Journal of Gastroenterology 12*, 18, 2830–2838.

Post-White, J., Lada, E. J., and Kelly, K. M. (2007) "Advances in the use of milk thistle (Silybum marianum)." *Integrative Cancer Therapies 6*, 2, 104–109.

Reiner, R. (dir.) (2007) *The Bucket List.* Warner Bros.

Riedl, A., Schmidtmann, M., Stengel, A., Goebel, M., *et al.* (2008) "Somatic comorbidities of irritable bowel syndrome: A systematic analysis." *Journal of Psychosomatic Research 64*, 6, 573–582.

Rome Foundation (2016) "Rome IV Criteria Appendix A: Rome IV Diagnostic Criteria for FGIDs, Esophageal Disorders—H3b. Nonretentive Fecal Incontinence." Accessed 9/23/22 at https://theromefoundation.org/rome-iv/rome-iv-criteria.

Sinclair, M. (2011) "The use of abdominal massage to treat chronic constipation, review." *Journal of Bodywork and Movement Therapy 15*, 4, 436–445.

Song, B. K., Cho, K. O., Jo, Y., Oh, J. W., and Kim, Y. S. (2012) "Colon transit time according to physical activity level in adults." *Journal of Neurogastroenterology and Motility 18*, 1, 64–69.

Staudacher, H. M. and Whelan, K. (2017) "The low FODMAP diet: Recent advances in understanding its mechanisms and efficiency in IBS." *British Medical Journal, Gut 66*, 8, 1517–1527.

Sultan, S., El-Mowafy, M., Elgami, A., Ahmed, T. A. E., *et al.* (2021) "Metabolic influences of gut microbiota dysbiosis on inflammatory bowel disease: Review." *Frontiers in Physiology 12*, 7, 1590.

Taneja, I., Deepak, K. K., Poojary, G., Acharya, I. N., Pandey, R. M., and Sharma, M. P. (2004) "Yogic versus conventional treatment in diarrhea-predominant irritable bowel syndrome: A randomized control study." *Applied Psychophysiology Biofeedback 29*, 19–33.

Tantawy, S. A., Karnel, D. M., Abdelbasset, W. K., and Eloghary, H. M. (2017) "Effects of a proposed physical activity and diet control to manage constipation in middle aged obese women." *Diabetes Metabolic Syndrome Obesity 10*, 513–519.

Teach Me Physiology (2022) "Defecation." Accessed 9/23/22 at https://teachmephysiology.com/gastrointestinal-system/large-intestine/defecation.

Zia, J. K., Barney, P., Cain, K. C., Jarrett, M. E., and Heitkemper, M. M. (2016) "A comprehensive self-management irritable bowel syndrome program produces sustainable changes in behavior after 1 year. Randomized controlled trial." *Clinical Gastroenterology Hepatology 14*, 2, 212-9. e1–2.

FURTHER RESOURCES

Chaudhary, K. (2022) Dosha Quiz. Accessed 4/1/2022 at https://drkulreetchaudhary.com/dosha-quiz.

Chaudhary, K. (2022) Gut IQ Quiz. Accessed 4/1/2022 at https://drkulreetchaudhary.com/gut-iq-quiz.

Constipation (2021) Mayo Clinic. Accessed 4/1/2022 at www.mayoclinic.org/diseases-conditions/constipation/diagnosis-treatment/drc-20354259.

Defecation (2022) Teach Me Physiology. Accessed 4/1/2022 at https://teachmephysiology.com/gastrointestinal-system/large-intestine/defecation.

Denhard, M. (2022) Digestive enzymes and digestive enzyme supplements. Health, Wellness and Prevention, Johns Hopkins Medicine. Accessed 4/1/2022 at www.hopkinsmedicine.org/health/wellness-and-prevention/digestive-enzymes-and-digestive-enzyme-supplements.

FODMAP Diet Chart (2022) IBS Diets. Accessed 4/1/2022 at www.ibsdiets.org/fodmap-diet/fodmap-diet-chart.

Kapoor, V. K. (2016) Upper GI Tract Anatomy. MedScape. Accessed 4/1/2022 at https://emedicine.medscape.com/article/1899389-overview#a4.

Your Digestive System & How it Works (2017) National Institute of Diabetes and Kidney Diseases. Accessed 4/1/2022 at www.niddk.nih.gov/health-information/digestive-diseases/digestive-system-how-it-works.

CHAPTER 11

Pelvic Health: Midlife into Elder Years

This chapter considers pelvic health challenges from midlife to elder years. Menopause, andropause, orthopedic surgeries, neurological diseases, and cancer are some of the many conditions which can impact pelvic floor dysfunction PFD in the aging population.

Many elder pelvic health problems may be helped by conservative care, including behavioral and lifestyle management training, such as maintaining fitness, optimum hydration, nutrition, and bowel regularity. Lifestyle factors that promote healthy aging will be profiled regarding optimizing pelvic health, and overall fitness and wellness.

As individuals age into their 40s and beyond, life experience grows, and wisdom may be gained in understanding self, and others. However, each decade has increased risks for health which may impact pelvic function.

PELVIC FLOOR DYSFUNCTION

The incidence of pelvic floor dysfunction (PFD) increases in the midlife to elder years (Deiter, Wilkins, and Wu 2015) (Box 11.1). The potential challenges of pelvic pain, pelvic organ prolapse, and bladder, bowel, and sexual function limitations are not typically addressed by providers. Individuals often suffer in silence, due to a lack of resources for care, as well as a lack of understanding regarding self-care and lifestyle habits that may be of benefit.

With aging, people need to become more comfortable with "being" rather than "doing" as they lose physical functioning.

(Nancy Olmsted Kaehr 2014)

> **Box 11.1 Optimize social and fitness activity**
> Health is wealth, and motion is lotion for the mind–body–spirit. Yet not everyone can remain active, and as physical function is lost, adjustments need to be made to lifestyle, such as preserving walking on flat surfaces versus hills, inclines, steps, and stairs, using assistive devices if needed, and maintaining social and community connections.

PFD AND AGING

Specific PFD that may occur includes urinary and bowel continence/storage issues, as well as problems with emptying, pelvic organ prolapse (POP), pelvic pain in the genitals, and other pelvic regions such as the coccyx. Sexual function loss and performance problems may occur. These conditions may have associated spine, hip, or knee pain. Medication and surgical intervention may be needed for PFD, which may help reduce symptoms and increase function. However, side effects from medical and surgical treatment may occur and cause or exacerbate PFD (Al Khaja *et al.* 2020; Bjerregaard *et al.* 2015).

Menopause and andropause

Female menopause and male andropause are two recognized transitions in declining midlife hormone production, with physiological changes that can be associated with PFD (Boxes 11.2–11.4). Declines in estrogen and testosterone occur, as well as generalized strength loss and declines in functional fitness (Brinton *et al.* 2015; Matsumoto 2002).

> **Box 11.2 Stages of menopause and symptoms**
>
> Perimenopause: Hormone fluctuations begin with variation in estrogen levels, as well as other hormones. Menstrual cycles become irregular and hot flashes, insomnia, memory problems, and depression may begin to occur.
>
> Menopause: Permanent cessation of fertility due to absent menstruation and ovarian function. Associated vasomotor symptoms: hot flashes, vaginal thinning or atrophy, and increased vaginal ph. Diagnosed by the absence of menses and by follicle stimulating hormone tests at 30 mIU/mL or higher and other tests.
>
> Post-menopause: The time frame following cessation of menses, and with increased risk for lowered bone density, muscle strength, and libido lowering. The risk for PFD increases at this time, as well as potential cognitive changes (Brinton *et al.* 2015; Makwana, Shah, and Chaudhary 2020; North American Menopause Society 2022).

The genital symptoms of menopause (GSM)

GSM may be experienced by 60 percent of women. Symptoms may include genital region pain, dryness, lack of lubrication, and painful sex (dyspareunia). Other GSM symptoms include urinary urgency, dysuria, recurrent urinary tract infections, vaginitis and vaginosis, lichen sclerosis, and other conditions. There may be changes in self-esteem and body image (North American Menopause Society 2022; Portman and Gass 2014).

> **Box 11.3 Hormone rollercoasters**
>
> Estrogen receptors are found throughout the body and changes in vascular, bone, joint, cognitive, and somato-emotional functions are associated with the menopause transition. In life, women may be challenged with an emotional rollercoaster associated with vacillating hormone levels, at the same time raising teenagers, who may also be on an emotional rollercoaster!

Male andropause and symptoms

> **Box 11.4 Andropause**
> Male andropause includes age related declines in testosterone levels, growth hormone, lowered muscle mass, reduced muscle strength and power, balance, lowered bone mineral density, and decreased skin thickness and body hair. Risks increase for type 2 diabetes, cardiovascular disease, hypertension, and fractures. Males have a slower transition towards hormone related aging compared to females, and can maintain fertility into elder years, yet erectile dysfunction typically occurs and the health of sperm may degrade (Matsumoto 2002; Schwarcz, Phan, and Willix 2011).

NEUROLOGICAL CONDITIONS AND PFD

Alzheimer's disease (AD) and Parkinson's disease (PD) are two of the most common neurological conditions that occur with aging. Urinary incontinence is a common finding in these diseases with prevalence rates of 22–84 percent in AD and 27–80 percent in PD, respectively (Na and Cho 2020; Sakakibara *et al.* 2015). Incontinence may occur due to a lack of inhibition or loss of regulatory control of the bladder detrusor muscle, and this is termed neurogenic detrusor overactivity. Also, problems sensing bladder filling and loss of bladder contractility may occur, leading to a slow stream and prolonged urination, characteristics more likely in PD. Functional incontinence may occur, and worsen as mobility declines, due to the inability to make it to the toilet.

Gastrointestinal disorders

Gastrointestinal (GI) disorders are common in the midlife to elder years and can be a source of great distress. In AD and PD, gut health is emerging as causative factors in systemic inflammation and disease progression in these conditions. Constipation, inflammatory bowel disease, irritable bowel syndrome, and other GI conditions have been found to significantly associate with these neurological diseases, with researchers recommending national governments "extend health plans to improve intestinal health to prevent potential neurological disorders" (Fu, Gao, and Yung 2020).

CANCER CHALLENGES AND PFD

Cancers may be localized and can be treated medically with observation, medication, or minimal surgery. Some cancers may be more widespread, requiring chemotherapy and/or complex surgeries with significant morbidity and mortality. PFD may occur from surgical, radiation, chemotherapy, medication, and hormone side effects. Generalized weakness, fatigue, lower mobility, chronic pain, and lymphatic-based swelling (lymphedema) can occur and cause or exacerbate PFD (Boxes 11.5–11.7). Anxiety and depression often occur after cancer diagnosis (Center *et al.* 2012; Linden *et al.* 2012; Torre *et al.* 2017).

> **Box 11.5 Lymphedema**
> Lymphedema is a condition of swelling that may be in the trunk or in the limbs. It is more obvious with increased limb volume. It is due to reduced function of the lymphatic system.

The lymphatic system is a series of channels of lymph vessels and nodes throughout the body which carry lymphatic fluid back to the heart, assist circulation, and also help with immune functions.

Visual screening for swelling may detect increased limb volume, reduced skin creases due to swelling, and there may be associated pain and limitation of motion. Lymph-based swelling may precede the recognition of ovarian cancer, where abdominal swelling and unilateral leg swelling can occur. Lymphedema may follow surgeries due to disruption or removal of lymph nodes. Lymphedema can also be idiopathic and congenital (MacLellan and Greene 2014). Swelling may also occur from heart, lung, or kidney problems.

> **Box 11.6 Cancer survivorship: shortened lives, or long lives**
> People may, and often do, live long lives following cancer diagnoses, yet some are cut abruptly short. Cancer can be called a "thief of time." Yet it can also help transform the remaining lifetime to a state of grace and appreciation, while cutting out meaningless activities in order to thrive through illness.

Prostate cancer and prostatectomy

Postoperative complications may include urinary tract infections, bowel and bladder incontinence, narrowing of the bladder outlet, erectile dysfunction, pelvic pain, and lymphocele (lymph cyst) formation (Prostatectomy 2022). Somato-emotional concerns include depression, with possible social isolation and lowered activity levels, especially if dependent on continence pads, with worry regarding odor and discomfort with pad use.

Complex PFD and cancer

> **Box 11.7 Patient case: Amelia**
> Amelia, age 58, suffered, through a breast cancer diagnosis, a radical mastectomy, lymphedema, chemotherapy, and hormone suppression therapy. She presented for therapy for urinary incontinence, and dyspareunia which had occurred over the recent years of her breast cancer treatment. She had recent bouts of constipation and associated pain with straining to empty. She had stopped her fitness walking and Pilates class due to low energy levels and some concern if her lymphedema would be aggravated by exercise. See Box 11.8 for her treatment.

Pelvic surgery

Surgeries specifically for PFD are most often required in midlife into elder years, and these may include:

- bladder suspensions or slings
- bowel/anal surgeries
- pelvic organ prolapse surgery
- prostate surgery, prostatectomies
- uterine ablation, and/or hysterectomies.

Pelvic surgery for urinary incontinence is common, as well as surgery for pelvic organ prolapse, with a lifetime risk of surgery for PFD of 20 percent by age 80 (Dieter *et al.* 2015). Adverse effects may occur post operatively, with the patient's expectations of a "fix" not being met, and a persistence of symptoms, a need for recurrent surgery and/or infection treatment, and having a sense of shame and/or personal failure, with impacts on lowered quality of life (Dunivan *et al.* 2019).

SPINE AND JOINT SURGERIES AND PFD

Surgery for spinal stenosis and hip and knee replacements are common surgeries in mid-life into senior years. Anesthesia, antibiotics, immobility, pain medications, catheterization, and potential urinary tract infections may set the stage for PFD (Al Khaja *et al.* 2020; Baba *et al.* 2014).

Functional losses postoperation

After spine surgery and/or lower extremity joint replacement, functional strength in moving out of bed, getting in and out of a chair, and negotiating steps and stairs is limited. Mobility challenges may be associated with PFD.

SCREENING FOR PFD

Sample questions that providers may ask are listed below. Providers can refer to appropriate professionals beyond their scope of practice as needed.

General screening questions for PFD (partial list)

- Are you generally well hydrated, with urine output every 2–3 hours?
- How is your bladder doing? Is it storing and emptying OK?
- Is there any leaking? Are any pads needed?

- Can you sleep through the night, or do you get up often to urinate?
- How are your bowels doing? Are you having daily or regular output with no pain or strain?
- Are you having constipation with very hard stools, or the opposite: are stools too loose?
- Are you having any bowel leaks?

Referring individuals for specialty care can help improve their quality of life.

TREATMENT FOR PFD

Condition specific treatment paradigms are presented in other chapters. Healthy adults can cooperate and comply with behavioral, lifestyle, nutrition, and exercise training.

Optimizing health: provider overview

- Provide condition specific rehabilitation for PFD.
- Optimize strength, coordination, balance, gait, and mobility training to optimize function at home, work, leisure, and recreational activities.

Specific PFD treatment may include:

- behavioral training: timed voiding, adequate fluid and fiber use, and avoidance of bladder triggers or irritants
- pelvic muscle synergy for urination: relaxed effort; and for defecation: abdominal wall firming and PFM relaxation, with ideally minimal bearing down
- manual therapy for sites of myofascial pain, organ specific visceral

mobilization, and treatment for a "short pelvic floor" if needed

- specific pelvic floor muscle training, with isolated PFM contractions as well as co-contractions with other muscle groups for functional tasks
- fitness training to optimize abilities at home, work, community, and possible recreation participation
- sexual health education and resource training
- nutritional education to optimize gut microbiome, assimilation, immunity, and energy production
- counseling support for somato-emotional aspects of loss of functions, as well as for support for self-care and interpersonal relationships.

Manual therapy

Manual work may help promote or restore sensory awareness, PFM strength, and PFM relaxation-stretch and function. Organ specific visceral mobilization can help restore balance in the vast array of myofascial, lymphatic, vascular, and neurological systems. Midlife to elder individuals may have never received bodywork, and inclusion of manual therapy for health can be a new self-care, relaxation, and vitality enhancing format for wellness.

POST PROSTATECTOMY REHABILITATION CONSIDERATIONS

- screening and treatment for urinary incontinence and perineal region pain
- instruction in temporary adaptive seating equipment such as donut cushions
- restoration of standing versus seated urination, the latter of which is used when large pads are needed
- support for relationships and sexual health options
- oncology supervision and survivorship

protocols including exercise, nutrition, and lifestyle factors.

(Center et al. 2012; Student et al. 2017)

Hormone replacement therapy: HRT

FEMALES

Treatment for genital symptoms of menopause (GSM) often includes the medical prescription of topical estrogen for those that are appropriate.

Hormone therapy (HT) remains the most effective treatment for vasomotor symptoms (VMS) and GSM and has been shown to prevent bone loss and fracture. The risks of HT differ depending on type, dose, duration of use, route of administration, timing of initiation, and whether a progestogen is used.

(Pinkerton *et al.* 2017)

Non-hormonal care interventions for the vasomotor symptoms of menopause include other medications, cognitive behavioral therapy, hypnosis, probiotics, red clover, acupuncture, and physical activity (Hickey, Szabo, and Hunter 2017; Javadivala *et al.* 2020).

MALES

Males in midlife to elder years may be treated with testosterone for symptomatic hypogonadism (Dandona and Rosenberg 2010; Kherea *et al.* 2014). Males are often targeted by marketing for "low T" and testosterone supplementation as a libido and sexual performance booster (Healthline 2022). HRT protocols are common trends in "anti-aging medicine" and require individualized care and medical supervision of health (Brinton *et al.* 2015; Kherea *et al.* 2014; Matsumoto 2002).

Complex cases and PFD

Individuals with PFD who have co-morbidities such as diabetes, cognitive decline, or neurological disease may have permanent losses of function with aging (Boxes 11.8–11.10). There may be a need for senior support services and housing due to health challenges including loss of physical and/or mental function. Social services and health care advocates can assist as expert providers in placement and supervision of aspects of long-term care.

Box 11.8 Patient case: Amelia's treatment

Amelia's PFD after cancer treatment included instruction to restart a fitness walking program to tolerance, restart her Pilates exercises, and then Pilates classes when ready. She was referred to a lymphedema specialist for lymphatic massage, lymphedema upper extremity garment fitting, lymphedema lifestyle education, and skin care guidelines. She received urinary continence, constipation, and sexual medicine treatment and home care habit training with physical therapy (PT). She was grateful for the ability to regain bladder control and bowel regularity, as well as to restore her fitness and sexual function. Her husband attended a few sessions to receive education in sexual medicine as well as to encourage couples' fitness with walking and hiking.

Box 11.9 Restoring health and vitality

Exercise for flexibility, strength, and endurance, and manual and visceral therapy, can help restore function and quality of life. It is a joy for therapists to be able to guide a transformation toward wellness and even vitality following cancer diagnosis and treatment.

Box 11.10 Patient case: Miguel

Miguel, age 42, was sent to PT for abdominal and pelvic pain following his colon cancer surgery. He had a temporary ostomy bag that was to be removed as his system recovered. He had stomach, back, lower abdominal, and gastrointestinal pains that worsened with eating, and he had lost 35 pounds through his cancer journey. He reported that he was shocked when he received his cancer diagnosis. In his initial session, he admitted he was in a depression over his loss of function and income earning; he was homebound with his pain and postoperative recovery. He had a son and daughter with whom he played basketball, and he was sad he could no longer play with them. His posture was flexed at the trunk, and he held his arms crossed over his abdomen. He needed to use his arms to push up out of a chair, he walked stooped, and he appeared older than his 42 years. His goal was to return to work as a machinist.

Screening and testing identified:

- increased thoracic kyphosis, a stooped gait with increased double support time
- limited spine, upper and lower extremity range of motion
- upper chest respiration, and an inability to perform diaphragm and lateral costal breathing
- tenderness to palpation and guarding around ostomy site, abdominal wall, spine, and external pelvic floor muscles
- visceral mobility testing identified tenderness and restricted motion from the pylorus to the ileal cecal valve and descending colon, and restrictions surrounding his ostomy site.

His rehabilitation care involved progressive increased exercise (see photo list), manual therapy and visceral mobilization, deep relaxation training, and an outline of the bereavement process and options for soma-to-emotional self-care (Russel, Gough, and Drosdowsky 2015). He was instructed to take two 10-minute walks per day, and to build towards 20–45-minute walks over the next few months to tolerance. He was provided with initial exercise (see sample below) and progressed to weightlifting, basketball, and agility training. Over four months' time he regained the ability to be active with his children and returned to work within the year. A critical factor in his recovery was education on participation in exercise and a restoration of his social life with his family and friends.

Restoration of leisure time physical activity is a key factor to lower mortality risk (Box 11.11). Survivors of colon cancer with seven or more hours of leisure time physical activity per week were found to have a 31 percent lower mortality risk compared to those with no leisure time physical activity (Arem *et al.* 2015).

Box 11.11 Aging well
How is it that some people age and maintain vibrancy, vitality, and joy and seem to have a sense of flow about their life, while others call themselves old and withdraw from activity and social life, while losing fitness and joy? Some people seem blessed with happiness and health, while others suffer depression and illness, and lose function. Health appears as the true asset with aging, regardless of socioeconomic status.

Exercise
Promotion of exercise for health can help mood, bone density, muscle strength, endurance, and balance and improve sexual function, restorative sleep, and wellbeing. A gentle program for midlife to senior health can include exercises as in the following photos (Figures 11.1–11.15).

SEATED

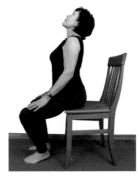

Figure 11.1 Cat-camel: lifting breastbone.

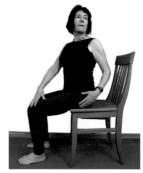

Figure 11.2 Trunk rotations.

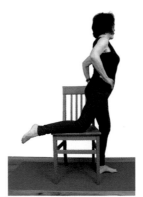

Figure 11.3 Hip flexor stretches off side of chair.

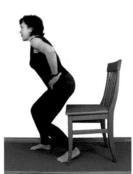

Figure 11.4 Sit to stand.

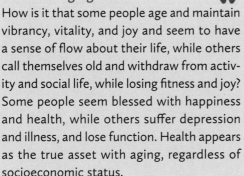

STANDING

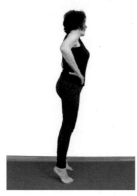

Figure 11.5A Heel raise.

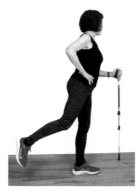

Figure 11.5B Heel raise with support.

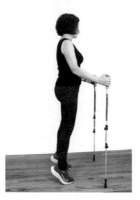

Figure 11.8A Hip flexion.

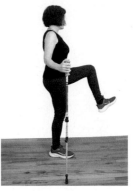

Figure 11.8B Hip flexion with support.

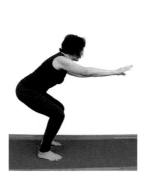

Figure 11.6A Mini squat.

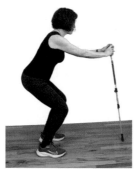

Figure 11.6B Mini squat with support.

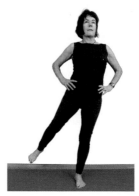

Figure 11.9A Hip abduction.

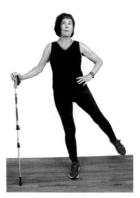

Figure 11.9B Hip abduction with support.

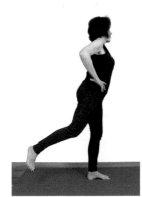

Figure 11.7A Hip extension.

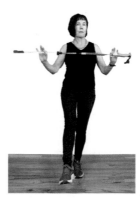

Figure 11.7B Hip extension with support.

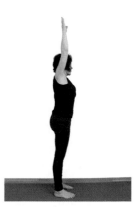

Figure 11.10 Leg lift front and balance.

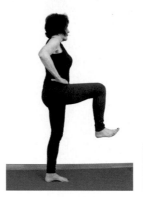

Figure 11.11 UE flexion, spine extension.

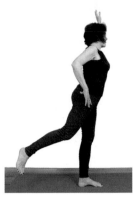

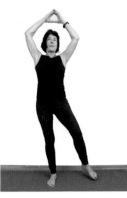

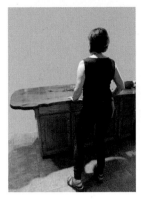

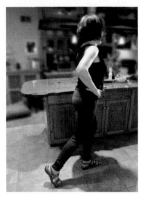

Figure 11.12 Alternate UE flexion and LE hip extension.

Figure 11.13 Single limb balance.

Figure 11.14 Side steps holding counter (resistance band if stable and more strengthening is needed).

Figure 11.15 Forwards, backwards walking holding counter (resistance band if stable and more strengthening is needed).

Wellness care ideally provides education and support for the prevention of illness, and we can consider positive health factors as listed below.

PREVENTATIVE HEALTH CARE

Positive health factors which promote wellness in midlife to elder years may lessen the occurrence or impact of PFD. Preventative health fitness and lifestyle factors are:

Fitness activity to:

- maintain cardiovascular fitness
- maintain strength for functional activities
- maintain bone health
- maintain flexibility
- maintain balance and postural control, coordination, and agility
- optimize mood and brain blood flow.

Lifestyle factors for health and longevity:

- optimum nutrition intake, including adequate fluid and fiber, vitamins and minerals, antioxidants, electrolyte balance, and anti-inflammatory foods
- maintain optimum body weight to prevent disease and illness, and stabilize blood sugar
- support for health with friends, coaches, trainers, bodyworkers, and fitness and medical professionals
- a sense of purpose, of being needed, being able to contribute towards the greater good
- social and community networks for emotional and psychological wellbeing
- intellectual stimulation, engaging the mind in learning over the lifespan.

(Buettner and Skemp 2016; Depp, Glatt, and Jeste 2007)

Count your age by friends, not years. Count your life by smiles, not tears.

(John Lennon)

Thriving

Blue zones are regions worldwide where we see exceptional longevity. Researchers find these blue zones have strong social support networks, regular lifestyle physical activity, and individual sense of purpose in a community, with these factors providing health benefits (Buettner and Skemp 2016; Depp *et al.* 2007). Aging, significant illness, and functional decline are not always associated. Providers treating PFD can help improve clients' health beyond condition specific treatment by referring individuals to social, volunteer, and fitness activities for health.

SUMMARY

PFD is a common condition in midlife to elder years. Health history factors such as parity, menopause, andropause, cancer, neurological disease, spine and joint surgeries, diabetes, obesity, smoking and alcohol use, and mental health status decline can be associated with PFD. Medical interventions for PFD may be necessary. However, there is vast potential for improving or eliminating PFD with conservative rehabilitation care.

Manual and/or visceral hands-on care, therapeutic exercise, movement practices, lifestyle habits, nutrition, and cognitive behavioral and wellness training can put the client in the driver's seat and encourage skills for self-care and health. The beauty of conservative therapy for PFD in the older population is that it can empower them with education and tools to manage their health and optimize function, thereby promoting lifelong wellness.

REFERENCES

Al Khaja, K. A. J., James, H., Veeramuthu, S., Tayem, Y., *et al.* (2020) "Prevalence of drugs with constipation-inducing potential and laxatives in community-dwelling older adults in Bahrain: Therapeutic implications." *International Journal of Pharmaceutical Practice 28*, 5, 466–472.

Arem, H., Pfeiffer, R. M., Engels, E. A., Alfano, C. M., *et al.* (2015) "Pre- and postdiagnosis physical activity, television viewing, and mortality among patients with colorectal cancer in the National Institutes of Health-AARO diet and health study." *Journal of Clinical Oncology 33*, 2, 180–188.

Baba, T., Homma, Y., Takazawa, N., Kobayashi, H., *et al.* (2014) "Is urinary incontinence the hidden secret after total hip arthroplasty?" *European Journal of Orthopedic Surgery and Traumatology 24*, 8, 1455–1460.

Bjerregaard, L. S., Bogo, S., Raaschou, S., Troldborg, C., *et al.* (2015) "Incidence of and risk factors for postoperative urinary retention in fast-track hip and knee arthroplasty." *Acta Orthopaedica 86*, 2, 183–188.

Brinton, R. D., Yao, J., Yin, F., Mack, W. J., and Cadenas, E. (2015) "Perimenopause as a neurological transition state." *Nature Reviews, Endocrinology 11*, 393–405.

Buettner, D. and Skemp, S. (2016) "State of the art reviews." *American Journal of Lifestyle Medicine 10*, 5, 318–321.

Center, M. M., Jemal, A., Lortet-Tieulent, J., Ward, E., *et al.* (2012) "International variation in prostate cancer incidence and mortality rates." *European Association of Urology 61*, 6, 1079–1092.

Dandona, P. and Rosenberg, M. T. (2010) "A practical guide to male hypogonadism in the primary care setting." *International Journal of Clinical Practice 64*, 6, 682–696.

Deiter, A. A., Wilkins, M. F., and Wu, J. M. (2015) "Epidemiological trends and future care needs for pelvic floor disorders." *Current Opinion in Obstetrics and Gynecology 27*, 5, v–vi.

Depp, C. A., Glatt, S. J., and Jeste, D. V. (2007) "Recent advances in research on successful or healthy aging." *Current Psychiatry Reports 9*, 1, 7–13.

Dunivan, G. C., Sussman, A. L., Jelovsek, J. E., Sung, V., *et al.* (2019) "Gaining the patient perspective on pelvic floor disorders' surgical adverse events." *American Journal of Obstetrics and Gynecology 22*, 2, 185.e1–185.e10.

Fu, P., Gao, M., and Yung, K. K. L. (2020) "Association of intestinal disorders with Parkinson's disease and Alzheimer's disease: A systemic review and meta-analysis. Abstract." *ACS Chemical Neuroscience 11*, 3, 395.

Healthline: Health conditions (2022) Can testosterone supplements improve your sex drive? Accessed 3/14/2022 at https://www.healthline.com/health/low-testosterone/do-testosterone-supplements-work.

Hickey, M., Szabo, R. A., and Hunter, M. S. (2017) "Non-hormonal treatments for menopausal symptoms." *British Medial Journal 359*. doi: 10.1136/bmj.j5101

Javadivala, Z., Allanhverdipour, H., Jafarabadi, M. A., and Emami, A. (2020) "An interventional strategy of physical activity promotion for reduction of menopause symptoms." *Health Promotion Perspectives 10*, 4, 383–392.

Kherea, M., Crawford, D., Morales, A., Salonia, A., and Morganthaler, A. (2014) "Collaborative review—andrology. A new era of testosterone and prostate cancer: From physiology to clinical implications." *European Urology 65*, 1, e31–e32.

Linden, W., Vodermair, A., MacKenzie, R., Greig, D., *et al.* (2012) "Anxiety and depression after cancer diagnosis: Prevalance by cancer type, gender, and age." *Journal of Affective Disorders 141*, 2–3, 343–351.

MacLellan, R. A. and Greene, A. K. (2014) "Lymphedema." *Seminars in Pediatric Surgery 23*, 4, 150972.

Makwana, N., Shah, M., and Chaudhary, M. (2020) "Vaginal pH as a diagnostic tool for menopause: A preliminary analysis." *Journal of Midlife Health 11*, 3, 133–136.

Matsumoto, A. M. (2002) "Andropause: Clinical implication of the decline of serum testosterone levels with aging in men." *The Journals of Gerontology: Series A 57*, 2, M76–99.

Na, H. R. and Cho, S. T. (2020) "Relationship between lower urinary tract dysfunction and dementia." *Dementia and Neurocognitive Disorders 19*, 3, 77–85.

North American Menopause Society (2022) "Expert Answers to Frequently Asked Questions about Menopause." Accessed 9/26/22 at https://www.menopause.org/for-women/expert-answers-to-frequently-asked-questions-about-menopause.

Pinkerton, J. V., Aguirre, S., Blake, J., Cosman, F., *et al.* (2017) "Abstract: The 2017 hormone therapy position statement of the North American Menopause Society." *Menopause 24*, 7, 728–753.

Portman, D. J. and Gass, M. L. S. (2014) "Genitourinary syndrome of menopause: New terminology for vulvo-vaginal atrophy from the International Society for the Study of Women's Sexual Health and the North American Menopause Society." *Journal of Sexual Medicine 11*, 12, 557–563.

Prostatectomy (2022) Mayo Clinic Patient Health Care and Health Information, Tests and Procedures. Accessed 6/13/2022 at https://www.mayoclinic.org/tests-procedures/prostatectomy/about/pac-20385198.

Russel, L., Gough, K., and Drosdowsky, A. (2015) "Psychological distress, quality of life, symptoms, and unmet needs of colorectal cancer survivors near the end of treatment." *Journal of Cancer Survivorship 9*, 462–470.

Sakakibara, R., Panicker, J., Finazzi-Agro, E., Iacovelli, V., *et al.* (2015) "A guide for management of bladder dysfunction in Parkinson's disease and other gait disorders." *Neurourology and Urodynamics 35*, 5, 551–563.

Schwarcz, E. R., Phan, A., and Willix, R. D. (2011) "Andropause and the development of cardiovascular disease presentation—more than an epi-phenomena." *Journal of Geriatric Cardiology 8*, 35–43.

Student, Jr, V., Vidlar, A., Grepi, M., Hartmann, I., *et al.* (2017) "Advanced reconstruction of vesicourethral support during robotic-assisted radical prostatectomy: One-year follow up outcomes in a two-group randomized controlled trial." *European Urology 71*, 5, E95–E96.

Torre, L. A., Islam, F., Siegel, R. L., Ward, E. M., and Jemal, A. (2017) "Global cancer in women: Burden and trends." *Cancer Epidemiology, Biomarkers and Prevention 26*, 4, 444–457.

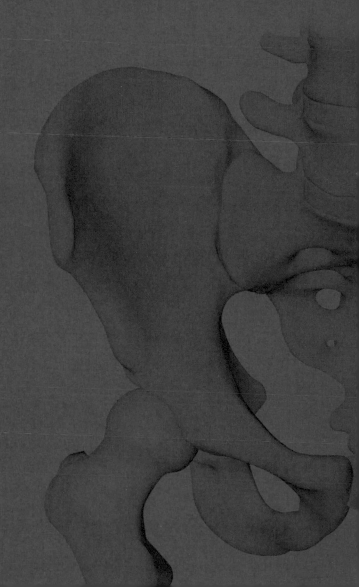

Section Four

INTEGRATED PROVIDER AND CLIENT CARE

CHAPTER 12

Mindfulness and Meditation for Pelvic Health

PAULINE LUCAS

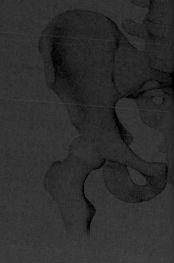

INTRODUCTION

Meditation and mindfulness are closely connected concepts and practices, originating in ancient Eastern philosophy. A secularized version became popularized in the West by pioneers like molecular biologist Jon Kabat-Zinn PhD, who founded the Stress Reduction Clinic, which later became the popular Mindfulness Based Stress Reduction (MBSR) program at Massachusetts Medical Center. Around that same time, in the late 1970s, Herbert Benson MD developed a program called "The Relaxation Response" at Harvard Medical Center. These programs consist of various techniques adapted from the original religious practices, in order to meet the standards and acceptance of Western medicine and science, while still offering the many benefits.

MINDFULNESS AND MEDITATION DEFINED

Mindfulness has become a household word, typically used in the context of general paying attention, as in "be mindful of your step." But the concept of mindfulness is actually a much more complex one and refers to paying attention in a specific way: intentional, in the present moment, with kind and curious focus, and without judgment. Besides a technique or skill that can be learned and practiced, the term also refers to a state of mind: having awareness of our own present moment experiences, and ultimately a way of living life. University of California Berkeley's Greater Good Science Center defines mindfulness as "maintaining a moment-by-moment awareness of our thoughts, feelings, bodily sensations, and surrounding environment, through a gentle, nurturing lens" (Greater Good Magazine 2022).

Presence, being in the moment, and mindful awareness are other ways to express the same concept. We can learn to bring mindful awareness to any activity or interaction. Meditation, however, is a deliberate and specific practice outside of our daily activities. It is described by the National Institutes of Health as "A mind and body practice that has a long history of use for increasing calmness and physical relaxation, improving psychological balance, coping with illness, and enhancing overall health and well-being" (NCCIH 2022).

Practicing mindfulness

Mindfulness practice is about using techniques to train the mind to stay engaged with what we are doing while we are doing it. Mindfulness can be a planned and deliberate activity like a meditation session, or it can be practiced during daily tasks like walking, eating, or having a conversation. Common mindfulness practices include seated mindfulness meditation, mindful walking, yoga, mindful eating, body scan practice, and breath awareness technique. As we develop our skills, we can bring an attitude of mindfulness to everything we do, and it becomes a way of living life. Someone who lives life in this mindful awareness is considered to be present.

Evidence for mindfulness/health benefits of mindfulness

Especially over the past ten years, mindfulness and meditation have gained popularity, which is evident by the explosion in scientific publications, the vast amounts of books and magazines available on the topic, an ever-expanding variety of apps, and the rapidly growing number of mindfulness training programs. Thousands of research studies on the topic have demonstrated benefits both in physical as well as psychosocial and cognitive domains accounting for the integration of mindfulness programs not only in health care institutions but in churches, schools, prisons, professional sports, and large businesses. Benefits of consistent and regular mindfulness and meditation practices include stress and anxiety reduction, better sleep, improved immune function, slowing of the aging process, better memory, and more. Studies on the effect on chronic pain have focused mostly on low back pain and are inconclusive about pain reduction but show that patients are less bothered by their symptoms; they cope better. A systematic review and meta-analysis of mindfulness interventions for chronic pain conditions such as headaches, rheumatoid arthritis, irritable bowel syndrome (IBS), and fibromyalgia found some evidence for pain reduction and significant evidence for reduced depression symptoms and improved quality of life (Hilton *et al.* 2017).

To date there is limited research specifically looking at the effects of mindfulness-based interventions on pelvic symptoms. Research has shown that an eight-week MBSR program significantly improved symptoms and quality of life in patients suffering with IBS with more than 70 percent of participants in this study reporting a reduction in the severity of their IBS symptoms, less anxiety, and improved quality of life following the training. These benefits continued three months after conclusion of the program. Stress is strongly correlated to symptoms of IBS and the researchers explained this very high success rate as the result of the participants practicing present moment awareness resulting in reduced worrying about the future or fretting about the past (Naliboff *et al.* 2020).

Mindfulness and pelvic health

Mindfulness-based interventions focus on two key ingredients: present moment awareness and acceptance. These are important components for the successful outcome of a program for pelvic health promotion. Our body communicates with us throughout the day. It signals when there is a need for eating or drinking, rest, movement, or to use the bathroom. With our busy lifestyle and many distractions, we often ignore these signals. Health care professionals and teachers, for example, are known to postpone emptying their bladder or defecating because they are not able to leave their patients or classrooms. Many other professionals are simply too busy to take a break to honor these needs. Over time, this can lead to a disconnect to where we lose awareness of these sensations, with consequences like constipation, incomplete voiding, or pelvic pain.

When working with clients with bowel, bladder, pain, and/or sexual problems, providers typically start with teaching them about the anatomy and function of their pelvic organs and pelvic floor. The client may be encouraged to explore and pay attention to what it feels like to have an urge to urinate or defecate, to empty the bladder or bowel, and the sensations afterwards. This awareness of sensations from inside the body is called *interoception*.

In the case of sexual challenges, providers may suggest they become aware of the body's response to thoughts about intimacy, changes in breathing, or any tension in the body, specifically in the pelvis, at the start and during an intimate encounter. This mindful awareness can be taught and practiced during a specialist pelvic examination.

During urination, defecation, and penetration, the pelvic floor muscles need to relax. In the case of pelvic pain, and when it is difficult to initiate the urine stream or bowel movement, and with painful penetrative sex, the pelvic floor muscles can be in a state of too much tension. One of the first steps to help the muscles relax is awareness of this muscular holding pattern.

BREATH

The breath is another component with these conditions, and learning to be aware of the breath makes it possible to identify and reduce tension. The breath tends to be fast and shallow when a person is stressed, and slower and deeper when relaxed. A calm, diaphragmatic breathing pattern can be used to create relaxation in the abdomen and the pelvic floor.

THOUGHTS AND SYMPTOMS

Additionally, it is important to become aware of stressful thoughts as they can contribute to a variety of symptoms (Box 12.1). In the case of an overactive bladder, for example, some people worry so much about finding a bathroom when they are out that it increases their sense of urgency and the likelihood of incontinence. Learning to identify this pattern and refocusing attention, or purposely taking relaxed breaths, will likely ease the urge. In patients with pain

conditions, the thought that the pain may never go away can add significant stress and worsen the symptoms. Becoming aware of these thoughts and questioning them can be a powerful healing skill and contribute to reduction in symptoms and chronic stress.

Box 12.1 Patient case: Linda's pelvic pain

Linda is a 29-year-old lawyer with severe vaginal pain when flying across the country, which she does for work at least three times per month. "When I arrive in Boston, I can barely make it to my hotel room and need to take pain medicine to get some sleep." Interestingly, she doesn't otherwise have much pelvic pain. She finds the meetings in Boston very stressful and always dreads the trip. During her first pelvic physical therapy visit it was identified during the vaginal examination that her pelvic floor muscles were very tight and tender to touch. Linda was quite surprised to feel the pain during this exam. With exploration of the sensations of contraction versus relaxation of the pelvic floor muscles, she was able to identify the difference in the first visit. When she returned for a follow up treatment, she was excited to share that while on the plane to Boston, when feeling the start of her familiar pain, she was able to identify that she was clenching her pelvic muscles and breathing very shallow. By resting her awareness on the sensation of tension, using yoga breathing and the relaxation techniques we discussed earlier that week, she had been able to relax her body and specifically the pelvic floor muscles and arrived at her destination without pain.

MEDITATION AND PHYSICAL PAIN

The practices of mindfulness and meditation offer tremendous benefits for people dealing with pain. We used to think of pain as a simple process of nerves in an injured body structure getting stimulated by an injury through mechanical and chemical processes (nociception). An example would be stepping on a piece of glass, in which case pain serves as a warning, to keep us safe. The logical treatment was to treat the injured body part, removing the pain trigger, for the pain to go away. With advances in neuroscience, it has become clear that pain, and especially persistent pain, is a much more complicated process, involving our emotional response and our thoughts about the pain. We have also learned that our nervous system can become sensitized and sometimes, even once the tissue injury has healed, the pain can remain. It has become apparent that our perception of pain has a great influence on our pain experience. For example, if someone with pelvic pain is convinced that there is something terribly wrong with their body, despite every medical test coming back "normal," they may falsely believe that medical professionals just haven't found the problem yet. In that case, the nervous system may stay on high alert, making sure to register every sensation to keep them focused and try to find the cause of the pain.

Mindfulness and meditation practices can provide insight into our response to pain and other challenging experiences (Boxes 12.2 and 12.3). It can also provide us with the awareness needed to skillfully observe and regulate our reactions to stress and pain and make choices that help reduce our suffering.

> **Box 12.2 Therapist insight**
> We can ask ourselves questions such as: "What are my beliefs about the pain, what do I think is going on, where does the pain start and where does it end, what does it feel like, and how would I describe the sensation without using the word pain?"

> **Box 12.3 Patient case: Mary, pain everywhere**
> When Mary, a 68-year-old woman, was asked where her pain was located, she answered, "Everywhere, my entire body hurts." She was further questioned, "There is no place in your body without pain?" "Correct," she replied. She was further queried about sensations in various body parts: "How does your right ear feel, how about your left ear, what sensations are present in the front of your neck?" and so on. During this guided body scan, Mary became aware that her pain was actually located in only a limited part of her body, across the lower abdomen. She had been very guarded and had tensed her entire body for quite a long time, which may have contributed to her experience of her entire body hurting.

Another aspect of the pain experience is "the story," which refers to the context of the pain. If we voluntarily engage in a painful experience (for example, getting a tattoo), the sensation of pain is likely significantly more manageable than when we are forced or someone else causes the same intensity of pain against our will. With mindfulness practices we can gain more awareness of the storyline and lessen its effect or even disconnect it from the uncomfortable sensations.

HOW AND WHERE TO LEARN

Information on learning mindfulness is widely available through apps, websites, books, and blogs. Although learning this way works for many, this author has found in 20 years as a meditation and mindfulness teacher that people often benefit from getting personalized guidance from a qualified instructor. Everyone's life circumstances are unique, and an instructor can address each person's specific needs and challenges and create a truly personalized mindfulness practice. The main issues frequently asked about are how to quiet a busy mind, how to deal with emotions or physical pain during meditation, and how to stay motivated when the benefits are not immediately noticeable. Learning in a group and hearing experiences and questions from other participants can be very enriching.

GETTING STARTED

When embarking on a meditation practice, it is important to plan ahead and have realistic expectations. Decide where, when, and how long to meditate, in what position, and what to focus on. Will you meditate with an app or other guidance, or guide yourself mentally, and how will you track the time? It might also help to have an intention for the practice; perhaps to find out for yourself what it's all about, to deepen your spiritual practice, to deal with pain and stress, or to sleep better.

- Timing: Traditionally, the ideal times for meditation are right after waking up in the morning when the mind is calm (RPM: rise, pee, meditate), and during the transition from daytime activities to evening ("happy hour"). However, with variety in circumstances, flexibility is key, and the meditation timing should be customized to each person's schedule. It is beneficial if there is consistency in time, duration, location, and techniques.
- Duration: Although various meditation schools recommend 20 minutes of meditation twice daily, for the novice it's recommended to practice for a shorter period, around 5 minutes, and gradually extend to 15 or 20 minutes once or twice daily. Researchers are still trying to figure out the minimal effective meditation time, and for now conclude that any time spent meditating is better than none. The use of a timer with a gentle sound to signal the end of the session helps with a gradual transition from meditation to waking state.

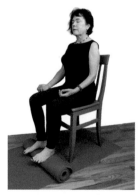
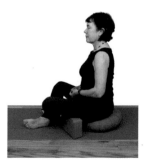

Figure 12.1 Seated meditation.

Figure 12.2 Seated on the floor (with supportive cushion and blocks).

- Posture: The position in which meditation is practiced is quite important and should be both comfortable and help the meditator stay awake and alert.

The ideal position is sitting, either on a comfortable chair with straight back (Figure 12.1), or if preferred, on the floor with legs crossed (Figure 12.2) or in hero pose (Figure 12.3). As sitting can be uncomfortable for people with pelvic symptoms, lying down (Figure 12.4), or even standing, might be a better alternative.

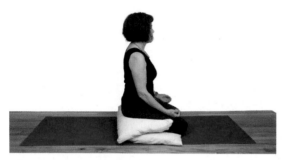

Figure 12.3 Hero pose.

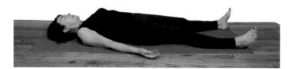

Figure 12.4 Lying down meditation pose.

- Body scan and breathing practices are often performed in a comfortable lying down position, and in the case of pelvic floor pain, we often use the "butterfly" position for the legs (Figure 12.5).

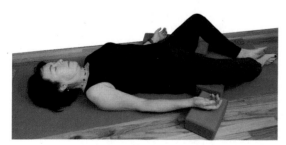

Figure 12.5 Butterfly position lying down.

- The eyes: meditation can be practiced with eyes open or closed or "capped," which means half closed and typically with downward gaze. The benefit of eyes closed is a reduction in input and distraction.

- Focus: Because the mind tends to wander as soon as one starts meditation, some type of anchor is needed for the mind to stay in the present moment. The breath is the most commonly used meditation focus. Others include body sensations (the body scan), a word or short phrase repeated mentally (mantra meditation), or visuals like a candle flame (trakata meditation). The attention should rest lightly on the anchor point ("like a butterfly resting on a flower"), and when the meditator finds the mind wandering, they gently bring it back to the object of attention. This consistently returning the awareness to the object of meditation is considered the *practice* of meditation.

- Guided versus non-guided meditation: Guided practices like those offered through many virtual platforms can be quite helpful at first but may not be ideal in the long run because they make one dependent on the guidance. Ideally you learn to also guide yourself without need for the external cues.

- Expectations: Novice meditators often have the false expectation of having a completely calm mind once they start their practice and get frustrated when they find their mind lost in thought throughout the meditation practice. It's therefore important to understand that the mind will likely continue to be busy with thinking and planning. Instead of fighting the thoughts, simply redirect the mind to the chosen anchor (i.e. breath, body sensations, mantra, etc.). This noticing and redirecting is the practice of meditation.

- Stick with it! Although some may find immediate benefit from their meditation practice, it typically takes a while. Just like brushing your teeth a few times a day without expectation for instant dental health change (and in hopes of a good dental check up every six months), the changes in meditation take time and diligent practice. Even if no change is apparent at first, sticking with a consistent practice will create many beneficial health changes. Although some sessions may feel more relaxing than others, our experience of each meditation is not an indication of how beneficial it was for our health and wellness. The beneficial changes in our nervous system and body happen over time.

SUMMARY

In summary, mindfulness and meditation have health benefits that are directly applicable to pelvic health challenges. Providing clients with mindfulness and meditation training can improve their health and wellness and promote the development of interoception and insight into their personal self-care.

REFERENCES

Greater Good Magazine (2022) *What is Mindfulness?* Accessed 3/13/2022 at https://greatergood.berkeley.edu/topic/mindfulness/definition.

Hilton, L., Hempel, S., Ewing, B. A., Apaydin, E., *et al.* (2017) "Mindfulness meditation for chronic pain: Systematic review and meta-analysis." *Annals of Behavioral Medicine 51*, 2, 199–213.

Naliboff, B. D., Smith, S. R., Serpa, J. G., Laird, K. T., *et al.* (2020) "Mindfulness-based stress reduction improves irritable bowel syndrome (IBS) symptoms via specific aspects of mindfulness." *Neurogastroenterology Motility 32*, 9, p.e13828.

NIH National Center for Complementary and Integrative Health (NCCIH) (2022) *Meditation and Mindfulness: What You Need to Know.* Accessed 3/13/2022 at www.nccih.nih.gov/health/meditation-in-depth.

CHAPTER 13

Sexual Health

This chapter presents topics on sexual health and wellness, dysfunction, and conservative care options. Information presented here can help individuals improve their sexual health, including communication with partners and care providers. For providers treating individuals with sexual health concerns, this information can inform, educate, and provide insights on aspects of sexual health and dysfunction.

A definition of sexual health (WHO 2015):

- "Sexual health today is a state of physical, emotional, mental, and social wellbeing in relation to sexuality."
- "Sexual health includes reproductive health, freedom from sexually transmitted infections (STI), freedom from sexual dysfunction, and freedom from the sequelae following sexual violence or female genital mutilation."
- "Sexual health includes 'the possibility for having pleasurable and safe sexual experiences, free of coercion, discrimination, and violence.'"

OVERVIEW

From the WHO definition we see that sexual health is a broad topic. Providers caring for individuals with sexual health challenges ideally have a solid education in the topics addressed in the definition. Provider cultural sensitivity and personal ethics are important, as follows.

Cultural sensitivity: client preferences

Cultural sensitivity is important in care provider interaction with individuals being seen for reproductive and sexual health concerns. Client religious, cultural influences, and personal history combine to produce a client's personal attitudes, beliefs, and sexual practices. The combination of these personal health, religious, and cultural factors can have a positive influence on sexual practices, as well as health care seeking and utilization of services. Or these personal health, religious, and cultural factors may provide a barrier to sexual health and seeking care. For example, a review finds that "Within all major religious traditions, Judaism, Christianity, Islam, Hinduism, Sikhism, and Buddhism, scholars have in one way or another reflected upon the meaning of sexuality, providing frameworks for good and bad sexuality, characteristics of male and female sexuality, and family planning strategies" (Arousell and Carlbom 2016).

An example of how personal health, religious, and cultural factors can intersect is in the consideration of the topic of virginity (Box 13.1). With a taboo on premarital sexual activity, and an associated value of the feminine in regard to chastity, purity, and honor, the life value of the female may be lost in the incidence of sexual trauma. Additionally, an elevation of the status of the hymen in defining virginity is medically complex and a clinically difficult item to measure. A lifelong sense of sexuality as a duty, and a sense of disconnect from the pelvic region, may follow suit for women, and this may lead to an unconsummated marriage and inability to be an active sexual partner, as well as enduring chronic pain with sex: dyspareunia (Happel-Parkins, Azim, and Moses 2020; Herman 2015; Rosenbaum 2022).

Box 13.1 Virginity

Certain religious cultures value virginity in determining the individual, family, community, and societal status of women (Mishori *et al.* 2019). A "loss" of virginity may be erroneously based on an examination of the hymen, and this practice, "virginity testing," has been condemned by health and human rights organizations. The researchers describe myths about the hymen that perpetuate medical, societal, and cultural harm towards females; the hymen is a varied membranous structure which is incongruous, difficult to visually screen or palpate, and not an indicator of a history of consensual or nonconsensual sexual experience (Kent 2019).

Avoiding bias: care providers

Provider interaction with clients and their personal health history, religious, and cultural influences ideally will consider individual differences and avoid bias and stereotyping. Some devout religious women, for example, may prefer a same sex gynecologist. Yet others may value their health care provider interaction and skill sets such as professionalism, competence, and being

treated with respect more than a preference for a same sex provider. And despite particular religious standards honoring virginity, clients with religious affiliation may seek health care for premarital sexual concerns, such as contraceptive planning, sexually transmitted disease screening, and pregnancy care (Arousell and Carlbom 2016).

Ethics and belief systems: care providers

Providers have varied opinions, preferences, and belief systems in whether they choose to offer certain services for sexual health. Due to provider cultural, religious, personal ethics, and belief systems, care providers may or may not agree on the following topics (Fiala and Arthur 2014) (Box 13.2):

- the right to sexuality outside of marriage
- pregnancy prevention care; access to contraception
- pregnancy termination options from the "morning after" pill to surgeries/abortion
- education for prevention and treatment of STI
- the possibility and acceptance of different sexual orientations
- gender confirmation hormone treatment and surgery.

Box 13.2 Code of ethics

Providers must follow their code of ethics, such as the American Physical Therapy Association's standards: code of ethics (APTA 2022).

Barriers to sexual health care

Socioeconomic and environmental barriers may exist which prevent access to care, such as lack of health insurance and funds to pay for care, disparities of care in minority, low-income regions, and inability to reach health care sites due to transportation barriers. These factors intersect with the broader issues of equity, race, justice, the law, and health (WHO 2015).

Sexual diversity, discrimination, and mental health

Sexual diversity ranges from lesbian, gay, bisexual, transgender, and queer (LGBTQ+) to other identities. The LGBTQ+ population suffers greater rates of mental health challenges, from anxiety and depression to suicide risk. Discrimination may be experienced in housing, public life, employment, and health care settings. Health service providers may benefit from training on gender affirming care, and community centers may provide a variety of needed services yet may be understaffed and underfunded (Su *et al.* 2016) (Box 13.3).

> **Box 13.3 Trans male experience** ♥
> Once known as Patricia, Patrick had transitioned to male, with hormone therapy which had caused a deepening of his voice, growth of facial hair, and enlarged genitalia, the clitoris, which he identified as his "little penis." He had slowly made the transition to trans male with the acceptance and support of his husband, still his partner, and his teenage children. He had decided to not seek "top surgery" (breast removal) or "bottom surgery" (phalloplasty). However, he had required a bladder suspension surgery a few years prior, before transitioning, and he had pelvic and abdominal pain, and urinary hesitancy following the procedure. He also had low back and hip pain related to work injuries. Before attending physical therapy (PT) he called the clinic to discern whether they were LGBTQ+ positive/affirmative. He told the therapist that he had prior traumatizing experiences with health care including negative attitudes by medical staff, mockery, and shaming, and since then he had a system to call and check before meeting new providers. He was informed that he would be treated with respect and professionalism, and this was a practice that welcomed diversity.

SEXUAL FUNCTION AND DYSFUNCTION

Terminology

- Sexual acts are behaviors involving the erogenous zones and the genitalia.
- Sex is considered as a primary drive, along with hunger, thirst, and pain avoidance (Trieschmann 1975).
- Sexuality is a combination of individual sex drive, sexual acts, and psychosocial factors involving attitudes, emotions, and relationships.

Sexual health boosters versus limiting factors

We can identify factors that support a healthy libido and sexual function versus factors that may lead to limitations in interest, arousal/libido, and sexual satisfaction (Table 13.1 and Boxes 13.4 and 13.5).

Table 13.1 Health factors, sexual health, and dysfunction

Positive factors for sexual health	Negative factors for sexual health
Exercise: regular fitness activity	No exercise: sedentary
Stress level: low	Stress level: high
Sleep: restorative, waking feeling refreshed	Sleep: nonrestorative, sleep apnea, insomnia
Psychosocial: no mood disorders	Psychosocial: anxiety and depression
Metabolic health: optimum blood pressure, blood sugar, body weight within normal limits	Metabolic health: periodontal disease, hypertension, diabetes, overweight or obese
No tobacco use	Tobacco use
Alcohol use: minimal	Alcohol use: high, alcoholism
Hormone status: balanced	Hormone status: unbalanced, menopause/andropause, thyroid disorders
No illicit drug use	Illicit drug use
Nutrition: anti-inflammatory Mediterranean diet	Nutrition: pro-inflammatory Western diet
Medications: no sexual side effects	Medications: sexual side effects
Health history: positive sexual experiences, no trauma, surgeries, or conditions affecting sexuality	Health history: negative sexual experiences, emotional, physical, and/or sexual trauma, and surgeries and/or conditions affecting sexuality
Cultural and/or religious affiliations: positive towards sexual health	Cultural and/or religious affiliations: negative towards sexual health

(*Jannini and Nappi 2018; La, Roberts, and Yafi 2018; McCabe et al. 2015; Mollaioli et al. 2020*)

Box 13.4 Sexual dysfunction can link to vascular problems

"Endothelial dysfunction, which can result from excess inflammation seen in metabolic syndrome and obesity, can lead to poor blood flow to genitourinary organs, thus providing a pathophysiological link between these diseases and sexual dysfunction."

(*Towe* et al. *2020*)

Box 13.5 Sex, or no sex, and intimacy

Not everyone needs to be interested or active in sex. Some individuals are asexual. Others may slowly lose interest with aging or illness. The problem arises if one partner has a high interest level and the other has no interest. And some couples have a high level of emotional intimacy, and physical intimacy, without sex.

Sexual response cycles

The sexual response cycle is viewed as a cyclical model, with variable starting points which may be a single or combined factors, including:

- a willingness to become receptive
- sexual stimuli
- desire
- arousal
- plateau of excitement
- orgasm or sexual satisfaction
- resolution/refractory phase.

Prior models of sexual responsiveness outlined a linear model, which started with arousal and desire. However, more recent research verifies that there are different starting points and reasons for engaging in sexual activity. These may include spiritual and emotional reasons, giving and receiving pleasure, to enhance emotional intimacy, as well as personal wellbeing (Basson 2005; Masters and Johnson 1966; Ogden 2013).

Gina Ogden's use of a medicine wheel exploring spiritual, emotional, mental, and physical aspects of self, and the self at different points in life, is a powerful and adaptable healing paradigm. This moves beyond sexuality as mere physiologic processes and allows individuals to explore and literally step into one quadrant or another in discovery, revelation, and renewal (Ogden 2013).

MALES

Male genital arousal occurs from the influence of testosterone, sensory stimulation of the genitalia, and physiologic and psychological factors. Erectile function is accompanied by external visual and proprioceptive changes (Figure 13.1).

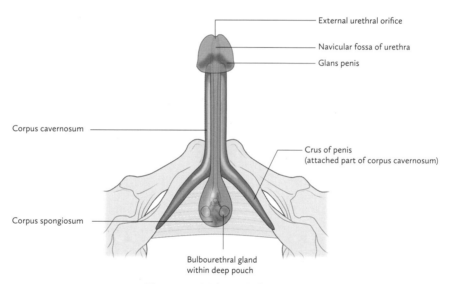

Figure 13.1 Male genital anatomy.

FEMALES

The female arousal response cycle is a relatively hidden process involving the structure of the clitoris and its associated parts—the bulb and the crus—as well as vaginal wall and uterine changes with arousal (Figure 13.2). Research expands our understanding of female sexual anatomy to include the clitoral–urethral–vaginal complex (CUV) and varied regional responses to clitoral or vaginal stimulation with sonography (Buisson and Jannini 2013; Jannini *et al.* 2014).

Genital functions required for penetrative penis-in-vagina (PIV) sexual intercourse

Male: Penile erection and firmness sufficient to sustain penetration

Female: PFM stretch, elasticity sufficient to allow penetration

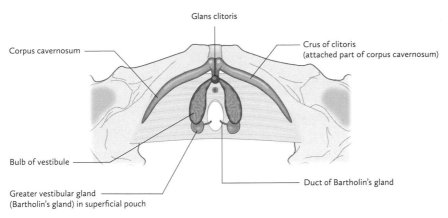

Figure 13.2 Female clitoral anatomy.

Anal intercourse requirements

Anal intercourse requires the use of lubrication and sufficient elasticity of the external and internal anal sphincter.

Reported use of anal intercourse by heterosexual couples is on the rise, and it is also a common practice among men that have sex with men (MSM). This practice is considered as taboo by some individuals, painful by many, and also may be a source of STD infection, such as chlamydia, herpes, HIV, or other infections. The practice may be pleasurable for some couples, yet it may be a part of nonconsensual activity and coercion as well (Marston and Lewis 2014). Typically, female partners experience pain, and may perform to please their partner, prevent pregnancy, and/or maintain virginity (El Feki 2013). Condom use for STD protection should be used, a lubricant, and the anal sphincter may require gradual stretching and preparation for penetration. Sexual toys can be used as a preparation, specifically those with a flange at the base so it will not be drawn up into the rectum. Rectal/colon retention of toys may require medical assistance or surgery. Rates of anal cancer are increasing and researchers consider rising rates of unprotected anal intercourse, HPV infection, and smoking as risk factors (Van der Zee *et al.* 2013).

EVALUATION FOR SEXUAL HEALTH

Sexual dysfunction: intake screening

Sexual dysfunction can involve problems from genetics, biological and physiologic functioning, and health history to psychosocial, attitudinal/ emotional, and/or relational concerns (Box 13.6). A team of providers is ideal to assess each unique individual, their concerns, needs, and challenges, and provide care to meet their goals (Goldstein *et al.* 2018). A sexual history intake may include screening factors such as:

- low libido, desire, and arousal difficulties

- anorgasmia: inability to achieve orgasm (Komisaruk, Beyer-Flores, and Whipple 2015; Nagoski 2015)
- dyspareunia: pain with sex, either superficial or deep (Goldstein, Clayton, and Goldstein 2011)
- pelvic pain with arousal, orgasm, positioning, or post relations
- persistent genital arousal disorder (PGAD) (Goldstein *et al.* 2011)
- priapism: uncontrolled, painful, sustained erections (Levey, Segal, and Bivalacqua 2014)

- premature or early ejaculation (Metz and McCarthy 2003)
- erectile dysfunction (Bø *et al.* 2015)
- penile malformation from trauma and/ or Peyronie's disease (NIDDK 2022; Stuntz *et al.* 2016)
- penile dysmorphic disorder (Marra *et al.* 2020)
- partner/relationship dynamics regarding sexuality (Konzen and Konzen 2016)
- infertility issues and treatments
- anxiety/depression related to sexual dysfunction
- sexual addiction and co-morbid alcohol or drug addiction
- trauma history: verbal, physical, or sexual (Emerson 2015; Khalaf 2019)
- medical factors affecting health and sexual function.

Many of these above listed factors overlap in categories including genetics, mind–body considerations (attitudes, belief systems, psychological and spiritual states), environmental and biological factors, and health history influence (McCabe *et al.* 2015) (Boxes 13.7 and 13.8). Interested readers may pursue textbooks on human sexuality and dysfunction, some with topic specific orientation, or broad topic texts, as listed: Bø *et al.* 2015;

Goldstein *et al.* 2011; Gunter 2019; Kerner 2010; Komisaruk *et al.* 2006; Konzen and Konzen 2016; Myss 1996; Nagoski 2015; and Northrup 2010.

Most people think other people are having more sex, and better sex, than they are.

(Dr. Holly Herman 2017)

Box 13.6 The female sexual function index

A validated outcomes form, the female sexual function index (FSFI), is useful in assessing problems related to sexual function, and monitoring changes in function over time. The domains of the FSFI include desire, arousal, lubrication, orgasm, satisfaction, and pain (Rosen *et al.* 2000).

Box 13.7 Love languages

Knowing a partner's "love language," as well as recognizing personal preference, can help strengthen relationships. The love languages are: words of affirmation, quality time, physical touch, acts of service, and giving gifts (Chapman 2004).

SEXUAL HEALTH CHALLENGES: PROFILES

Exact descriptors of problems provide clues as to necessary treatments. Health history screening may reveal factors such as an unconsummated marriage due to vaginismus, premature ejaculation, or erectile dysfunction. An unconsummated marriage may also be due to a lack of communication, and knowledge of sexual practice options to enhance partner comfort and pleasure. At the other end of the spectrum, a client may have an obsessive-compulsive based sexual addiction history, or a penile dysmorphic disorder, and/or

pelvic pain due to pelvic/genital trauma (Karila *et al.* 2014). Client goals may be varied from a desire to reduce pain, a desire to consummate a marriage to attain pregnancy, a desire to achieve an orgasm, or a desire to please a partner with sexual performance. There may be a goal to rehabilitate sexual and other pelvic functions, or postoperative and associated bladder and bowel dysfunction concerns. Factors which may be examined to delineate problems include (a limited list):

- flexibility of the spine, extremities, and PFM
- strength of the spine, extremities, and PFM
- sensation in nerve zones supplying the back, hips, pelvic area: normal, sensitized, or are neuralgias present?

- tone in the myofascial system: guarded, clenching, normal, or low tone?
- medical: lab tests for blood sugar, hormone levels, thyroid, and psychological profiles for assessment of mood, relationship dynamics, and other issues.

TREATMENT

Following intake screening, a treatment plan is composed to meet client goals. Typical programming paradigms may include the items below.

Client education

Education can be provided with encouragement towards positive health enhancing factors to improve sexual function (Table 13.1). Anatomy education and physiological aspects of hormone influence, libido, desire, arousal, and orgasm can be discussed with the use of anatomical charts and models to help clients understand their conditions. Referral to sexual health resources such as specialist providers can help to enhance biological, physiological, somato-emotional, psychological, and spiritual aspects of sexuality.

Safety and pleasure

Education regarding foundational aspects of safety and pleasure can provide ground rules for sexual activity. Sexologist Heather Howard (2013) advises three questions for boundaries in sexual behavior:

- Is it safe?
- Can you hurt yourself?
- Can you hurt someone else?

Communication between partners: emotional intimacy

Safety and pleasure require respect and communication between partners, belief systems of equality, decision sharing, and sensitivity. In this regard, activities should be safe from potential sexually transmitted disease (STD), have options of pregnancy prevention, as well as be pain free, or pain minimizing. The partner in pain is ideally able to communicate and stop activities as needed. Individuals with low self-esteem, or a sense of "duty" to "service" a partner, may expect and accept discomfort as part of the experience. Others may simply want to improve their comfort and reduce pain. And finally, some individuals seeking care require information and therapeutic intervention to help them have a positive sexual experience, pleasure, and to achieve orgasm. Who can help with these interventions? Providers with specialty training and certifications may provide care, as listed:

- psychologists, psychiatrists, sexologists
- gynecologists, OBGYN, internal medicine, urologists, nurses, nurse practitioners, pharmacists, physical therapists, midwives, osteopaths.

Specialty sexual medicine providers may be trained with, or affiliated with, professional medical organizations as listed below:

- ASSECT: American Association of Sexuality Educators, Counselors and Therapists
- ISSWSH: International Society for the Study of Women's Sexual Health
- American College of Sexologists

- International Professional Surrogates Association
- American Physical Therapy Association, Institute of Pelvic Health.

Outercourse

"Outercourse" is a helpful option for sexual activity, and partners using outercourse may agree to the terms of no penetrating activity, such as penis in vagina (PIV) intercourse. Outercourse can spare those in pain from having to "have sex" with a pain experience to comfortable and pleasurable intimacy (Happel-Parkins *et al.* 2020). Sexual function is often not addressed in relation to illness, and those in partnered relationships can benefit from education and counseling (Konzen and Konzen 2016; Rosenbaum 2022).

PLISSIT model for education

Education for recovery after illness or surgery can enhance sexual function for couples and/ or individuals. The PLISSIT model for sexual education includes involving *p*ermission, *l*imited *i*nformation, *s*pecific *s*uggestion, and *i*ntensive *t*herapy (Keshavarz *et al.* 2021). The PLISSIT model has been shown to improve FSFI and quality of life (QOL) in patient populations. The PLISSIT model and FSFI have been used to validate improved sexual functioning in status post breast cancer (Faghani and Ghaffari 2016) and these methods are applicable to a wide population.

Orthopedics and sexual function

For sex with pelvic girdle, hip, or low back pain, individuals may need adaptive positioning with pillows or bolsters, the use of a sacroiliac belt, partner instruction, and possible abstinence from penetrative intercourse in cases of pain (Herman 2017). A detailed chart for adaptive intercourse positioning is available for providers and clients: *Orthopedic Considerations for Sexual*

Activity (Herman and Wallace Pelvic Rehabilitation Institute 2021).

> ### Box 13.8 Neurological and orthopedic considerations
> Any condition of the thoracic, lumbopelvic hip can impact sexual function. Males with herniated lumbar discs and reported sexual dysfunction have demonstrated improved functioning postoperatively (Panneerselvam *et al.* 2021). Clients ideally can be treated for neuromuscular and orthopedic limitations affecting sexual function.

Sensate exercises

Progressive steps to enhanced intimacy may be instructed and help provide options for enjoyable physical and/or sexual contact. Sensate exercises can reduce pressure for performance and provide options for new methods for sensory discovery, communication, and practice. Nonverbal feedback is used, with touching and movement of hands to communicate yes or no. Phase one instructs partners to explore body contact yet avoid genitals and breasts. Phase two involves tactile contact of genitals and breasts. Phase three and beyond may involve intercourse if both parties are willing and comfortable (Weiner and Avery-Clark 2014). A guide for couples' nonverbal communication is available (Howard 2010).

Anyone who is observant, who discovers the person they have always dreamed of, knows that sexual energy comes into play before sex even takes place. The greatest pleasure isn't sex, but the passion with which it is practiced. When the passion is intense, then sex joins in to complete the dance, but it is never the principal aim.

(Paulo Coelho)

MANUAL THERAPY AND EXERCISE

Manual therapy and exercise provided by a licensed provider have great application for improving sexual function. Education in anatomy with "mapping" and "saying hello" to the PFM and associated leg, hip, spine, and respiratory muscles can help tune in to areas of comfort, or of discomfort/pain, and associated body tension with breath holding or other problems. Associated nervous system and somato-emotional responses can be addressed and directed to empower the client. There should always be client choices regarding the techniques being performed, i.e. external or internal manual, or the use of other treatments such as exercise, guided meditation, and other modalities.

The short, tight pelvic floor may compress the spermatic cord, pudendal nerve, or simply not allow an up–down motion of myofascial structures to sustain arousal, climax, and resolution. Visceral restrictions from the round ligament into the labia, hernia repairs, and restrictions at the spermatic cord (or other scar tissue) may be associated with pain. Manual therapy is a nonsexual, health care professional method for myofascial release and pain therapy. Ideally this is practiced with trauma sensitive techniques as discussed in earlier chapters.

Individuals can learn to perform self-myofascial release to tender and trigger points, to relax-release with breath practices and "letting go" the PFM. They can learn comfort and pleasure in safe single sexual activity at home, including an optional intention for self-stimulation to produce orgasm. Or this may be a partnered activity, with guidelines for communication for safety and trauma prevention.

Exercise

Exercise is found to enhance blood flow to the genitalia, and support cardiovascular health via blood sugar and blood pressure regulation. It also promotes stress management, nervous system homeostasis, improved gut microbiome, and positive self-esteem. Target exercises for PFM strengthening have been found to enhance male erectile function and female sexual function in reviews of literature (Bø *et al.* 2015). Exercise induced experience of sexual pleasure, including orgasms, have been reported in women. An online survey found 51.4 percent of the respondents experienced exercise induced orgasms, yet also with the experience of feeling self-conscious (Hebenick and Fortenberry 2012).

SEXUAL HEALTH EQUIPMENT AND LUBRICANTS

Sexual health equipment: sex toys

Sexual health equipment, also known as "sex toys," are numerous. Sex toys are gaining recognition in public perception, social mores, and in a broader acceptance of sexual health in the media. Vibrators and an assortment of external as well as penetrative devices are sold at local and online shops. The toys offer an option for partnered or solo sexual activity. Those with relationship problems and pain/sexual dysfunction may have difficulties with these toys, whereas some individuals and couples may have positive experiences, including first experiences of orgasm with the use of toys.

Lubricants

Lubricants can be essential for comfort during penetrative sexual activity. Females may have desire and arousal yet have vaginal dryness. J. Michelle Martin advises postpartum clients that they may use "a vaginal lubricant to address dryness and discomfort. These may be Water based

(Slippery Stuff, Intimate Rose), Silicone based (Uberlube, Momentum), Oil based (coconut oil, Coconu), or Aloe based (Good Clean Love)" (J. Michelle Martin Health Solutions, personal communication, December 2021). For use with sexual equipment or toys, silicone-based toys break down with silicone lubricant, and oil-based products break down latex condoms. Water-based products are necessary for latex condom use. Oil-based lubricant is safe for stainless steel and glass-based toys (see goodcleanlove.com).

SUMMARY

A sexual wellbeing model includes fertility regulation, sexually transmitted infection prevention and management, prevention of sexual violence, and the presence of sexual desire and arousal (Casado-Espada *et al.* 2019; Mitchell *et al.* 2021). Sex and interest in who is doing what, with whom, and how often are basic human-interest items. Sexuality and sexual practices are diverse and there are many misconceptions and sexual health problems as addressed in this chapter. Providers can help optimize client sexual health and wellness with education, counseling, and medical intervention including contraceptive services and STD screening and treatment, hormone treatment, manual therapy exercise, and PFM training modalities. This subject can fill an entire book itself, and readers are directed to books, research articles, and internet resources.

REFERENCES

American Physical Therapy Association (APTA) (2022) *Code of Ethics for the Physical Therapist.* Accessed 3/17/2022 at www.apta.org/siteassets/pdfs/policies/codeofethicshods06-20-28-25.pdf.

Arousell, J. and Carlbom, A. (2016) "Culture and religious beliefs in relation to reproductive health." *Best Practice and Research Clinical Obstetrics and Gynecology 32,* 77–87.

Basson, R. (2005) "Women's sexual dysfunction: Revised and expanded definitions." *Canadian Medical Association Journal 172,* 10, 1327–1333.

Bø, K., Berghmans, B., Morkved, S., and Van Kampen, M. (2015) *Evidence-Based Physical Therapy for the Pelvic Floor: Bridging Science and Clinical Practice.* Edinburgh: Churchill Livingstone.

Buisson, O. and Jannini, E. A. (2013) "Pilot echographic study of the differences in clitoral involvement following clitoral or vaginal sexual stimulation." *Journal of Sexual Medicine 10,* 11, 2734–2740.

Casado-Espada, N. M., de Alcaron, R., de Iglesia-Larrad, J. I., Bote-Bonaechea, B., and Montejo, A. L. (2019) "Hormone contraceptives, female sexual dysfunction, and managing strategies: A review." *Journal of Clinical Medicine 8,* 6, 908.

Chapman, G. (2004) *The Five Love Languages: The Secret to Love That Lasts.* Chicago: Northfield Publishing.

El Feki, S. (2013) *Sex and the Citadel: Intimate Life in a Changing Arab World.* New York: Pantheon Books, Random House.

Emerson, D. (2015) *Trauma-Sensitive Yoga in Therapy: Bringing the Body into Treatment.* New York: W. W. Norton and Company.

Faghani, S. and Ghaffari, F. (2016) "Effects of sexual rehabilitation using the PLISSIT model on quality of sexual life and sexual functioning in post-mastectomy breast cancer survivors." *Asian Pacific Journal of Cancer Prevention 17,* 11, 4845–4851.

Fiala, C. and Arthur, J. H. (2014) "'Dishonorable disobedience'—Why refusal to treat in reproductive health care is not conscientious objection." *Woman-Psychosomatic Gynecology and Obstetrics 1,* 12–23.

Goldstein, A., Pukall, C., and Goldstein, I. (2011) *When Sex Hurts: A Woman's Guide to Banishing Sexual Pain.* New York: Perseus Books.

Goldstein, I., Clayton, A. H., Goldstein, A. T., Kim, N. N., and Kingsberg, S. A. (2018) *Textbook of Female Sexual Function and Dysfunction, Diagnosis and Treatment,* 1st ed. Hoboken, NJ: John Wiley and Sons Ltd.

Gunter, J. (2019) *The Vagina Bible: The Vulva and the Vagina—Separating Myth From Legend.* New York: Citadel Press.

Happel-Parkins, A., Azim, K. A., and Moses, A. (2020) "'I just beared through it': Southern US Christian women's experiences of chronic dyspareunia." *Journal of Women's Health Physical Therapy 44,* 2, 72–86.

Hebenick, D. and Fortenberry, J. D. (2012) "Exercise induced orgasm and pleasure among women." *Sexual and Relationship Therapy 21,* 4, 2631–2640.

Herman, H. (2015) "Sexual medicine for men and women: A rehabilitation perspective." Herman and Wallace Pelvic Rehabilitation Institute, San Deigo, CA.

Herman, H. (2017) Male pelvic health seminar. Function-Smart Physical Therapy, San Diego, CA.

Herman and Wallace Pelvic Rehabilitation Institute (2021) "Orthopedic Considerations for Sexual Activity." Available to purchase from https://hermanwallace.com/products/orthopedic-considerations-for-sexual-activity.

Howard, H. (2010) *Reduce Sexual Pain: A Guide for Couples.* Accessed 4/10/2022 at https://heatherhoward.com/DrHeatherHoward-sexual_pain_guide-for_couples.pdf.

Howard, H. (2013) "Sexual health toolkit: Ergoerotics and sexual concerns for the pelvic disorder patient," seminar. San Diego, CA, June 22–23, 2013.

Jannini, E. A. and Nappi, R. E. (2018) "Couplepause: A new paradigm in treating sexual dysfunction during menopause and andropause." *Sexual Medicine Reviews 6*, 3, 384–395.

Jannini, E. A., Buisson, O., and Rubio-Casillas, A. (2014) "Beyond the G-spot: Clitourethralvaginal complex anatomy in female orgasm." *Nature Reviews, Urology 11*, 9, 531–538.

Karila, L., Wery, A., Weinstein, A., Cottencin, O., *et al.* (2014) "Sexual addiction or hypersexual disorders: Different terms for the same problem? A review of the literature." *Current Pharmaceutical Design 20*, 4012–4020.

Kent, C. (2019) *Myths About the Hymen.* Accessed 4/10/2022 at https://sexualbeing.org/blog/3-myths-about-the-hymen-that-really-need-to-die.

Kerner, I. (2010) *She Comes First: The Thinking Man's Guide to Pleasuring a Woman.* New York: Collins.

Keshavarz, Z., Karimi, E., Golezar, S., Ozgoli, G., *et al.* (2021) "The effect of PLISSIT based counseling model on sexual function, quality of life, and sexual distress in women surviving breast cancer: A single-group pretest–posttest trial." *BMC Women's Health 21*, 417.

Khalaf, M. A. (2019) "The relationship between female genital mutilation and post-traumatic stress disorder: Implications for trauma-sensitive informed social work." *Egyptian Journal of Social Work 8*, 1–40.

Komisaruk, B. R., Beyer-Flores, C., and Whipple, B. (2006) *The Science of Orgasm.* Baltimore, MD: Johns Hopkins University Press.

Konzen, T. and Konzen, J. (2016) *The Art of Intimate Marriage: A Christian Couple's Guide to Sexual Intimacy.* San Diego: Konzen Publishing.

La, J., Roberts, N., and Yafi, F. A. (2018) "Diet and men's sexual health." *Sexual Medicine Reviews 6*, 1, 54–68.

Levey, H. R., Segal, R. L., and Bivalacqua, T. J. (2014) "Management of priapism: An update for clinicians." *Therapeutic Advances in Urology 6*, 6, 230–244.

Marra, G., Drury, A., Tran, L., Veale, D., and Muir, G. H. (2020) "Systematic review of surgical and non-surgical interventions in normal men complaining of small penis size." *Sexual Medicine Review 8*, 1, 158–180.

Marston, C. and Lewis, R. (2014) "Anal heterosex among young people and implications for health promotion: A qualitative study in the UK." *BMJ Open Sexual Health Research 4*, 8, e004996.

Masters, W. H. and Johnson, E. J. (1966) *Human Sexual Response.* Toronto; New York: Bantam Books.

McCabe, M. P., Sharlip, I. D., Atalla, E., Balon, R., *et al.* (2015) "Risk factors for sexual dysfunction among women and men: A consensus statement from the fourth international consultation on sexual medicine." *Journal of Sexual Medicine 13*, 2, 144–152.

Metz, M. E. and McCarthy, B. W. (2003) *Coping with Premature Ejaculation: How to Overcome PE, Please Your Partner and Have Great Sex.* Oakland, CA: New Harbinger Publications.

Mishori, R., Ferdowsian, H., Naimer, M., and McHale, T. (2019) "The little tissue that couldn't—dispelling myths about the hymen's role in determining sexual history and assault." *Reproductive Health 16*, 74.

Mitchell, K. R., Lewis, R., O'Sullivan, L. M., and Fortenberry, J. D. (2021) "What is sexual wellbeing and why does it matter for sexual health?" *The Lancet Public Health 6*, 8, e608–e613.

Mollaioli, D., Ciocca, G., Limoncin, E., DiSante, S., *et al.* (2020) "Lifestyles and sexuality in men and women: The gender perspective in sexual medicine." *Reproductive Biology and Endocrinology 18*, 1, 10.

Myss, C. (1996) *Anatomy of the Spirit: The Seven Stages of Power and Healing.* London: Bantam Books.

Nagoski, E. (2015) *Come As You Are: The Surprising New Science That Will Transform Your Sex Life.* New York: Simon and Schuster.

National Institute of Diabetes and Digestive and Kidney Diseases (NIDDK) (2022) *Penile curvature (Peyronie's disease).* Accessed 4/10/2022 at https://www.niddk.nih.gov/health-information/urologic-diseases/penile-curvature-peyronies-disease#sec1.

Northrup, C. (2010) *Women's Bodies, Women's Wisdom: Creating Physical and Emotional Health and Healing.* London: Bantam Books.

Ogden, G. (2013) *Expanding the Practice of Sex Therapy. An Integrative Model for Exploring Desire and Intimacy.* Abingdon, UK: Taylor and Francis.

Panneerselvam, K., Kanna, R. M., Shetty, A. P., and Rajasekaran, S. (2021) "Impact of acute lumbar disc herniation on sexual function in male patients." *Asian Spine Journal 16*, 4, 510–518.

Rosen, R., Brown, C., Heiman, J., Leiblum, S., *et al.* (2000) "The female sexual function index (FSFI): A multidimensional self-report instrument for the assessment of female sexual function." *Journal of Sex and Marital Therapy 26*, 2, 191–208.

Rosenbaum, T. Y. (2022) *Sexual health resources.* Accessed 4/10/2022 at https://tallirosenbaum.com/articles/#.

Stuntz, M., Perlaky, A., des Vignes, F., Kyriakides, T., and Glass, D. (2016) "The prevalence of Peyronie's disease in the United States: A population-based study." *PLOS One 11*, 2, e0150157.

Su, D., Irwin, J. A., Fisher, C., Ramos, A., Kelley, M. *et al.* (2016) "Mental health disparities within the LGBTQ population: A comparison between transgender and nontransgender individuals." *Transgender Health 1*, 1, 12–20.

Towe, M., La, J., Khatib, F. E., Roberts, N., Yafi, F. A., and Rubin, R. (2020) "Diet and female sexual health." *Sexual Medicine Reviews 8*, 2, 256–264.

Trieschmann, R. B. (1975) "Sex, sex acts, and sexuality." *Archives of Physical Medicine and Sexuality 56*, 8–9.

Van der Zee, R. P., Richel, O., de Vries, H. J. C., and Prins, J. M. (2013) "The increasing incidence of anal cancer: Can it be explained by trends in risk groups?" Netherlands Review. *The Journal of Medicine 71*, 7, 401–411.

Weiner, L. and Avery-Clark, C. (2014) "Sensate focus: Clarifying the Master and Johnson model." *Sexual and Relationship Therapy 29*, 3, 307–319.

World Health Organization (WHO) (2002) "Sexual health, technical consultation." Accessed 9/23/22 at https://www.who.int/health-topics/sexual-health#tab=tab_2.

World Health Organization (WHO) (2022) *Sexual and Reproductive Health and Research (SRHR)*. Accessed 6/15/2022 at www.who.int/teams/sexual-and-reproductive-health-and-research/key-areas-of-work/sexual-health/defining-sexual-health.

FURTHER RESOURCE

Human Rights Campaign (2022) *Glossary of Terms.* Accessed 4/10/2022 at www.hrc.org/resources/glossary-of-terms.

CHAPTER 14

Integrative Pelvic Health Care

MAUREEN MASON AND JESSICA DRUMMOND

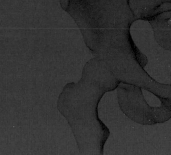

INTRODUCTION

This chapter addresses pelvic health promotion with multiple holistic care strategies. Nutrition, the gut microbiome, and the influence of co-morbidities in pelvic health will be profiled, with a view towards resiliency and transformation.

An integrative healing approach can provide optimum health care in the complicated world of pelvic health problems, with symptoms often presenting with interrelated conditions. Providers must consider and provide treatment for clients within their scope of practice, which may include deciphering the root triggers or causes for the presenting condition(s). This may include blood tests screening for parasites, viruses, bacteria, fungi, yeast, and metabolic profiles (Drummond and Sarna 2020). Genetic tests may reveal methylation challenges or other metabolic and enzymatic weaknesses. Stool testing may screen for the presence and absence, or dysbiosis, of key microbial species in the colon (at least some layers of the colon environment) to assess intestinal diversity and health. Detailed nutrition analysis can discern inflammatory triggers and deficits. The biomes from the mouth to the small intestine, large intestine, bladder, urethra, prostate, penis, or vagina may be harboring species that can trigger inflammation and disease. The biomes are emerging as key health foundations that interact with the environment and genetics.

As stated in Kau *et al.* (2011): "the time is right and the need is great to understand better the relationships between diet, nutritional status, the immune system, and microbial ecology in humans at different stages of life, living in distinct cultural and socioeconomic settings." And Pflughoeft and Versaloc (2012) state: "More detailed knowledge of the human microbiome will yield next-generation diagnostics and therapeutics for various acute, chronic, localized, and systemic human diseases."

In the optimum scenario, an individual may be "transformed" into health and vitality by expert care that addresses the whole person and their diagnoses, concerns, and challenges, and empowers self-care (Boxes 14.1–14.3). Complex cases that utilize multiple approaches and demonstrate marked improvement over time do not make the mainstream evidence-based journals. The scientific method used to discern efficacy relies on a single or limited set of interventions and outcome screenings. However, stories of health transformation abound in books by integrative practitioners, and these books may be recommended to clients desiring inspiration of what is possible. Holistic healing is profiled in books such as Chaudhary (2016), O'Bryan (2016), Porter (2018), and Tatta (2017).

Box 14.1 Patient case:
Allison's story: multiple
pelvic health problems

Allison, age 24, presented to physical therapy (PT) for dyspareunia, and she also suffered from interstitial cystitis (IC), fibromyalgia, reflux, and irritable bowel syndrome (IBS), constipation dominant (IBS-C). Her referring diagnosis was pelvic pain. She was underweight and experienced frequent nausea and a low appetite. Her symptoms began over the past two years starting with three episodes of food poisoning, recent increased sexual activity with frequent bladder infections, and multiple courses of antibiotics. She was using weekly bladder instillations for pain relief for IC. She had low back and hip pain, which started in gymnastics as a teen. She had suffered military sexual trauma, with a resultant diagnosis of post-traumatic stress disorder (PTSD), as well as describing childhood trauma with a high adverse childhood experience (ACE) score. She had anxiety and depression, and non-restorative sleep. She did sporadic cross-fit workouts that resulted in a few days of pelvic, hip, and back pain flares. Her main goal was pain reduction, with pain-free intercourse. (See Allison's treatment in Box 14.10.)

Box 14.2 Mutual respect:
providers and clients

A therapeutic team which regards the client as an equal partner in health care is a foundation of integrative care.

Box 14.3 Integrative
care principles

The Academy of Integrative Health and Medicine (AIHM) is a leader in integrative care, with the founding principles:

- Prevention is the best intervention, integration of healing systems is effective
- Holistic medicine is relationship-centered care, care should be individualized
- Teach by example
- Healing powers are innate
- All experiences are learning opportunities
- Embrace the healing power of love
- Optimal health is the primary goal.

(Riley et al. 2016)

All providers can benefit from considering these principles in their customized care plans for individuals.

OVERVIEW: HEALTH AND DISEASE

Co-morbidities and pelvic health

Co-morbid health conditions that can contribute to a pelvic health condition can include, but are not limited to, allergies and asthma, autoimmune inflammation (Ngo, Steyn, and McCombe 2014), acute and chronic infections (i.e. Lyme disease or Epstein-Barr virus), irritable bowel syndrome, Crohn's and celiac disease, depression and anxiety, non-restorative sleep, sleep apnea, respiratory conditions, thyroid disorders, oncology disease, and other conditions.

Substance use and addiction can occur due to attempts to self-manage stress and pain and can contribute to poor health and disease aggravation. Substance abuse can be related to a physical addiction to prescription pain medication, and/ or the need for better options for emotional support.

The socioeconomics of health

Individuals with lower socioeconomic status tend to live in areas where they are exposed to more air and water pollution, as well as stress with noise, social crowding, and crime. Anxiety and depression, and a high adverse childhood experience (ACE) score that is not addressed, will likely perpetuate pain and other limited self-care practices (Hughes *et al.* 2017; Merrick *et al.* 2017). Discrepancies exist with regards to access to health care education and training, and access to medical care. Preventative and wellness care are often the least well-funded.

CONCIERGE CARE

Wealthier individuals can access independent fee for service providers for specialty tests and services, also termed "concierge care." Many concierge providers fall under the realm of "functional medicine," considering in-depth lab testing, personalized nutrition therapy, and supplement targeting to support optimum health. Medical health systems (hospitals and community care clinics) tend to limit or not provide preventive care; the emphasis is on condition treatment and disease interventions, often with pharmaceutical-focused best practice protocols.

AUTOIMMUNE ILLNESS

People with higher socioeconomic status tend to live in areas where there is a greater burden of autoimmune diseases. The "hygiene hypothesis" suggests that the immune system that is not exposed to infection may overreact in response to immune challenges and present as autoimmune illness and allergies (Okada *et al.* 2010).

The nervous system and health

The nervous system optimally shifts from sympathetic functioning to parasympathetic. A heightened, prolonged sympathetic state is counterproductive to gastrointestinal motility, relaxed bladder storage and emptying, and sexual functioning. Individual variances exist in emotional resiliency and adaptability. Somatic therapists, trauma therapists, and other providers can be critical holistic providers in the pelvic health field, by recognizing signs and symptoms of sympathetic nervous system up-regulation and creating dialogue and opportunities for rehabilitation (van der Kolk 2014).

THE MICROBIOME IN HEALTH AND DISEASE

The microbiome is the collection of specific microbes and their genomes that are present in an ecosystem (Figure 14.1). Human microbiomes exist in specific locations such as the skin, nose, mouth, esophagus, stomach, small and large intestine, bladder, prostate, urethra, and vagina. The DNA signatures of the microbes present are specifically analyzed as the genome or genetic code.

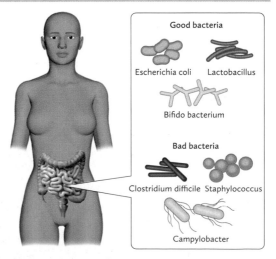

Figure 14.1 Gut microbiome.

MICROBES

The microbes that inhabit the gut, or gut microbiome (GM), are emerging as vital factors in health and immunity. Our GM evolved in humanity over eons, and the number of cells in our GM outnumber our human cells by ten to one and exist optimally in a symbiotic relationship within the body. GM species are critical in immune system modulation, mood management via neurotransmitter production, vitamin production (B and K), short-chain fatty acid production, and regulation towards leanness or obesity. Microbial species inhabiting the gut include bacteria, viruses, yeast, fungi, archaea, and phages, the latter two of which are least understood but interact with the other microbes in health and disease (Cani 2018; Lynch and Pederson 2016).

Prebiotics and probiotics

Prebiotics are nutritional items that form a base for microbial growth, such as non-digestible fiber in asparagus, bananas, blueberries, chia seeds, ground flaxseed, oats, onions, garlic, psyllium, Jerusalem artichoke, spinach, and many other items. These items supply nutrients and also help our intestinal lining to have a robust inner barrier that prevents pathogens from leaking out into the entire body (Box 14.4).

Probiotics are live microbes in nutritional items that are beneficial for the host. These are best known in yogurt and include acidophilus and bifidus organisms, as well as other species beyond the scope of this text. Symbiotics are items that have a mix of prebiotics and probiotics (Lynch and Pederson 2016). To stay alive in an environment, probiotics require a prebiotic type of substance as a base.

Box 14.4 Prebiotics
and probiotics
Recent research demonstrates symptom reduction in specific pelvic health conditions with the administration of prebiotics and probiotics. Gut dysbiosis and the associated bloating and constipation or diarrhea can aggravate pelvic pain, urinary incontinence, and gastrointestinal complaints. The biome is a key safeguard in our immunity, energy, and hormone production, and as such warrants medical attention for optimizing health. Yet sufficient research is lacking in targeting pre- and probiotics in individualized health care in mainstream medicine, and most individuals must explore the use of probiotics on their own or utilize concierge or private providers for testing and treatment. Urogynecologists may recommend the probiotic Culturelle® for preventing urinary tract infections, as well as acidophilus and bifidus. Males with chronic prostatitis have been shown to benefit from probiotic use VSL#3, following a course of antibiotics (Vicari et al. 2017).

Readers should consult their health care provider for direction and guidance.

Biomes

Microbial types that inhabit specific biomes are numerous, and their presence or absence in specific sites is now known to typify specific medical conditions and diseases. Profiles of the biome have been identified in acute gastroenteritis, inflammatory bowel disease, recurrent abdominal pain and irritable bowel syndrome, obesity, ulcerative colitis, bacterial vaginosis, and other conditions (Pflughoeft and Versaloc 2012).

Gut–brain axis

The effect of the GM and interaction with other body systems is being investigated for biologic signaling in health and disease, such as the gut–brain axis (Figure 14.2). A medical misconception has been to consider a blood–brain barrier that protects the brain from nutrient and foreign invader influence. Research is now showing the GM as a precipitating factor in illness, and lack of a blood–brain barrier as previously thought.

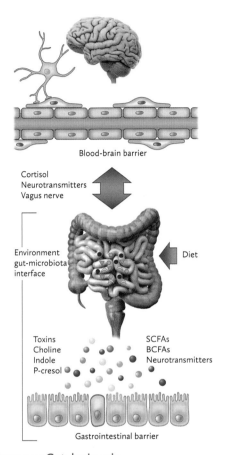

Figure 14.2 Gut–brain axis.

Neurodegenerative diseases

Many older clients presenting with pelvic disorders have co-morbid neurodegenerative diseases (NDD), such as Alzheimer's and Parkinson's diseases. Rosario *et al.* (2020) make a point for individualized dietary therapy in NDD, stating: "We reviewed direct and indirect pathways through which the microbiota can modulate the bidirectional communication of the gut–brain axis, and explored the evidence of microbial dysbiosis in Alzheimer's and Parkinson's diseases."

Researchers find that the biome with an abundant species profile typifies robust immunity and health. Research and testing methods are developing to sample the biomes more accurately as well as to elucidate the role of biomes in health and immunity (Lynch and Pederson 2016; Mashhadi *et al.* 2019; Pamer 2016; Wu and Wu 2012).

Gut dysbiosis occurs when there is a predominance of certain species in the small and large intestine, and a lack of adequate beneficial organisms. Gut dysbiosis and the associated bloating and constipation or diarrhea can aggravate pelvic pain and urinary incontinence, as well as gastrointestinal complaints and autoimmune illness (Mu *et al.* 2017).

Leaky gut

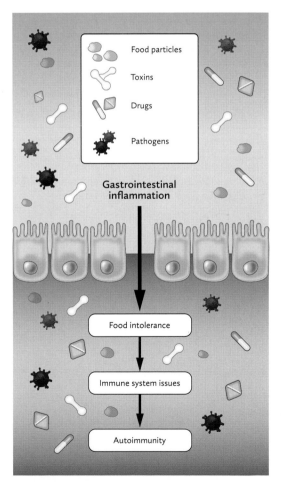

Figure 14.3 Leaky gut.

Leaky gut is a condition where the epithelial layer of cells in the inner lining of the intestine is no longer intact, and the disrupted cellular lining allows digestive products to leak out into the abdomen, and consequently the entire body (Figure 14.3). This can lead to systemic inflammation. An intact epithelial layer in the GM is described as having "tight junctions" that protect the body from pathogens and, when disrupted, the gut becomes leaky, allowing bacteria, viruses, antigen–antibody complexes, and pathogens to spread into the body and cause dysfunction or, possibly in chronic cases, disease. Our biomes function optimally when we have a positive emotional state, sufficient exercise and sleep, a healthy pre- and probiotic profile, and nutritional status free from irritants, infections, and biome disrupters.

MICROBIOME DISRUPTERS

Factors that disrupt the microbiome range from nutrition imbalances to food additives, antibiotics and other medications, hormone imbalances, environmental pollution, stress, and inadequate exercise (Zaura *et al.* 2015). One of the most common scenarios for individuals with chronic pelvic pain and dysfunction is the repeated use of antibiotics and subsequent gut dysbiosis.

Autoimmune illness and disease in pelvic health

Research studies have traced the development of autoimmune health conditions to inflammatory markers increasing years before disease diagnosis. In some cases, the use of antibiotics that disrupt the gut microbiome, and/or the pro-inflammatory Western diet, contribute to inflammation (O'Bryan 2016; Orbuch and Stein 2019; Tatta 2017).

Autoimmune diseases are common in those presenting for care with pelvic health conditions. Autoimmune diseases are characterized by the body "attacking" its cells and tissues, and can lead to disordered body function, pathological changes, and inflammation, and lead to illness or even contribute to mortality. Autoimmune conditions may be either organ specific, or systemic. Symptoms may range from mild to debilitating.

Autoimmune conditions that may present with pelvic symptoms include celiac and Crohn's diseases, endometriosis, fibromyalgia, Graves' disease, Hashimoto's thyroiditis, inflammatory bowel disease, interstitial cystitis, lichen planus, lichen sclerosus, lupus, Lyme disease, peripheral neuropathy, psoriasis, rheumatoid arthritis, scleroderma, type 1 diabetes, and many other conditions.

Iatrogenic influence: medication side effects

Medications for pelvic symptom management can have negative sequelae on health.

While antibiotics can be life-saving, their overuse has led to an exacerbation of illness as well as antibiotic-resistant bacteria. Many clients receive antibiotic therapy as a shotgun-type approach to kill off potential bacteria, yet this can disrupt the gut, bladder, and bowel GM homeostasis that is a foundation for the immune system, as well as impair neurotransmitter production, mood, metabolism, and weight (Lynch and Pederson 2016; Wu and Wu 2012). *C. difficile* infection is an example of post-antibiotic illness and colitis; the development of megacolon and possible death may ensue (29,000 US deaths in 2011) (Theriot and Young 2015).

Ideally, gut dysbiosis and a GM rebuilding post-antibiotic course can be addressed by health care professionals, yet current standards of care typically do not address biome changes after pharmaceutical treatment. Research is ongoing to investigate the optimum probiotics to restore depleted microbiomes (Grazul, Kanda, and Gondek 2016; Pamer 2016).

Hormonal birth control and antidepressants

Hormonal birth control (b.c.) is a beneficial tool for pregnancy prevention and reducing pain in some pelvic health conditions, such as endometriosis. The hormone suppressive properties of b.c. include limited endometrial growth and limiting or stopping menses and associated cramping. Side effects from b.c. can contribute to vulvar atrophy, vulvar pain, dyspareunia, depression, and osteopenia. Similarly, antidepressants can reduce neuropathic pelvic pain but can aggravate bowel and bladder symptoms, as well as cause weight gain and sexual side effects.

ENVIRONMENTAL TOXINS AND HEALTH

Environmental exposure to toxins and hormone disruptors, as well as infectious agents, dietary factors, and genetic susceptibility, combine to manifest in autoimmunity and the presence of signs and symptoms of varied illnesses, with an eventual diagnosis of disease (Dutta, Verma, and Nair 2019; O'Bryan 2016; Orbuch and Stein 2019; Tatta 2017).

Environmental toxins are abundant in the modern world and include air, water, and soil pollution, as well as items in our households, cosmetics, furniture, clothing, food, and beverages (EWG 2022). The impact of toxin exposure is compounded by the dose, cumulative exposure to all toxins, individual genetic predisposition to disease, as well as multigenerational influences. Environmental toxins and exposure to carcinogens such as radiation (ionizing and ultraviolet) are extrinsic factors that interact with host intrinsic factors resulting in changes in cell division, mutation, and the possible development of diseases including cancer. Researchers suggest that extrinsic factors appear to be the predominant influence for carcinogenesis (Wu *et al.* 2016).

Exposure to environmental toxins can disrupt pelvic health in males and females from exposure in utero with disrupted gene signaling and subsequent altered anatomical development of sexual organs and their metabolism (Box 14.5). Altered gene signaling can create multigenerational effects. Recent alarming rates of declining male fertility have led researchers to study genetic signaling and its disruption by environmental toxins as a major influence (Skakkebaek *et al.* 2015). In females, older maternal age, cigarette smoking, diabetes, pelvic inflammatory disease, sexually transmitted disease history, and exposure to endocrine-disrupting chemicals are associated with infertility and female reproductive disorders (Moghadam, Delpisheh, and Khosravi 2013; Zama and Uzumcu 2010).

> ## Box 14.5 Chemical exposure, and cancers
>
> The endocrine-disrupting chemicals of perfluorooctanoic acid (PFOA), polychlorinated biphenyls (PCB), persistent organic pollutants (POP), and polyfluoroalkyl acids (PFAS) have been shown to affect the male reproductive tract from anatomic development to metabolism and fertility (Pallotti *et al.* 2020). The aforementioned environmental toxins (PFOA, PCB, PFAS, and POP) are linked to cancers of the reproductive organs and other cancers, including endometrial cancer (Mallozzi *et al.* 2017) and brain, breast, kidney, lung, and pancreatic cancers (Fucic *et al.* 2012). PFOA exposure is linked to kidney and testicular cancer (Barry, Winquist, and Steenland 2013). Organophosphates are linked to thyroid, breast, and ovarian cancers

(Lerro *et al.* 2015). These items are known under the general headings of plasticizers, pesticides, artificial fragrances, and antimicrobial products. These pollutants mimic our natural hormones and the feedback with metabolic processes, including immune system function, and can therefore disrupt our immune system.

Glyphosate herbicide is used in genetically modified crops (GMO) which are fed to animals in commercial feedlots, and also consumed in commercial food crops including soy, wheat, oats, corn, and many other crops. Glyphosate exposure has been linked to Parkinson's disease and other degenerative conditions, with the authors of a toxicology study suggesting that it could be a key factor in Western disease development (Kruger *et al.* 2014) (Box 14.6). Chronic exposure in low doses may occur and affect the microbe population in the soil, in plants, and animals, and may produce antibiotic resistance to fungal and bacterial challenges (Van Bruggen *et al.* 2018). The insecticide chlorpyrifos and the herbicide glyphosate have both been found to induce changes in the species array in the gut biome in animal and human studies (Roca-Saavedra *et al.* 2017).

Box 14.6 Epigenetics,
genotoxins, and disease
Kruger *et al.* (2014) review evidence that autism, Alzheimer's disease, depression, diabetes, gastrointestinal diseases, heart disease, infertility, and obesity are associated with the Western diet. They cite multiple sources with evidence for a disturbance of the gut microbiome, and genotoxic and teratogenic effects are associated with glyphosate.

Epigenetics is emerging as a new tool to study the interaction of species and environmental triggers for health or disease. Idiosyncrasies in DNA and gene coding can be protective against disease, or place individuals at risk for illness. These predispositions can exist towards the manifestation of an organ or systemic illnesses. Epigenetics informs us in regard to pelvic health conditions and beneficial versus detrimental environmental influences. Research has identified genetic markers and environmental influences in the expression of pelvic disorders in the case of endometriosis (Borghese *et al.* 2016), bladder pain syndrome (Li *et al.* 2022), infertility (Zorrilla and Yatsenko 2013), and other conditions. Genotoxins are poisonous substances that can damage DNA and cause mutations, trigger cancer cells to grow (a carcinogen), as well as causing birth defects (teratogen). Epigenetics explains the changes at the metabolic and cellular levels that are due to the influence of genotoxins on the presentation of the disease. Ideally, studies in epigenetics and health can drive optimal global standards in environmental safety and regulations while preserving economic sustainability.

STANDARD AMERICAN DIET (SAD) AND POOR HEALTH

Nutritional influences may be hidden epigenetic triggers for disease in the case of food additives and subsequent inflammation. While preserving food storage, reducing spoilage, and enhancing flavor and appearance, the food industry has created some great tasting, shelf-stable food. Yet highly processed foods include additives that promote gut dysbiosis, which can be a root factor in disease. The Standard American diet (SAD) and its nutritional influences may be hidden epigenetic triggers for disease in the case of food additives and inflammation. Clients may be overwhelmed by this information if they have a lifestyle featuring fast food consumption and highly processed, packaged foods. Health care providers optimally can consider client interest, choice, health care literacy, and behavior change models in providing education and treatment including providing samples of new recipes.

Sweeteners

A list of additives that can create dysbiosis by altering gut permeability and promoting bacterial overgrowth includes non-nutritive sweeteners such as stevia, sucralose, saccharin, and aspartame. Both animal and human studies show an association of increased calorie consumption and tendencies towards weight gain in individuals using these sweeteners to reduce caloric intake (Roca-Saavedra *et al.* 2017).

Food emulsifiers

Another common food additive is food-emulsifying agents. Emulsifiers in food perform the function of improving the consistency and "mouthfeel" of products and the overall texture, yet the effect on the biome is disadvantageous. The emulsifiers carboxymethylcellulose and polysorbate 80 have been found to disrupt the gut mucosal barrier and, in fact, may be linked to exacerbation of Crohn's disease (Roca-Saavedra *et al.* 2017). The review by Lerner and Matthias (2015) traces the correlation between rising autoimmune diseases and increasing consumption of seven modern food industry additives (glucose, salt, emulsifiers, organic solvents, nanoparticles, microbial transglutaminase, and gluten) that contribute to intestinal junction porosity and illness.

The negative effects of these food additives are bacteriostatic, which contributes to the growth of bacteria detrimental to health.

Additionally, these additives can disrupt the tight junctions or barrier in the lining of the small intestine, with changes in cellular, lymphatic, and immune system functioning.

Common foods that may be gut disruptors

Dairy products and wheat (gluten) are recognized by many health care professionals as key contributors to gut dysbiosis and illness (Guerreiro *et al.* 2018; O'Bryan 2016; Onitveros, Hardy, and Chavez 2015). Screening and treatment are likely best provided by nutrition specialists. The specifics of nutritional intervention can be complex; for example, in the case of inflammatory bowel disease, the case can be made for dairy as an intervention for treatment (Aaron and Torsten 2018) or dairy as pro-inflammatory (Orel *et al.* 2017).

Gluten has been found to disrupt the gut microbiome cellular layer via the protein gliadin, which is also present in barley, oats, spelt, and rye. Gluten intolerance is extreme in the full manifestation of celiac disease, with intestinal villi disruption. Individuals with celiac disease may experience cramping, pain, and watery diarrhea after ingesting gluten, and the response may be within minutes of ingestion.

In non-celiac gluten sensitivity (NCGS), the symptoms may be more subtle than in celiac disease. Symptoms of NCGS may include pains in bones, joints, and muscles, arm or leg numbness, brain fog, depression, and skin rashes. NCGS sensitivity has also been implicated in the development of autoimmune diseases such as fibromyalgia and spondylarthritis (Catassi *et al.* 2013).

Elimination diets

Corn, soy, and eggs are also common food items that can cause inflammation, as well as sugar consumption. Wheat, dairy, corn, soy, and eggs commonly trigger individuals with autoimmune and pelvic health conditions, and with every food group that must be avoided, new options are available for those that can shift to a new way of eating (Box 14.7).

> ### Box 14.7 Caution in restricting food groups
>
> It's important to be mindful of eating disorder risk in some clients who struggle with food sensitivities. Taking away a food item, such as bread, may be their main caloric intake.

Elimination diets and health and symptom tracking are optimally guided by a medical professional, yet some individuals may be able to progress themselves with education, discipline, and a process of self-assessment and discovery in learning new food choices recipes and self-care. Nourishing Meals, for example, is an online site with free healthy eating recipes founded by nutrition professional Alissa Segersten, and it is a good resource for individuals to gain an education, including links to recommended recipes (Nourishing Meals 2020; Segersten and Malterre 2016). Online coaching, as well as health and nutrition education, are emerging as resources for individuals to connect globally for information and health care, including GM analysis and care (Drummond 2019; Drummond and Sarna 2020; Garner 2016). Individuals with limited to no access to care may practice an elimination diet (Arscott and Rindfleisch 2018; Porter 2018). Of note is that wheat, corn, soy, and eggs have high exposure to glyphosate in many countries, therefore the combined effects of food intolerances and pesticide exposure may create a double whammy of health disruption.

Nutritional deficiencies

Vitamin and mineral deficiencies are implicated in many diseases and are present in over three billion individuals worldwide (Roca-Saavedra *et al.* 2017) with low zinc, iron, and vitamin A. These deficiencies are correlated with impaired gut microbiome status, impaired immune functions, as well as limitations in growth and development.

Low levels of vitamin D have been associated with multiple autoimmune conditions (Silverberg *et al.* 2010). Low vitamin D is correlated with pelvic floor disorder symptoms (Autry *et al.* 2012), and a vitamin D receptor has been found on the bladder wall (Crescioli *et al.* 2005). Vitamin D is receiving attention for its critical role in health, and vitamin D deficiency is a risk factor for strength loss (Visser, Deeg, and Lips 2003).

The polyunsaturated fatty acids (PUFA) are essential nutrients for biological membrane integrity and other vital functions and must be consumed as they are not produced by the body. In modern diets, there is an abundance of pro-inflammatory omega 6 versus omega 3 fatty acids, which are anti-inflammatory (Calder 2017). An ideal ratio is suggested for the consumption of omega 6 to omega 3 fatty acids at a 1:1 level (Tatta 2017), although opinions vary. Individuals with a balance of omegas 6 and 3 have reduced risk factors for the inflammatory conditions of obesity, cardiovascular disease, and cancer. Positive metabolic effects of omega 3 consumption include reduced visceral fat, improved lipid homeostasis, and reduced inflammatory markers. Additionally, EPA and DHA, byproducts of omega 3 consumption, play a role in reducing pro-inflammatory cytokines and hepatic liver fat infiltration which can lead to liver disease (Khadge *et al.* 2018). "Saturated fatty acids, trans-fatty acids, high-GI carbohydrates, and a high omega 6 to omega 3 polyunsaturated fatty acid ratio are associated with increased levels of inflammation" (Galland 2010).

An extensive nutrition review concluded that "consumption of magnesium, fiber, omega 3 and polyunsaturated fatty acids, flavonoids, and carotenoids from food is associated with decreased levels of inflammatory markers in serum" (Galland 2010). The anti-inflammatory diet has anti-depressive, anti-cancer, cardioprotective, and neuroendocrine benefits. "Habitual dietary pattern appears to have a moderate influence on chronic, low-grade systemic inflammation, an important risk factor for diseases of aging and industrialization" (Galland 2010).

Anti-inflammatory diets

Dietary choices can reduce inflammation in the body, such as the anti-inflammatory or Mediterranean diet (MD) (Martinez-Gonzalez et al. 2015). The MD includes ample fruit and vegetables, protein, and fats from sources such as olive oil, nuts, and seafood. This is the most popular, medically mainstream nutrition approach that can be customized to those with pelvic health challenges. Tailoring an MD diet to a pelvic rehabilitation client would depend on the unique profile of client diagnoses and conditions, such as an individual with IBS-D needing less fruit, more cooked vegetables, and limited to no onions and garlic. A client with an overactive bladder may benefit from a low acid diet, reducing citrus and caffeine, or a celiac client eliminating gluten, and gluten-related items such as oats, barley, and many other items. A client with endometriosis may benefit from reducing soy due to its estrogenic effects, as well as the elimination of the pro-inflammatory effects of gluten, corn, eggs, and sugar (Orbuch and Stein 2019).

Dietary choices also include the ketogenic (keto) diet, which is a low-carbohydrate, low to moderate protein, and high fat diet, which promotes ketosis or a fat-burning state in the body. This diet is sugar- and practically carbohydrate-free, and it helps to reduce or in some cases eliminate sugar craving. Application of the keto diet by an individual with Crohn's disease demonstrated improvement in several parameters in the case report by Tóth et al. (2016), including the improved status of the intestinal lumen on MRI analysis.

The paleo or ancestral diet is a whole food, grain- and legume-free diet, and includes limited fruit and starchy vegetables, grass-fed meat and wild-caught fish, and no dairy or gluten. Both keto and paleo diets avoid processed foods and may help reduce inflammation and pain, yet potentially have a high carbon-footprint due to the high consumption of animal protein.

Herbs and spices

Herbs and spices are natural antioxidant sources that humans have used throughout history (Box 14.8). They possess flavonoids which are scavengers of free radicals, as well as phytochemical compounds that inhibit food break down and rancidity. An analysis of herbs and spices demonstrated multiple antioxidant compounds found in most herbs, with allspice, basil, cinnamon, clove, mint, oregano, thyme, rosemary, and sage scoring the highest (Embusco 2015).

> **Box 14.8 Herbal medicine**   ∞
> Herbal medicine is an ancient field of health care existing throughout human history, with herbalists utilizing complementary herbs to create balance and efficacy for targeted health conditions. The combination approach for formulations used by herbalists is at odds with evidence-based medicine which requires standardized extracts in isolation and testing in vitro (petri dish) or in vivo (animal or human model). Current in vivo studies are primarily utilizing mouse models and demonstrate the potential for topical application distillates of thyme, oregano, and wild mustard for herpes simplex infections (Rad Sharifi 2017).

Essential oils distilled from herbs are known to have beneficial effects against disease, and their effects may be antiseptic, antiparasitic, antifungal, antibacterial, antiviral, and insecticidal.

Additionally, their effects may also be analgesic, and possibly anticarcinogenic, and they may help spare components of the biome during oncology treatment (Bakkali *et al.* 2008; Kumar *et al.* 2020; Roca-Saavedra *et al.* 2017; Romm 2018). Oil of oregano has properties that inhibit the growth of yeast, such as *candida albicans*, in in vitro testing (Adams *et al.* 2011).

Recent research demonstrates the antiviral activity of geranium and lemon essential oils in human cells in a study targeting viral receptor site binding. Human interaction with herbal medicine products depends on the individual's constitution, genetics, and even microbiome. For safety on botanical medicine, individuals should consult certified herbalists who are fluent with the Botanical Safety Handbook, which identifies classes 1–4 guidelines for use from ingestion, topical application, avoidance with pregnancy or nursing, and other guidelines (Gardner and McGuffin 2013).

Ayurveda

Ayurvedic therapy, dating back 3,000 years, recognizes the protective as well as health-enhancing benefits of dietary routines and nutrition, including herbs/spices such as ashwagandha, boswellia, ginger, trifala, and turmeric. Ayurveda considers the dosha, or individual physical and constitutional attributes (Vata, Pitta, Kapha) and customized programming. Ayurvedic providers offer multi-faceted lifestyle, nutrition, and nutraceutical intervention for clients. Research on efficacy in disease states is in its infancy yet there are promising results from studies, and more research is needed (Chaudhary 2016; Kamali *et al.* 2012; Pandey, Rastogi, and Rawat 2013; Vishal, Mishra, and Raychaudhuri 2011).

Nutrient supplementation for healing

Nutrient supplementation can be a vital component for pelvic healing, in addition to optimum food choices, and integration of botanical approaches and/or ayurvedic therapy.

For example, probiotics, L-glutamine, and zinc can support the linings of the intestines and the bladder. Additionally, antioxidants and anti-inflammatory nutrients such as vitamins C and E, N-acetyl cysteine, glutathione, and curcumin in therapeutic doses can support liver function and scavenge free radicals.

Sleep quality and health

Sleep quality is a primary factor in health status, with poor sleep quality related to increased incidence of cardiovascular disease, obesity, diabetes, and cancer (Knutson and Cauter 2008; Von Ruesten *et al.* 2012). Poor sleep quality is often a factor in chronic pain. Ashworth, Davidson, and Espie (2010) analyzed a chronic pain population and poor sleepers demonstrated increased pain ratings, disability, depression, and anxiety in comparison to good sleepers with chronic pain.

In women, increased levels of the inflammatory marker C-reactive protein are present in association with poor sleep, and this marker is correlated with blood vessel and cholesterol markers of cardiovascular disease (Liu *et al.* 2014). Women tend to have more challenges with sleep due to several factors, with researchers concluding:

> *Sex differences in sleep begin at a very early age and women report poorer sleep quality and a have a higher risk for insomnia than do men. Sleep may be affected by variation in reproductive hormones, stress, depression, aging, life/role transitions, and other factors.*
>
> (Nowakowski, Meers, and Heimbach 2013)

Addressing factors to improve sleep, or "sleep hygiene," can improve restorative sleep and also help improve health status (Box 14.9). Strategies that can promote restorative sleep include limiting exposure to light an hour before bed, a bedtime routine of meditation/mindfulness, a consistent sleep and waking schedule, daytime exercise, and limiting or eliminating consumption of caffeine and alcohol. Additionally, eliminating noise and light at night, as well as maintaining a cool bedroom temperature, improves sleep quality.

> ### Box 14.9 Promoting restorative sleep
> Neurotransmitters that cycle into sleepiness and restorative random eye motion sleep periods do not occur in many individuals with poor sleep. Some individuals may also need pharmacological intervention. Optimum nutrition intake has been associated with improved sleep quality in some research and can help the production of melatonin and other transmitters (Sanlier and Sabuncular 2020).

Nutraceutical and vitamin supplements have been found to promote relaxation and lower muscle tension and anxiety, and therefore may help with sleep. Supplements that have historically been used for relaxation and sleep promotion include, in a limited list, ashwagandha, chamomile, hops, kava kava, lavender, lemon balm, lobelia, magnesium, melatonin, passionflower, St. John's Wort, theanine, and valerian root (Erland and Saxena 2017; Mason 2001; Romm 2018; Taavoni, Nazeem, and Haghani 2013).

Note: Any supplement herb, spice, pre- or probiotic, vitamin, or mineral item listed in this chapter should be used under the guidance of a health care provider.

INTEGRATIVE MEDICINE SUMMARY

Medical testing is emerging to assess the biomarkers for disease beyond physical examination and bloodwork, with some providers utilizing stool and urine sampling with an analysis of the microbiomes. Diseases and the associated biome disruption are emerging as signature patterns based on current research, from autism spectrum disorder to interstitial cystitis, obesity, prostatitis, and Parkinson's disease. Specialized lab testing by integrative practitioners may look for signs of viral, yeast, fungal, and/or bacterial overgrowth, and use pharmaceutical, nutritional, nutraceutical, and environmental approaches to shift the microbiome to a state of reduced inflammation and homeostasis. Identifying root causes and offering treatment can reduce morbidity as expressed in clients with pelvic health symptoms. Optimizing the environment, sleep, nutrition, and exercise status, and reducing stress and improving self-care, social support, and exercise, are all key spokes in the wheel of health care for chronic pelvic health conditions.

Team rehabilitation

Integrative rehabilitation for pelvic health and healing can include strategies such as acupuncture, exercise and myofascial treatment, nutritional, nutraceutical, psychological, and pharmaceutical care, and surgery as indicated, with options for a multitude of therapies based on client choice for self-discovery and care (Box 14.10). Metabolic factors such as stabilizing blood sugar and lowering inflammation with nutrition can have cascading positive effects in other areas. Ultimately, one of the best gifts therapists with an integrative perspective can give their clients is support for their commitment to regular self-care with attention to quality movement, bodywork, rest, and nourishment.

Box 14.10 Patient case: ♥
Allison's healing team

Allison was referred by her PT to a nutritionist, a trauma care-oriented psychologist, and patient support groups, as well as to websites, blogs, and books to help her improve her health. In over one and a half years of treatment she sought help in each of her areas of concern. She became "virtually pain-free and full function," and provided a summary of her healing protocols as a resource for others, including:

- pelvic PT, including internal and external pelvic myofascial and visceral work, a self-care program with vaginal dilators, and sexual medicine guidelines for comfort
- orthopedic PT: lumbopelvic hip manual therapy, exercise, posture, and ergonomics training
- GI mapping and mindfulness to notice the influence of nutrition, stress, and mood on pain, or feeling well
- the anti-inflammatory diet, including gluten, refined sugar, and dairy reductions
- regular use of Desert Harvest® aloe vera pills, bromalin, and quercetin to help her digestion, omega 3 vitamins, a broad-spectrum probiotic, and frequent green juicing with apple juice
- a shift from self-catheterizing "weekly rescue instillations" to posterior tibial nerve stimulation, acupuncture, bodywork, meditation, and CBD/THC (medical use of cannabinoids) topically to the pelvic region (Carey and As-Sanie 2016)

- trauma therapy including counseling, eye movement desensitization, and a self-care myofascial pain workbook
- support and information synthesis from a patient support group
- participation in post-traumatic stress disorder (PTSD) free programs for health and relaxation, including kayaking with veterans for heroes.

She finished her final therapy visit with an expression of gratitude, with a printout for her therapist: "I have no choice but to live a peaceful life." This was a statement the therapist had spoken to her while providing storytelling about a veteran with PTSD, and improvements over time in that client's pelvic problems and digestion, with a multimodal treatment approach. Allison reported that the therapist had given her permission to enjoy her life and to choose peace.

Compassion-based care is imperative for the success of any intervention, and the principles of functional medicine provide analysis and health care protocols that address the biopsychosocial aspects of each individual. Offering clients choices in interventions towards their key interest areas and team care can engender a locus of control and self-efficacy. Utilizing a team system can also help prevent provider compassion fatigue and burnout from trying to help the client address all their health needs as a sole provider. Individuals seeking pelvic health care may be offered online resources, books, support groups, and options for tracking change, to help promote behavior change and compliance, in addition to, or instead of, in-office care.

REFERENCES

Aaron, L. and Torsten, M. (2018) "The salutogentic effects of cow's milk and dairy products in celiac disease." *Journal of Clinical and Cellular Immunity 9*, 2.

Adams, A., Kumar, S., Clausen, M., and Sahi, S. (2011) "Anti-yeast activities of *orignanum* oil against human pathogenic yeasts." *Advances in Bioscience and Technology 2*, 103–107.

Arscott, S. and Rindfleisch, A. (2018) "The elimination diet." University of Washington Integrative Health, School of Public Medicine and Health. Accessed 6/16/2022 at www.fammed.wisc.edu/files/webfm-uploads/documents/outreach/im/handout_elimination_diet_patient.pdf.

Ashworth, P. C. H., Davidson, K. M., and Espie, C. A. (2010) "Cognitive behavioural factors associated with sleep quality in chronic pain patients." *Behavioural Sleep Medicine 8*, 1, 28–39.

Autry, C. Y. P., Markland, A. D., Ballard, A. C., Gunn, D., and Richter, H. E. (2012) "Vitamin D status in women with pelvic floor disorder symptoms." *International Urogynecology Journal 23*, 12, 1699–1705.

Bakkali, F., Averbeck, S., Averbeck, D., and Idamar, M. (2008) "Biological effects of essential oils—a review." *Food and Chemical Toxicology 46*, 2, 446–475.

Barry, V., Winquist, A., and Steenland, K. (2013) "PFOA exposures and incident cancers among adults living near a chemical plant." *Environmental Health Perspectives 121*, 11–12.

Borghese, B., Zondervan, K. T., Abrao, M. S., Chapron, C., et al. (2016) "Recent insights on the genetics and epigenetics of endometriosis." *Genetics 91*, 254–264.

Calder, P. C. (2017) "Omega-3 fatty acids and the inflammatory processes: From molecules to man." *Biochemical Society Transactions 45*, 5, 1105–1115.

Cani, P. (2018) "Human gut microbiome: Hopes, threats, and promises." *Gut 67*, 9, 1716–1725.

Carey, E. T. and As-Sanie, S. (2016) "New developments in the pharmacotherapy of neuropathic chronic pelvic pain." *Future Science OA 2*, 4, FSO148.

Catassi, C., Bai, J., Bonaz, B., Bouma, G., et al. (2013) "Non-celiac gluten sensitivity: The new frontier of gluten related disorders." *Nutrients 5*, 10, 3839–3853.

Chaudhary, K. (2016) *The Prime: Prepare and Repair Your Body for Spontaneous Weight Loss*. New York: Harmony Books.

Crescioli, C., Morelli, A., Adorini, L., Ferruzzi, P., et al. (2005) "Human bladder as a novel target for vitamin D receptor ligands." *Journal of Clinical Endocrinology and Metabolism 90*, 962–972.

Drummond, J. (2019) *Nutrition for Relieving Pelvic Pain: Fueling the Patient/Practitioner/Healing Partnership*. Pennsauken, NJ: BookBaby.

Drummond, J. and Sarna, S. (2020) The Microbiome Rescue Summit. Accessed 6/16/2022 at https://7day.healthmeans.com/mcr20.

Dutta, S. K., Verma, S., and Nair, P. (2019) "Parkinson's disease: The emerging role of gut dysbiosis, antibiotics, probiotics, and fecal microbiota transplantation." *Journal of Neurogastroenterology and Motility 25*, 3, 363–376.

Embusco, M. E. (2015) "Spices and herbs: Natural sources of antioxidants—a mini review." *Journal of Functional Foods 18*, 811–819.

Erland, L. A. E. and Saxena, P. (2017) "Melatonin natural health products and supplements: Presence of serotonin and significant variable of melatonin content." *Journal of Clinical Sleep Medicine 13*, 2, 275–281.

EWG (2022) "Toxic chemicals." Accessed 9/26/22 at https://www.ewg.org/areas-focus/toxic-chemicals.

Fucic, A., Gamulin, M., Ferencic, Z., Katic, J., et al. (2012) "Environmental exposure to xenoestrogens and oestrogen related cancers: Reproductive system, breast, lung, kidney, pancreas, and brain." *Environmental Health 11*, Suppl 1, S8.

Galland, L. (2010) "Diet and inflammation." *Nutrition in Clinical Practice 25*, 6, 634–640.

Gardner, Z. and McGuffin, M. (2013) *American Herbal Products Associations' Botanical Safety Handbook*. Boca Raton, FL: CRC Press.

Garner, G. (2016) *Medical Therapeutic Yoga*. London: Handspring Publishing.

Grazul, H., Kanda, L., and Gondek, D. (2016) "Impact of probiotic supplements on microbiome diversity following antibiotic treatment of mice." *Gut Microbes 7*, 2, 101–114.

Guerreiro, C. S., Caldo, A., Sousa, J., and Fonseca, J. E. (2018) "Diet, microbiota and gut permeability—the unknown connection." *Frontiers in Medicine, Rheumatology 5*, 349.

Hughes, K., Bellis, M., Hardcastle, K. A., Sethi, D., et al. (2017) "The effect of multiple adverse childhood experiences on health; a systematic review and meta-analysis." *The Lancet Public Health 2*, 8, e356–e366.

Kamali, S. H., Khalai, A. R., Hasani-Ranibar, S., and Esfehani, M. M. (2012) "Efficacy of 'Itrifal saghir,' a combination of three medicinal plants in the treatment of obesity: A randomized controlled trial." *DHARU Journal of Pharmaceutical Science 20*, 1, 33.

Kau, A. L., Ahern, P., Griffin, N. W., Goodman, A. L., and Gordon, J. I. (2011) "Human nutrition, the gut microbiome and the immune system." *Nature 474*, 327–336.

Khadge, S., Sharp, G., Thiele, G., McGuire, T., et al. (2018) "Dietary omega-3 and omega-6 polyunsaturated fatty acids modulate hepatic pathology." *Journal of Nutrition and Biochemistry 52*, 92–102.

Knutson, K. and Cauter, E. (2008) "Association between sleep loss and increased risk of obesity and diabetes." *Annals of the New York Academy of Science 1129*, 287–304.

Kruger, M., Schledorn, P., Schrodl, W., Hoppe, H. W., Lutz, W., and Shehata, A. A. (2014) "Detection of glyphosate residues in animals and humans." *Journal of Environmental and Analytical Toxicology 4*, 2.

Kumar, S. K. J., Vani, G. M., Wang, C. S., Chen, C. C., et al. (2020) "Geranium and lemon essential oils and their active compounds downregulate angiotensin converting enzyme (ACE 2), a SARS-CoV-2 spike receptor-binding domain, in epithelial cells." *Plants 9*, 770.

Lerner, A. and Matthias, T. (2015) "Changes in intestinal tight junction permeability associated with industrial food additives explain the rising incidence of autoimmune diseases." *Autoimmune Review 14*, 479–489.

Lerro, C. C., Koutros, S., Andreotti, G., Friesen, M., *et al.* (2015) "Organophosphate insecticide use and cancer incidence among spouses of pesticide applicators in the Agricultural Health Study." *Occupational and Environmental Medicine 72*, 10, 736–744.

Li, K., Cehn, C., Zeng, J., Wen, Y., *et al.* "Interplay between bladder microbiota and overactive bladder symptom severity: A cross-sectional study." *BMC Urology 22*, 39.

Liu, R., Liu, X., Zee, P. C., Hou, L., *et al.* (2014) "Association between sleep quality and C-reactive protein: Results from national health and nutrition examination survey, 2005–2008." *PLOS One 9*, 3, 1–7.

Lynch, S. and Pederson, O. (2016) "The human intestinal microbiome in health and disease." *New England Journal of Medicine 375*, 24, 2369–2379.

Maghadam, A. D., Delpisheh, A., and Khosravi, A. (2013) "Epidemiology of female infertility: A review of literature." *Sciences Biotechnology Research Asia 10*, 2, 559–567.

Mallozzi, M., Leone, C., Manurita, F., Belleti, F., and Caserta, D. (2017) "Endocrine disrupting chemicals and endometrial cancer: An overview of recent laboratory evidence and epidemiological studies." *International Journal of Environmental Research and Public Health 14*, 334.

Martinez-Gonzalez, M. A., Salas-Salvado, J., Estruch, R., Corella, J., *et al.* (2015) "Benefits of the Mediterranean diet: Insights from the PREDIMED study." *Progress in Cardiovascular Diseases 58*, 50–60.

Mashhadi, R., Taheri, D., Mousavibahar, S. H., Ashaii, M., *et al.* (2019) "Association of microbiota and overactive bladder: A mini literature review." *Translation Research in Urology 1*, 2, 54–59.

Mason, R. (2001) "200 mg of Zen, L-Thianine boosts alpha waves, promotes alert relaxation." *Alternative and Complementary Therapies 7*, 2, 91–95.

Merrick, M., Ports, K., Ford, D., Afifi, T. *et al.* (2017) "Unpacking the impact of adverse childhood experiences on adult mental health." *Child Abuse and Neglect 69*, 10–19.

Mu, Q., Kirby, J., Reilly, C. M., and Luo, X. M. (2017) "Leaky gut as a danger signal for autoimmune disease." *Frontiers in Immunology 8*, 598.

Ngo, S. T., Steyn, F. J., and McCombe, P. A. (2014) "Gender differences in autoimmune disease." *Frontiers in Neuroendocrinology 35*, 347–369.

Nourishing Meals (2020) "Basic Elimination Diet." Accessed 9/26/22 at https://nourishingmeals.com/diet/basic-elimination-diet.

Nowakowski, S., Meers, J., and Heimbach, E. (2013) "Sleep and women's health." *Sleep Medicine Research 4*, 1, 1–22.

O'Bryan, T. (2016) *The Autoimmune Fix: How to Stop Hidden Autoimmune Damage That Keeps You Sick, Fat, and Tired Before it Turns into Disease.* New York: Rodale.

Okada, H., Kuhn, C., Feillet, H., and Bach, J.-F. (2010) "The 'hygiene hypothesis' for autoimmune and allergic disease: An update." *Clinical and Experimental Immunology 160*, 1, 1–9.

Onitveros, N., Hardy, M. Y., and Chavez, C. F. (2015) "Assessing of celiac disease and nonceliac gluten sensitivity." *Gastroenterology Research and Practice*, Article no. 723954.

Orbuch, I. K. and Stein, A. (2019) *Beating Endo: How to Reclaim Your Life from Endometriosis.* New York: Harper Wave.

Orel, R., Benedik, E., Erzen, J., Orel, A., and Urlep, D. (2017) *Nutritional Therapy for Inflammatory Bowel Disease.* http://dx.doi.org/10.5772/intechopen.73259.

Pallotti, F., Pelloni, M., Gianfrilli, D., Lenzi, A., *et al.* (2020) "Mechanism of testicular disruption form exposure to bisphenol A and phthalates." *Journal of Clinical Medicine 9*, 2, 471.

Pamer, E. G. (2016) "Resurrecting the intestinal microbiota to combat antibiotic-resistant pathogens." *Science 352*, 6285, 535–538.

Pandey, M. M., Rastogi, S., and Rawat, A. K. S. (2013) "Indian traditional ayurvedic system of medicine and nutritional supplementation." *Evidence-Based Complementary and Alternative Medicine*, Article ID 376327.

Pflughoeft, K. and Versaloc, J. (2012) "Human microbiome in health and disease." *Annual Review of Pathology: Mechanisms of Disease 7*, 99–122.

Porter, V. (2018) *Resilient Health: How to Thrive in a Toxic World.* Boston: Enlighten Health Media.

Rad Sharifi, J., Salehi, B., Schinitzler, P., Ayatollahi, S. A., *et al.* (2017) "Susceptibility of herpes simplex virus type 1 t-monoterpenes thymol, carvacrol, P-cymene and essential oils of sinapis arvensis L, Lallemantia royleana Benth, and pulocaria vulgaris gaertn." *Cellular and Molecular Biology 63*, 8, 42–47.

Riley, D., Anderson, R., Blair, J. C., Crouch, S., *et al.* (2016) "The academy of integrative health and medicine and the evolution of integrative medicine practice, education and fellowships." *Integrative Medicine 15*, 1, 38–41.

Roca-Saavedra, P., Mendez-Vilabrille, V., Miranda, J. M., Lamas, A., *et al.* (2017) "Food additives, contaminants, and other minor components: Effects on human gut microbiota—a review." *Journal of Physiology and Biochemistry 74*, 69–83.

Romm, A. (2018) *Botanical Medicine for Women's Health.* London: Elsevier.

Rosario, D., Boren, J., Uhlen, M., Proctor, G., *et al.* (2020) "Systems biology approaches to understand host-microbiome interactions in neurodegenerative disease." *Frontiers in Neurosciences 14*, 716.

Sanlier, N. and Sabuncular, G. (2020) "Relationship between nutrition and sleep quality, focusing on the melatonin biosynthesis." *Sleep and Biological Rhythms 18*, 89099.

Segersten, A. and Malterre, T. (2016) *Nourishing Meals: Healthy Recipes from The Whole Life Nutrition.* New York: Harmony Books.

Silverberg, J. I., Silverberg, A. I., Malka, E., and Silverberg, N. B. (2010) "A pilot study assessing the role of 25 hydroxy vitamin D levels in patients with vitiligo vulgaris." *Journal of the American Academy of Dermatology 62*, 6, 937–941.

Skakkebaek, N. E., Raijpert-De Meyts, E., Louis, M. B. G., Toppari, J., *et al.* (2015) "Male reproductive disorders and fertility trends: Influences of environment and genetic susceptibility." *Physiological Reviews 96*, 1, 55–97.

Taavoni, S., Nazeem, N., and Haghani, H. (2013) "Valerian/lemon balm use for sleep disorders during menopause." *Complementary Therapies in Clinical Practice 19*, 4, 193–196.

Tatta, J. (2017) *Heal Your Pain Now: The Revolutionary Program to Rest Your Brain and Body for a Pain Free Life.* Boston: Da Capo Press.

Theriot, C. M. and Young, V. B. (2015) "Interactions between the gastrointestinal microbiome and clostridium difficile." *Annual Review Microbiology 69*, 445–461.

Tóth, C., Dabóczi, A., Howard, M., Miller, N., and Clemens, Z. (2016) "Crohn's disease successfully treated with the paleolithic ketogenic diet." *International Journal of Case Reports and Images 7*, 9, 570–578.

Van Bruggen, A. H. C., He, M. M., Shin, K., Mai, V., *et al.* (2018) "Environmental and health effects of the herbicide glyphosate." *Science of the Total Environment 616–617*, 255–268.

van der Kolk, B. (2014) *The Body Keeps the Score: Brain, Mind, and Body Healing of Trauma.* London: Penguin Books.

Vicari, E., Salemi, M., Sidoti, G., Malaguarnerna, M., and Castiglionne, R. (2017) "Symptom severity following rifaximin and the probiotic VSL#3 in patients with chronic pelvic pain syndrome (due to inflammatory prostatitis) plus irritable bowel syndrome." *Nutrients 9*, 11, 1208.

Vishal, A. A., Mishra, A., and Raychaudhuri, S. P. (2011) "A double blind, randomized placebo controlled clinical study evaluates the early efficacy of Aflapin™ in subjects with osteoarthritis of knee." *International Journal of Medical Science 8*, 7, 615–622.

Visser, M., Deeg, D. J. H., and Lips, P. (2003) "Low vitamin D and high parathyroid hormone levels as determinants of loss of muscle mass (sarcopenia): The longitudinal aging study, Amsterdam." *Journal of Clinical Endocrinology and Metabolism 88*, 12, 5766–5772.

Von Ruesten, A., Weikert, C., Fietze, I., and Boeing, H. (2012) "Association of sleep duration with chronic diseases in the European prospective investigation into cancer and nutrition (EPIC)—Potsdam study." *PLoS One 7*, 1, e30972.

Wu, H. J. and Wu, E. (2012) "The role of gut microbiota in immune homeostasis and autoimmunity." *Journal of Gut Microbes 3*, 1, 4–14.

Wu, S., Powers, S., Zhu, W., and Hannun, Y. A. (2016) "Substantial contribution of extrinsic risk factors to cancer development." *Nature 529*, 7584, 43–47.

Zama, A. M. and Uzumcu, M. (2010) "Epigenetic effects of endocrine-disrupting chemicals on female reproduction: An ovarian perspective." *Frontiers in Neuroendocrinology 31*, 4, 420–439.

Zaura, E., Brandt, B. W., Teixerira de Mattos, M. J., Buijs, M. J., *et al.* (2015) "Same exposure but two radically different responses to antibiotics: Resilience of the salivary microbiome versus long-term microbial shifts in feces." *American Society for Microbiology 6*, 6, e01693–15.

Zorrilla, M. and Yatsenko, A. (2013) "The genetics of infertility: Current status of the field." *Current Genetics Medicine Reports 1*, 247–260.

List of Acronyms

Abdominal hypopressive technique: AHT

Active straight leg raises: ASLR

Adverse childhood experiences: ACE

American Physical Therapy Association: APTA

American Urogynecological Society: AUGS

Association for Pelvic Organ Prolapse Support: APOPS

Autism spectrum disorder: ASD

Biopsychosocial model: BPS

Bristol stool scale: BSS

> A graphic illustration and written descriptions of stool types #1–7, useful for client education and tracking results of nutrition changes. BSS #3 and #4 are optimum output. Clients with difficulties emptying often have stools that are too firm, BSS #1 or #2, or too loose, BSS #5–7.

Chronic pelvic pain: CPP

Clinical practice guidelines: CPG

> CPG are expert evidence-based guidelines for management of patients with specific conditions. The CPG utilize the World Health Organization's international classification of functioning, disability, and impairment (ICF) terminology to define and classify conditions, and recommend the interventions based on the highest available levels and grades of evidence. CPG use evidence-based medicine as their foundation. Current CPG for physical therapy is available at www.apta.org/patient-care.

Diastasis rectus abdominis: DRA

Dyssynergia: A lack of coordination between the pelvic and respiratory diaphragms for functions such as respiration, or attempted pelvic floor muscle contraction, relaxation, or bearing-down bulging maneuvers.

Evidence-based medicine: EBM

Levels of evidence for EBM

Ranking Foundation

I High quality randomized controlled trials, prospective cohort studies, prognostic studies, meta-analysis, and level I studies summarized in systematic reviews

II Lesser quality randomized controlled studies, retrospective cohort studies, diagnostic studies, or systematic reviews of level II studies

Studies may have not been the best design due to lack of blinding, inadequate follow up or improper randomization, and weaker diagnostic standards or criteria

III Case controlled studies, or systematic review of level III studies

IV Case series, or poorly ranked cohort studies or reference standards

V Expert opinion without critical appraisal, or based on physiology, or use of "first principles"

Grades of evidence

A Strong

B Moderate

C Weak

D Conflicting

E Theoretical, foundational

F Expert opinion

Levels of evidence data-based guides

CINAHL Complete: The Cumulative Index to Nursing and Allied Health Literature

Cochrane Database of Systematic Reviews, cochranelibrary.com

Physiotherapy evidence database: PEDRO, pedro.org.au

PubMed-National Library of Medicine-NIH, pubmed.gov

Female sexual function index: FSFI

Fermentable oligosaccharides, disaccharides, monosaccharides, and polyols: FODMAP

FODMAP items are short-chain carbohydrate components of foods.

Gastrointestinal: GI

Generalized joint laxity: GJL

Gut microbiome: GM

Incontinence quality of life instrument: I-QOL

International classification of functioning, disability, and health: ICF

International index of erectile function: IIEF

Interstitial cystitis: IC

Interstitial cystitis help: ICHELP, www.ichelp.org

This link is the professional resource for IC/overactive bladder patient education.

Irritable bowel syndrome: IBS

Levator ani: LA

Low back pain: LBP

Lumbopelvic hip: LPH

Menstrual distress questionnaire: MDQ

Mindfulness-based stress reduction: MBSR

Numeric pain rating scale: NPRS

Oswestry disability index: ODI

Pelvic floor distress inventory: PFDI

Pelvic floor dysfunction: PFD

Bladder, bowel, pain, and/or sexual function challenges.

Pelvic floor impact questionnaire: PFIQ-7

Pelvic floor muscles: PFM

Pelvic girdle pain: PGP

Pelvic girdle questionnaire: PGQ

Pelvic organ prolapse: POP

Pelvic organ prolapse questionnaire: POPQ

Physical therapy: PT

Polycystic ovarian syndrome: PCOS

Pregnancy related pelvic girdle pain: PRPGP

Premenstrual dysphoric disorder: PMDD

Premenstrual syndrome: PMS

Premenstrual syndrome scale: PMSS

Quality of life: QOL

Real time ultrasound: RUSI

Relative energy deficiency in sport (RED-S)

Sacroiliac: SI

Short form health survey: SF-36, www.physio-pedia.com/Category:Outcome_Measures

Single limb stance: SLS

Symphysis pubis dysfunction: SPD

Transverse abdominis: TRA

The deepest abdominal core which blends with myofascia into the spinal multifidus, the pelvic floor muscles, and the latissimus dorsi fascia.

Urinary distress inventory: UDI

Urinary incontinence: UI

Vaginal atrophy: VA

Subject Index

Note: illustrations are referenced by page numbers in *italics*

Author Index

Acknowledgments

I wish to thank my parents Thomas and Louise, who lived with passion and style: my dad, a neurosurgeon, avid sportsman, and aspiring singer, and my mom, who included everyone as family, raised eight children with love and devotion, and gifted her flowers to neighbors, nursing home patients, and friends. And I thank my brothers and sisters for their time shared in work and play, with favored hikes, and Zooms over Covid times to stay connected, heart to heart, across the US.

I am grateful for my teachers from Boston University, Arcadia College, the American Physical Therapy Association, and the Herman and Wallace Institute. I have developed my mind and skills with coursework thanks to the talented clinician-educators Holly Herman, Kathe Wallace, Shirley Sahrmann, Tracy Spitznagle, Gail Wetzler, Ramona Horton, Holly Tanner, Jenni Gabelsberg, Elizabeth Hampton, Tracy Sher, Yousef Ghandour, Neil Sturman, Diane Lee, Irwin and Sue Goldstein, Heather Howard, and countless other teachers.

Osteopaths John Upledger, Ken Lossing, Michael Kurisu, Jean Pierre Barral, and MaryAnn Morelli, thank you for demonstrating how the fascial body has resilience and how healers can "listen" and promote ease, comfort, and balance. Integrative medicine pioneers Bernie Siegal, Andrew Weil, Deepak Chopra, Mimi Guarneri, Kulreet Chaudhary, and Valencia Porter, thank you for your books and online offerings which provide pearls and insights into the nuances of health, wellness, and healing in mind, body, and spirit.

I appreciate being nudged to take a class on continence by Joseph Marty, and encouraged in coursework and opportunities for program development for patient care by Mike Ryder, Cindy Furey, and Renee Cinco. And for the opportunity to work in research, I thank Emily Lukacz of UCSD, and Lori Tuttle of SDSU. My yoga teachers Dustienne Miller, Ginger Garner, and Shelly Prosko, I thank you all for modelling the ways yoga can be a lifestyle, and an adaptable format for client care. My co-authors J. Michelle Martin and Pauline Lucas, thank you for carving out time to contribute wise words to this book, and Jessica Drummond, for your editing pearls in the final chapter.

Sarena Wolfaard, former editor at Handspring, thank you for attending my talk on "The secret world of pelvic physical therapy," and commissioning this book, as well as helping me to find my voice from strictly medical and factual to include my opinions and insights to reach a larger audience. And the staff at Singing Dragon: Maddy Budd, Masooma Malik, Claire Wilson, Victoria Peters, and Carole McMurray, thank you for your editorial expertise and support, and gratitude also to illustrator Bruce Hogarth.

To all my patients over the years, thank you for the opportunity to share laughter and tears, and the hard work, discipline, and patience required in the rehabilitation journey, from simple conditions to more complex and troubling challenges. You are my teachers.

Finally, I thank my husband and daughters for their support over the years as I have travelled for courses, to and from the clinic, and for their sense of humor as I have instilled "too much information" (TMI) in my desire to optimize their health literacy and self-care action plans.